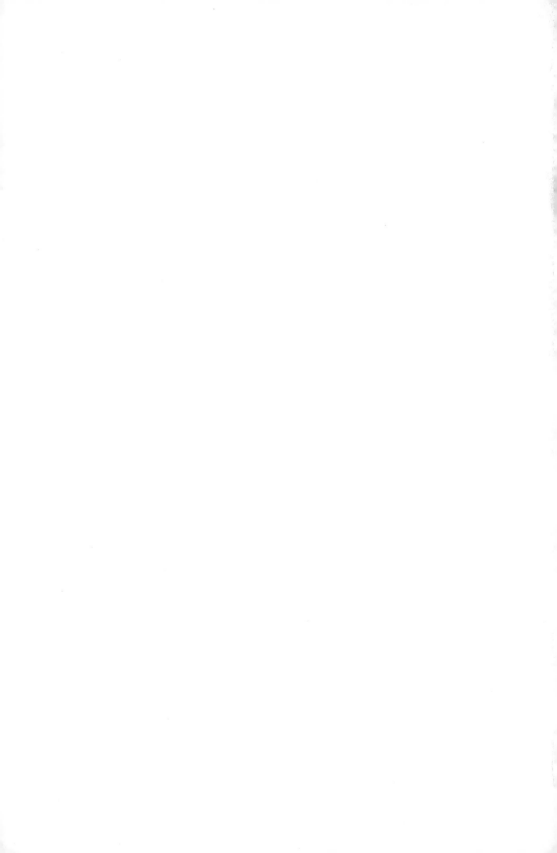

Praise for *The Supplement Pyramid*

"Doctor as teacher is a foundational principle that I believe in and practice by. *The Supplement Pyramid* can assist people in learning how and which dietary supplements to take in a clear and understanding way."

—Holly Lucille, N.D., R.N., Author, TV Host, and Lecturer

▲

"If you're having difficulty determining which dietary supplements are right for you, *The Supplement Pyramid* is a necessary guide to enhancing your health and wellness program."

—Dr. Sherill Sellman, N.D., Psychotherapist,
Health Researcher, and Author

▲

"Dr. Smith is a frequent guest expert on our radio program. Our listeners tell us that his presentation always makes them want to get healthy. *The Supplement Pyramid* will do the same for you."

—Paul Rodgers, Host and Producer, Full
Disclosure Advocates Radio

▲

"The health quizzes Dr. Smith has created helped me understand how I need to change my nutrition regimen. It's given me a road map to better personal health."

—Pete Croatto, Manager, Supplement Perspectives

THE
Supplement
Pyramid

HOW TO BUILD YOUR PERSONALIZED NUTRITIONAL REGIMEN

Michael A. Smith, M.D.
with Sara Lovelady
Foreword by Suzanne Somers

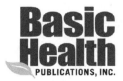

Basic
Health
PUBLICATIONS, INC.

The information in this book (and any accompanying material) is not intended to replace the attention or advice of a physician or other qualified health-care professional. Anyone who wishes to embark on any dietary, drug, exercise, or other lifestyle change intended to prevent or treat a specific disease or condition should first consult with and seek clearance from a physician or other qualified health-care professional. Pregnant women in particular should seek the advice of a physician before using any suggested nutrient listed in the book. This book is intended for adults only, unless otherwise specified. Product labels may contain important safety information and the most recent product information provided by the product manufacturers should be carefully reviewed prior to use to verify the dose, administration, and contraindications. National, state, and local laws may vary regarding the use and application of many of the therapies discussed. The reader assumes the risk of any injuries. The authors and publisher, their affiliates and assigns are not liable for any injury and/or damage to persons arising from this book and expressly disclaim responsibility for any adverse effects resulting from the use of the information contained herein.

This book raises many issues that are subject to change as new data emerge. None of the suggested nutrients can guarantee health benefits. The author and LE Publications, Inc., have not performed independent verification of the data contained in the referenced materials, and expressly disclaim responsibility for any error in the literature.

Basic Health Publications, Inc.
28812 Top of the World Drive
Laguna Beach, CA 92651
949-715-7327 • www.basichealthpub.com

Library of Congress Cataloging-in-Publication Data

Smith, Michael A., author.
    The supplement pyramid : how to build your personalized nutritional regimen /
Michael A. Smith, M.D.
        pages cm
    Includes bibliographical references and index.
    ISBN: 978-1-59120-383-4
1. Dietary supplements. 2. Self-care, Health. I. Title.
    RM258.5.S62   2014
    613.2—dc23

                                        2013050766

Editor: Carol Killman Rosenberg
Typesetting/Book design: Gary A. Rosenberg
Cover design: Harby Bonello

Printed in the United States of America

10   9   8   7   6   5   4

Contents

Acknowledgments, vii

Foreword by Suzanne Somers, ix

1. Why Take Nutritional Supplements?, 1

2. The Supplement Pyramid Overview, 27

3. Choosing High-Quality Supplements, 35

4. The Foundation Level, 51

5. The Personalization Level, 73

6. The Optimization Level, 139

7. Disease Supplement Pyramids, 147

8. Personalized Supplement Pyramid Case Studies, 219

9. Your Own Personalized Supplement Pyramid, 235

Conclusion, 237

Appendices

A. Recommended Nutritional Supplement Companies, 239

B. Recommended Nutrients, 245

Endnotes, 271

Index, 311

About the Author, 323

Acknowledgments

I would like to express my gratitude to the many people who saw me through this book; to all those who provided support, talked things over, read, wrote, offered comments, allowed me to quote their remarks, and assisted in the editing, proofreading, and design.

I would like to thank Kira Schmid, N.D., Steven Joyal, M.D., and Richard A. Stein, M.D., Ph.D., for reviewing the scientific content and providing expert and invaluable suggestions. All of you are a joy to work with, and I am honored to call you my colleagues and my friends.

Thanks to Basic Health Publications and Carol Killman Rosenberg for providing edits and comments—without which the book would not be as easy to read and understand—and who enabled me to publish this book.

To my focus group of friends and colleagues who helped edit the medical inventories and quizzes: Sandy Edgcumbe, Sherena Barton, Jessica Koehler, Deborah Lemery, Charles Widry, Sandra Rowe, Kathy Markell, Lee Anna Hicks, and Cindy Smith Maylin.

Thanks to Vladimir Polyak and Luis Fajardo—without both of you, this book would have never been developed for the Web. I want to also thank my dear friend Carrie Speno for simply being at my side and my family, who supported and encouraged me throughout the writing process. My dog, Edy, was a big stress reliever as well—good girl.

To my writing partner, Sara Lovelady: you're awesome! You effortlessly took my left-brained ideas and turned them into a story that's so easy to read. To my friend and Life Extension's PR director, Sheldon Baker, and my boss (and friend too), Rey Searles: your encouragement throughout the writing of this book is beyond words. Thank you!

I beg forgiveness of all those who have been with me over the course of the years and whose names I have failed to mention.

Last and not least, thank you God for Your grace, love, peace, and abundant blessings. May you be glorified in all I do.

Foreword

by Suzanne Somers

This book is better than going to the doctor.

Anyone who has ever stood in the aisle of a local health food store, stared at rows and rows of supplements, and walked out frustrated with only a lonely bottle of multivitamins will appreciate a thorough explanation of why supplementation can benefit you.

What are your deficiencies? What specifically do you need to operate at the max? What are your family genetics . . . and how do you maneuver around them so you won't suffer the same fate? For example, if your mother had heart disease, then taking daily fish oil and pomegranate supplements makes sense for you.

Because of government regulations, vitamin bottles are not allowed to tout the benefits of each particular nutrient on their labels. If they could, the process would be so much easier. Instead, the average person has to guess, armed at best with information they have read in the latest magazine . . . or gleaned from a report about the most recent find from the rain forest.

Today, poor health is the norm. So, out of necessity, people seek out new information about how they can feel better. Luckily, supplementation has become extremely advanced and sophisticated. While your parents and grandparents could brag that they never had to take a vitamin in their lives, they also lived on a different planet. In the last fifty years the Earth has sadly undergone profound negative changes due to the introduction of chemicals . . . pesticides on our food, chemicals in our food, toxic household cleaners, toxic hair care products, makeup filled with preservatives and dangerous parabens, plastic bottles leaching chemicals into our water (in the form of phthalates, dioxins, and other unpronounceables). The result of this massive toxic assault is a downgrade in the health of our nation and the global population. Our precious soil no longer holds within it the nutrients, minerals, and life-sustaining, life-giving components so vital to our health.

We have to question why 53 percent of the bees are gone. As the bees go, so do we. It's a sobering thought.

So . . . what to do? Clearly, each of us can try our best to clean up our living quarters by eliminating foods in our pantries and cupboards that contain chemicals, changing the household cleaning products we use, and eventually switching to organics in every area of our lives. We can also install reverse osmosis filters to try our best to eliminate the carcinogenic fluoride imposed on our water supplies, but the assault is pervasive and massive. It takes hundreds of years (maybe even longer) for pesticides and chemicals to dissipate . . . making even organic food suspect.

Nutrition is fuel for the human body. Nutrition is what determines how well our individual machinery works. To do nothing is to accept the status quo of heart disease, cancer, Alzheimer's disease, and more.

This is your worst nightmare. There is a general feeling of hopelessness. What are we supposed to do? How do we combat this invisible ninja warrior?

It seems everyone is going down, and we don't know how to stop it.

This is where supplementation steps in. It's a simple concept. Just put back what's missing in your body to make it operate optimally. Take advantage of being able to add in that which has never been due to family genetics.

Supplementation is no longer being scoffed at and disregarded as "expensive urine" by the medical establishment. Instead, it is now crucial for survival. Technology today keeps us alive longer than ever recorded in the history of humanity. But good health is a distant memory at best.

Who doesn't have some weirdness happening in their bodies? The gastrointestinal tract usually takes the first hit. The GI tract (also called the second brain) is crucial for health. If your gut isn't healthy, you're not healthy. Yet how can intestinal health be possible when your gut is struggling to process toxins never meant for human consumption? Cancer, intestinal inflammation, and autoimmune diseases are all increasing at alarming rates. Heart disease is expected and, sadly, Alzheimer's disease seems to dominate the end stage of life . . . and no one has an answer.

Dr. Michael Smith's book offers both hope and a solution. The need for supplementation is explained, then broken down ingredient by ingredient . . . providing the benefits of each, and connecting the dots between your symptoms and your needs.

I've wanted a book like this for a long time. A reference journal. A book to refer to over and over.

Dr. Smith lays out the basic requirements for all of us in his pyramid . . . what we require daily (those building blocks the human body cannot live without) . . . and progresses to a process of points. Then he helps you pinpoint where you are personally at risk based on your family genetics, and explains how to use supplements that can prevent or reverse your family dynamics. Finally, he provides you with the latest discoveries for age reversal and disease prevention. In this way, his pyramid enables you to prioritize according to your budget as well as your needs.

Doctors will use this book as a reference bible and lay people will become empowered to take charge of their health in ways never before possible.

Don't want atherosclerosis? Take vitamin K_3 to keep your arteries soft and pliable.

Stressed out? Take L-theanine, nature's tranquilizer.

Can't sleep? Take melatonin.

Libido gone? Take a maca and cordyceps extract.

Foggy brain? Take coenzyme Q_{10}.

These are just a few examples of the value of owning this manual.

Dr. Smith has done all the work for you . . . backed up by years of research and critical thinking.

Bottom Line: Supplementing your deficiencies, restoring what's missing, circumventing genetic predispositions are all possible when you know what's out there to accomplish these changes. Supplementation with knowledge gives peace of mind that you have taken charge of your health regardless of the reckless damage imposed on our planet.

This book is essential for good health and a long life.

Suzanne Somers has been dubbed a health pioneer by the *Wall Street Journal* and "crazy smart" by Dr. Mehmet Oz. She is the author of twenty-four books, including the #1 *New York Times* bestsellers *Sexy Forever; Knockout; Ageless; Suzanne Somers' Fast and Easy;* and *Get Skinny on Fabulous Food,* and the *New York Times* bestsellers *Bombshell; Breakthrough; Keeping Secrets; Eat Great, Lose Weight; Eat, Cheat, and Melt the Fat Away; Slim and Sexy Forever;* and *The Sexy Years.* Suzanne received an Emmy nomination as host of Lifetime's weekly morning talk show *The SUZANNE Show.*

CHAPTER 1

Why Take Nutritional Supplements?

As a doctor who specializes in nutritional supplementation, one of the most common questions I hear from people is: "I eat a pretty healthy diet. Do I really need to take supplements?" My answer is always a resounding "Yes!"

In this chapter, we'll cover some of the reasons why even the healthiest diets fall short in terms of supplying the optimal amount of nutrients you need not just to survive, but to thrive! We'll also discuss how your health is threatened on a daily basis by hidden "ingredients" in the food you eat, by environmental toxins right inside your home, and by the effects of chronic stress on your body. My hope is that after reading this chapter, you'll understand why I'm so emphatic that nutritional supplements aren't just a good idea in today's modern world—they're essential!

INADEQUATE FRUIT AND VEGETABLE INTAKE

It's no secret that fruits and vegetables are some of the healthiest foods on earth. Your risk of getting just about any disease you can think of—cancer, heart disease, diabetes, you name it—goes down the more produce you eat. For this reason, the U.S. government has tried to encourage Americans to eat more fruits and veggies for decades.

Currently, the U.S. Department of Agriculture (USDA) recommends that most women eat $2^1/_2$ cups of vegetables and $1^1/_2$ cups of fruit daily. (Salad lovers take note: 2 cups of leafy greens only count as 1 cup of vegetables.) Most men have to eat even more: 3 cups of vegetables and 2 cups of fruit.

That may sound doable, until you really break it down. A sample menu for a woman trying to meet the USDA recommendation looks like this: $1/2$ cup of blueberries with breakfast, 2 cups of salad greens and $1/2$ cup of cucumber with lunch, a snack of 1 small apple and 16 grapes, and dinner accompanied by 1 medium carrot and 1 small red bell pepper. Realistically, how often do you eat like that?

I can't answer for you personally, but I can share an eye-opening statistic with you. According to a recently published study, only 11 percent of Americans meet the USDA guidelines for fruit and vegetable consumption.[1] Can you honestly say you're that one in ten?

BOTTOM LINE: *You're probably not eating enough fruits and vegetables to fulfill your daily nutritional needs.*

POOR SOIL QUALITY

Now say you're in the minority that really does eat 4–5 cups of fruits and vegetables daily. You might assume with all the produce you're downing that you don't need to take a multivitamin/mineral or antioxidant supplements. But you'd be overlooking one important fact: A plant is only as nutritious as the soil it was grown in. It doesn't matter how many fruits

OVERFED AND UNDERNOURISHED

In 2005, the U.S. Department of Agriculture (USDA) issued a report analyzing the adequacy of nutrient intake from food alone in the United States. The percentages of Americans with inadequate nutrient intake from food are shocking and highlight the need to supplement to ensure optimal nutrition:

- 93% of Americans have an inadequate intake of vitamin E.
- 56% of Americans have an inadequate intake of magnesium.
- 44% of Americans have an inadequate intake of vitamin A.
- 31% of Americans have an inadequate intake of vitamin C.
- 14% of Americans have an inadequate intake of vitamin B_6.
- 12% of Americans have an inadequate intake of zinc.
- 8% of Americans have an inadequate intake of folate.

and vegetables you're eating if they're grown in nutrient-poor soil. And the unfortunate truth is that the nutrient content of our soil—and thus our crops—has been steadily declining for decades.

The first U.S. soil surveys were completed in the 1920s. They all concluded that our soil was depleted of key nutrients like nitrates and carbonates, which are necessary for the growth of healthy crops and, ultimately, nutrient-dense food. *And that was way back in the 1920s.* Things have only gotten worse since then.

Soil Interventions

Sure, some steps have been taken to improve the condition of our soil. In the 1930s and 1940s, following the Great Dust Bowl, farmers planted soy as a cover crop to reinvigorate topsoil. (Soybeans are nitrogen-fixing, meaning they extract nitrogen from the air and convert it into compounds that other plants can use to grow.) During the late 1990s, local governments initiated soil rejuvenation programs, which also included the planting of soybeans. These programs helped to some extent, but certainly not to the degree needed.

Today, commercial agriculture routinely incorporates synthetic fertilizers made from petroleum into the soil to rapidly improve growth potential. While this does help grow crops, it doesn't necessarily help grow *healthy* crops. In fact, according to Dr. Donald R. Davis, a former research associate with the Biochemical Institute at the University of Texas, the increase in crop yield achieved by synthetic fertilizers has a nasty side effect: a *decrease* in mineral content.[2]

Even more troubling, synthetic fertilizers actually degrade the soil further by hastening the degradation of organic matter. Once that happens, the soil loses its ability to store nitrogen, so it's actually *worse* off than before the fertilizer was added![3] This creates the need for—you guessed it—more synthetic fertilizer. Not only that, when soil loses its organic matter, it starts to become more compacted. Soil compaction leads to soil erosion. And if enough soil erodes, you can wind up with a Dust Bowl scenario.

BOTTOM LINE: *Because our soil is so nutrient-depleted, the fruits and vegetables you're eating probably aren't as nutritious as you think they are.*

Organic Produce versus Conventional Produce

So what about organic produce? Isn't that a more nutritious choice? While I certainly encourage you to eat organic because it drastically reduces your exposure to pesticide residue, organic food isn't necessarily nutrient-dense. Remember, our soil has been depleted of nutrients since the 1920s. All food—whether organic or conventional—is being grown in the same nutrient-deficient soil. Organic farmers do tend to practice more sustainable agricultural practices, such as planting cover crops, rotating crops, and adding compost to the soil. But these steps are not enough to overcome the poor condition of our soil.

That said, several (though not all) studies have found that organic fruits and vegetables do have a better nutritional profile than their conventional counterparts. For example, Rutgers University published a study showing wide discrepancies in the amounts of essential minerals occurring in vegetables grown in organic versus inorganic soil, as measured in millequivalents.

TABLE 1.1. MINERAL DENSITY OF VEGETABLES GROWN IN ORGANIC VERSUS CONVENTIONAL SOIL, IN MILLIEQUIVALENT				
CALCIUM	**MAGNESIUM**	**POTASSIUM**	**MANGANESE**	**COPPER**
Snap Beans 41-organic	60-organic	100-organic	60-organic	69-organic
16-conventional	15-conventional	29-conventional	2-conventional	3-conventional
Cabbage 60-organic	44-organic	148-organic	13-organic	48-organic
18-conventional	16-conventional	54-conventional	2-conventional	1- conventional
Lettuce 71-organic	49-organic	177-organic	169-organic	60-organic
16-conventional	13-conventional	54-conventional	54-conventional	3-conventional
Tomatoes 23-organic	59-organic	148-organic	69-organic	53-organic
5-conventional	5-conventional	57-conventional	1-conventional	1-conventional
Spinach 96-organic	294-organic	257-organic	117-organic	0-organic
46-conventional	47-conventional	84-conventional	1-conventional	0-conventional

WHEN IS ORGANIC NOT ORGANIC?

Organic soil may not be as "organic" as you think. Pesticides can have long half-lives, in some cases hundreds of years. As a result, soil can contain chemical residues years after it was converted to organic agriculture. This explains why studies have repeatedly shown that organic produce sometimes contains trace amounts of pesticides. Organic regulations also vary by country, and not all countries require soil testing for pesticide residues.

But keep in mind, millequivalents are tiny amounts. So just because produce grown in organic soil has more millequivalents of minerals than produce grown in conventional soil doesn't mean it has enough!

BOTTOM LINE: *The amount of essential minerals present in organic produce falls far short of what you need to optimize your health.*

The Nutritional Decline of Food

Dr. Bernard Jensen was a world-renowned clinical nutritionist who once said that a tomato today is not the same as a tomato from a hundred years ago. He was right, as a recently published scientific paper by Dr. Davis, the retired biochemist from the University of Texas that I mentioned earlier, illustrates.

Dr. Davis compiled and analyzed the results of three previous studies documenting nutrient declines in different groups of vegetables and fruits over the past fifty to seventy years. What he found was shocking: "In each study, about half of the studied nutrients showed large enough declines to be statistically significant," said Dr. Davis in an interview.[4] In fact, the average vegetable had lost from 5 to 40 percent (or more) of its mineral value.[5] Copper was particularly hard-hit, suffering a decline of 80 percent! What this means in practical terms is that you now have to eat five times as many vegetables to meet your copper needs as you did just a few decades ago.

It's not just minerals we've lost though. One study Dr. Davis cites shows that from 1950 to 1999, our vegetables also lost about 6 percent of their protein content, 20 percent of their vitamin C, and 38 percent of their riboflavin (vitamin B_2).[6]

BOTTOM LINE: *The amount of nutrients in our fruits and vegetables has declined rapidly in just fifty to seventy years, making it even more difficult for you to get all of your nutrients from food.*

SICK FOOD CHAIN

I'd like to tell you that it's just produce that's the problem. But unfortunately, our entire food chain is devoid of the nutrition your body needs—and polluted with junk it doesn't.

Are You Eating Real Food or Processed Food?

Let's start by looking at the processed food that makes up so much of the American diet. There's a lot of confusion around what even constitutes a processed food. Luckily, I have a very easy way to distinguish between real, whole foods and processed, refined foods. Ready? Here it is: If it goes bad quickly, it's real. If it goes bad slowly (or never!), it's processed.

Real food is fresh fruits and vegetables; lean meats, poultry, and fish; dairy products; nuts and seeds; and beans and whole grains. Processed food is crackers, cookies, chips, candies, sodas, packaged baked goods, preserved meats, and even some granola and nutrition bars.

Industrially produced foods are bad for obvious reasons. They're nutritionally bereft, because they've been stripped of all the good stuff whole foods naturally contain, while being augmented with excess sugar, oil, and salt. But there's a more insidious concern with processed foods: the hidden ingredients they contain.

What keeps these prepackaged foods "fresh" for months, when a homemade version of that food would go bad in a matter of days? Shelf-life enhancers, such as trans fats and preservatives. What makes them taste so good, even when they're sugar-free? Artificial sweeteners, such as saccharin, aspartame, and acesulfame. And what gives them their bright, unnatural hues? Artificial colors, such as Red No. 40 and Yellow No. 5. As you'll see, all of these hidden ingredients pose dangers to your health.

Trans Fats

There are few things worse for you in today's modern food chain than trans fats. These fats are magically turned from liquids to solids by infusing them with hydrogen, which is why they're also known as "partially hydrogenated" oils.

You've probably heard that saturated fats are bad for you, but trans fats are way worse. They make your good cholesterol go down and your bad cholesterol go up, increasing your risk of cardiovascular disease. They also muck up your brain, interfering with the ability of your brain cells to communicate and form memories.[7,8,9] They're so bad that a group of scientists at the Institute of Medicine, who got together to develop a safe daily level of trans fats consumption, said that there is none: any level above zero is harmful.[10]

The food industry loves trans fats, because they're terrific at keeping foods from going bad. That's why they're ubiquitous in margarine, fried foods, baked goods, and fast food. But food is *supposed* to go bad. And the fact that trans fats are long lasting means they last a long time in *you*!

Processed foods are required by law to disclose how much trans fat they contain. But there's a serious loophole: if a serving contains less than 0.5 grams of the stuff, it can legally be labeled "zero trans fats." Now half a gram may not seem like much, but you know how small recommended serving sizes can be. And if you eat several servings of several different foods, all containing 0.49 grams of trans fats, you're actually ingesting a lot of this toxic fat. Read your food labels and avoid anything that has the words "partially hydrogenated" in the list of ingredients. Here's some good news: the FDA is finally making a move to eliminate trans fat from our food.

Artificial Preservatives

Another way to keep foods fresh for unnaturally long periods of time is through the addition of artificial preservatives. Far from being benign, these artificial ingredients wreak havoc with your body.

Eating foods preserved with sodium nitrate (also called sodium nitrite)—such as processed meats and smoked fish—is linked to cancer.[11] BHA (butylated hydroxyanisole), used to keep fats from spoiling, is listed as one of *Time* magazine's "Top 10 common household toxins" because it may promote cancer in lab animals.[12] And finally, propyl gallate, which also protects fats from going bad, is associated with asthma attacks, stomach and skin irritation, and liver and kidney damage.[13,14,15] Oh, and it, too, may increase the risk of certain cancers.[16]

Artificial Sweeteners

Artificial sweeteners seem like attractive alternatives to sugar since they add virtually no calories to your diet. Contributing to the allure, you only need to use a fraction compared to the amount of sugar you'd normally use for adding sweetness. But there's a seriously big catch—they're dangerous. And they're showing up everywhere.

Artificial sweeteners are widely used in processed products, including tabletop sweeteners, baked goods, soft drinks, powdered drink mixes, candy, puddings, canned foods, jams and jellies, dairy products, and scores of other foods and beverages. What's really scary is that these fake sugars have also become popular at home. More and more home cooks are enthusiastically using artificial sweeteners, thinking that they're healthy alternatives to regular table sugar. Unfortunately, nothing could be further from the truth.

Despite serious safety concerns, five artificial sweeteners have been approved by the Food and Drug Administration (FDA) for use in foods and beverages: saccharin, aspartame, acesulfame potassium, sucralose, and neotame (the successor to aspartame). I could write a whole book about the many dangers of artificial sweeteners, but the biggest controversy surrounding them is whether or not they cause cancer.

For over twenty years, saccharin was officially considered a "probable human carcinogen" by the U.S. government, because animals fed the substance were more likely to develop cancer of the bladder, uterus, ovaries, skin, and other organs.[17] Some large case-control studies in humans have since found a significantly increased risk of bladder cancer among people who use the little pink packets.[18] However, others have not. That inconsistency was enough for the FDA to delist saccharin from the federal government's Report on Carcinogens in 2001.

According to the National Cancer Institute (NCI), "Human epidemiology studies...have shown no consistent evidence that saccharin is associated with bladder cancer incidence."[19] Personally, the fact that *some* studies have shown saccharin does cause bladder cancer is enough for me not to eat the stuff. And what about the other cancers that saccharin caused in animals but that were never studied in humans?

It's a similar story with aspartame. A 2005 study caused alarm when it showed that rats fed aspartame had higher rates of leukemia and lymphomas.[20] But since a study published the next year found no link between aspartame-sweetened beverages and these cancers in humans, the sweetener remains on the market.[21]

What concerns me, as well as other medical professionals, is that this human study only followed participants for five years. Cancer can have a very long latency period, sometimes not showing up for twenty years after exposure to a carcinogen. How many of these aspartame-chugging folks will have cancer by 2020?

Chances are we'll never find out, because the study is over. But the results of another study are telling. Just recently, the longest study conducted to date on aspartame, spanning twenty-two years, was published. It found the sweetener was associated with an increased risk of non-Hodgkin's lymphoma in men[22] That's enough evidence for me!

Then there's acesulfame. Amazingly, the FDA approved the safety of this synthetic sweetener based on three animal studies conducted in the 1970s. The first was considered inconclusive. The second was disregarded as unreliable. That leaves one last study.

Since the safety of acesulfame rests on this one study, you would think it did not find an association between the fake sugar and increased cancer risk, right? But that's not what happened. Rats fed acesulfame developed more tumors than rats fed regular rat chow. But the acesulfame execs argued that the reason the control rats didn't develop as many tumors was because they were unusually healthy—not because acesulfame is a carcinogen. And the FDA bought it.[23]

Those are just the cancer concerns. Some medical experts believe that certain artificial sweeteners, such as aspartame, are excitotoxins, meaning they cause excessive firing of brain neurons. In fact, a recent study concluded that eating large amounts of aspartame may lead to neurodegeneration—in other words, brain cell death.[24] This could explain why many people complain of headaches, migraines, dizziness, blurred vision, ringing in the ears, and other neurological symptoms after eating it.

Other potential adverse effects of artificial sweeteners include hyperinsulinemia (elevated insulin levels) and insulin resistance; gastrointestinal disturbance such as nausea, diarrhea, bloating, and gas; and hyperactivity in kids.

I include high-fructose corn syrup (HFCS) along with the five "official" artificial sweeteners. As much as the National Corn Growers Association would like to convince you that HFCS is natural, don't believe it for a second. Sure, this syrupy liquid may start with corn, but HFCS is so highly processed that its chemical bonds are actually broken and

TABLE 1.2. POTENTIAL ADVERSE EFFECTS OF POPULAR ARTIFICIAL SWEETENERS		
ARTIFICIAL SWEETENER	**BRAND NAME**	**POTENTIAL ADVERSE EFFECTS***
Acesulfame potassium	Sweet One; Sunett	Cancer; Hyperinsulinemia; Insulin Resistance
Aspartame; Neotame	Equal; Nutrasweet; Canderel	Cancer; Blurry Vision; Ringing in the Ear (Tinnitus); Headaches and Migraines; Hyperactivity in Kids
Saccharin	Sweet'N Low; SugarTwin	Cancer; Nervousness
Sucralose	Splenda	Nausea; Diarrhea; Bloating and Gas; Nervousness
High-fructose corn syrup		Insulin Resistance; Type 2 Diabetes; Non-Alcoholic Fatty Liver Disease; Gout (Hyperuricemia); High Triglycerides

*Source: Kovacs, Betty. Artificial Sweeteners. *MedicineNet*. Last reviewed Dec. 13, 2010.
http://www.onhealth.com/artificial_sweeteners/article.htm

rearranged—something that would never happen in nature. The reason HFCS is popular is because it's cheap and readily available, period. No chef in their right mind would ever use it otherwise.

Too much sugar is bad for you, but HFCS is worse. Both of them are composed of fructose and glucose, but whereas sugar contains a fifty-fifty mixture, HFCS contains 55 percent fructose and 45 percent glucose. That doesn't sound like a big deal, until you realize how bad for you isolated fructose really is. (Fructose naturally occurring in whole fruits is fine.)

Glucose and fructose are metabolized very differently by the body. Most glucose goes straight into the bloodstream and then into the cells, where it's burned as fuel. Most fructose, on the other hand, goes straight to the liver, where it's turned into triglycerides—artery-clogging fats. In fact, a recent study found that when obese people drank fructose-sweetened beverages with their meals, their triglycerides shot up nearly 200 percent over a twenty-four-hour period![25] No wonder people who eat large amounts of fructose are two to three times more likely to have non-alcoholic fatty liver disease.[26]

But that's not all fructose does. It's more likely than glucose to make you insulin-resistant—the first step toward developing diabetes.[27] It raises your blood pressure more than glucose does.[28,29] It makes you put on dangerous belly fat, while glucose makes you put on harmless subcutaneous (under the skin) fat.[30] Oh, and it may give you gout, because unlike other sugars, fructose increases uric acid levels in the blood.[31,32]

Artificial Colors

Recently, while dining out, I watched my nephew inhale a hot fudge sundae topped with a beautiful, bright-red, mysterious syrup. I asked the server what the syrup was made of, and she said it was a natural strawberry puree. I didn't believe her. When I got home, I did a quick Internet search and found that the restaurant in question wasn't using natural strawberries. They were using FD&C Red No. 40.

This piqued my curiosity. I wondered how many chain restaurants were using artificial colors in popular menu items. Much to my dismay, I found the answer is *a lot*! But what I discovered next was really surprising: The same restaurant chain that uses FD&C Red No. 40 to color its sundae topping in the United States uses red beet juice to do the job in Europe. Why? Because the European Medicines Agency has declared most chemical food dyes dangerous.

Most people don't realize this, but artificial colors are derived from coal tar. So it's not exactly surprising that they may have untoward health effects. Unfortunately, thanks to the powerful Big Food lobby, the United States is behind the European Union in outlawing them.

It is true that the federal government has banned eight synthetic colors since 1938, leaving only seven remaining.[33] Gone is Orange No. 1, which sickened many children during the Halloween of 1950. Also ousted is Red. No. 2, after it was found to cause tumors in rats. Yellows No. 1 through 4 are also history. But the FDA still allows red and orange and yellow dyes. It's just that now, instead of Red. No. 2, a confirmed carcinogen, we have Red. No. 40, a possible carcinogen. Not a great swap, if you ask me.

In fact, of the sevenapproved artificial food colorings left, five are possible carcinogens. Five may contribute to childhood asthma. Three may cause thyroid problems. Two are suspected of inciting hyperactivity in kids. Two provoke allergic reactions in some individuals. And one has been reported to cause dermatitis.

But unlike the European Union, which operates on the precautionary principle (that is, if a substance is suspected to cause harm, it should be pulled from the market until proven otherwise), the United States operates on the innocent-until-proven-guilty principle (that is, a substance cannot be banned until it has been *proven* to cause harm—that is, after it's too late). In the meantime, synthetic dyes, like artificial sweeteners, are everywhere. There are the obvious brightly colored products, like candy and popsicles and Jell-O. But they even find their way into everyday goods, like yogurt, pudding, sauces, chips, and meat. Even orange peels are routinely colored with Citrus Red No. 2.

Here's my take: Don't wait for your government to tell you that food dyes are dangerous. There's enough evidence right now to make that decision for yourself. Artificial food dyes might make your food look prettier, but they add no flavor and they're really bad for your health. You don't need a panel to come to this conclusion, so please don't wait for one.

TABLE 1.3. ARTIFICIAL FOOD DYES AND NATURAL ALTERNATIVES

Artificial Food Dye	The Potential Dangers*	The Natural Alternatives
FD&C Red No. 40	Possible Carcinogen; Potential Hyperactivity (kids); Potential Behavioral Problems (kids)	Annatto (seed of the achiote)—E160b; Beet Juice; Pomegranate Juice; Saffron—E160a; Paprika—E160c; Cochineal—E120
FD&C Red No. 3	Possible Carcinogen; Reported Thyroid Problems	Annatto (seed of the achiote)—E160b; Beet Juice; Pomegranate Juice; Saffron—E160a; Paprika—E160c; Cochineal—E210
FD&C Yellow No. 5	Reported Allergies; Reported Thyroid Problems; Potential Asthma (kids); Potential Hyperactivity (kids)	Turmeric—E100; Dried Mustard Seed Powder
FD&C Yellow No. 6	Possible Carcinogen; Reported Allergies; Reported Thyroid Problems; Potential Asthma (kids)	Turmeric—E100; Dried Mustard Seed Powder

TABLE 1.3. continued

Artificial Food Dye	The Potential Dangers*	The Natural Alternatives
FD&C Green No. 3	Possible Carcinogen	Chlorella—E140
FD&C Blue No. 1	Potential Asthma (kids)	Butterfly Pea; Elderberry Juice
FD&C Blue No. 2	Potential Asthma (kids)	Butterfly Pea; Elderberry Juice
D&C Yellow No. 11	Reports of Dermatitis	Turmeric—E100; Dried Mustard Seed Powder
Orange B	Reported Allergies; Potential Asthma (kids)	Annatto (seed of the achiote)—E160b; Saffron—E160a + Turmeric
Citrus Red No. 2; (red-orange)	Cancer in Animals	Saffron—E160a + Turmeric; Saffron—E160a; Paprika—E160c

*Sources:

1. Summary of color additives for use in the United States in foods, drugs, cosmetics, and medical devices. U.S. Food and Drug Administration. Updated Feb. 26, 2013. http://www.fda.gov/ForIndustry/ColorAdditives/ColorAdditiveInventories/ucm115641.htm

2. http://www.druglead.com

3. Kleinman RE, et al. A research model for investigating the effects of artificial food colorings on children with ADHD. *Pediatrics* 2011 Jun; 127(6):1575–84.

4. Kanarek RB. Artificial food dyes and attention deficit hyperactivity disorder. *Nutr Rev* 2011 Jul; 69(7):385–91.

5. Potera C. The artificial food dye blues. *Environ Health Perspect* 2010 Oct; 118(10):A428.

6. McCann D, et al. Food additives and hyperactive behaviour in 3-year-old and 8/9-year-old children in the community: a randomised, double-blind, placebo-controlled trial. Lancet 2007 Nov 3; 370(9598):1560–7.

7. Food Standards Agency. www.food.gov.uk. Sept. 11, 2007. Retrieved April 10, 2008.

8. Oplatowska M, et al. The potential for human exposure, direct and indirect, to the suspected carcinogenic triphenylmethane dye Brilliant Green from green paper towels. *Food Chem Toxicol* 2011 Aug; 49(8):1870–6.

9. Food additive code breaker colors E100-E181. NAC Allergy Forum. http://nac.allergyforum.com/additives/colors100–181.htm

BOTTOM LINE: *There is plenty of scientific evidence showing that trans fats, artificial preservatives, fake sweeteners, and chemical food dyes all pose serious health dangers. What's convenient for the food industry is toxic for you!*

What's Lurking in Your Meat, Poultry, and Dairy Products?

If you eat a typical slab of steak from the supermarket, you're ingesting a lot more than meat with every bite. You're also consuming hormones, antibiotics, and pesticides. Same goes with the typical glass of milk you drink. That's because big agriculture has taken every step possible to squeeze the most profit out of the animals it farms, regardless of the effects those steps have on your health (or the welfare of the animals).

Hormones

In today's large factory farms (or "concentrated animal-feeding operations," as the industry likes to call them), hormones are widely administered to cattle in order to artificially accelerate their growth and increase their milk production. In fact, it's estimated that two-thirds of cows raised in this country have been injected with hormones.[34]

Cows treated with hormones produce 15 percent more milk than regular cows, and they grow 20 percent faster, so that's a great incentive for the factory farmer. But it has no benefits for you and actually poses a significant threat to your health. That's because many cancers are hormone-related—such as breast cancer in women and prostate cancer in men—and excess hormones in your food may increase your risk. Hormones in meat and dairy are also a prime suspect in the quest to explain why children are entering puberty at a younger age than they did just a generation ago.

Antibiotics

Antibiotics are powerful, life-saving drugs. They are intended to be used short-term as a specific treatment for specific illnesses, namely bacterial infections. But that's not how antibiotics are typically used in this country. In fact, it might surprise you to find out that 80 percent of the antibiotics sold in the United States are fed to farm animals, the vast majority of which are healthy.[35]

Why? Three reasons. First, because antibiotics spur growth, and since beef, pork, and poultry are sold by the pound, larger animals mean larger profits. Second, animals raised in large factory farms are crammed together in unsanitary conditions, making bacterial infections common. And third, cows' bodies are meant to eat fibrous plants such as grasses, yet they are typically fed a grain-based diet, which literally makes them sick. Pretreating with antibiotics helps curtail what might otherwise be a massive tide of disease.

One effect of indiscriminately feeding livestock antibiotics is that the meat, milk, and eggs that they produce—and that you eat—contain traces of these drugs. I don't know about you, but I don't want to be eating drugs in my food!

Perhaps even more disturbing, this overuse of antibiotics has created a slew of antibiotic-resistant "superbugs." As a result, the next time you go to the doctor with a routine infection, the standard antibiotics you're prescribed may no longer do the trick.

This is serious life-threatening stuff. Before antibiotics, an infected wound or a simple case of sinusitis could mean death. It's not surprising, then, that Glenn Morris, director of the Emerging Pathogens Institute at the University of Florida, was quoted in a *New York Times* article as saying, "The single biggest problem we face in infectious disease today is the rapid growth of resistance to antibiotics."[36]

Pesticides

How many pounds of pesticides do you think are used each year in the production of grains used for animal feed? A few hundred? A few thousand? Try 167 million.[37] (That's more than the weight of 50,000 small cars combined!)

Inevitably, some of those pesticides remain on the grains. When animals eat these grains, they also eat the pesticide residue. And when you eat those animals, so do you. Since pesticides accumulate in the fatty portions of plants and animals, foods such as red meat, butter, and cheese are pesticide magnets.

Surely laws must be in place to ensure our meat doesn't contain dangerous levels of pesticide residues, you might be thinking. But our own government admits otherwise. According to a 2010 audit by the USDA's Office of Inspector General, the Environmental Protection Agency (EPA) has failed to set limits for many pesticides or adequately test for them. As a result, beef tainted with harmful pesticides is routinely sold to the public.[38]

Better Alternatives

All animal-based products fall somewhere along a spectrum of healthfulness. On one end of the spectrum, you have factory-farmed animals doped up on hormones and antibiotics, raised in cages or cramped conditions, and fed an unnatural diet laced with pesticides. On the other end of the spectrum, you have pasture-raised animals allowed to grow at their own pace, given plenty of room to wander and graze, and fed a pesticide-free diet their systems were designed to digest. There are also options in between.

To help you understand all of the choices in front of you, it's helpful to break down some definitions.

Natural: It would be perfectly reasonable for you to assume that if your meat is labeled "natural," it doesn't contain any of the bad stuff. Unfortunately, that's not true. By law, meat that is labeled "natural" simply means it's been minimally processed and doesn't include any artificial ingredients or preservatives. Accordingly, "natural" meat can still contain hormones, antibiotics, and pesticides. Who knew?

No Antibiotics: This one is pretty straightforward. In order for meat and poultry to be labeled "no antibiotics," the producer has to provide documentation to the USDA showing that the animals were raised without antibiotics.

No Hormones: This one is also clear-cut. It's illegal to administer hormones to hogs and poultry. So it's only cows and sheep you need to worry about. In order for beef to be labeled "no hormones," the producer has to provide documentation to the USDA showing the animals weren't given hormones.

Cage-free: This term has no legal definition, but is commonly used to refer to poultry raised without the battery cages frequently seen in factory farming operations. Instead, the birds are usually raised in large henhouses. Unfortunately, these houses may be extremely crowded, and the hens may or may not have outdoor access. So there's no guarantee of a healthy bird with this label.

Free-range: Federal standards require that poultry and eggs labeled "free-range" be allowed access to the outdoors. That's a step up from cages and henhouses, but it doesn't mean the birds will be out roaming native grasslands. The outdoor area may be dirt or gravel. And when it comes to other animals, the word "free-range" isn't regulated.

Organic: Thanks to the National Organic Program, the word "organic" has a very specific definition. Organic meat and eggs are raised without the use of hormones and antibiotics. Their feed must be 100 percent organic. And they have to be given access to the outdoors. This is one of the most rigorous labels out there.

Grass-fed: If they could choose their own diets, cows would eat grass for breakfast, lunch, and dinner. Most conventional (and some organic) beef, though, comes from cows raised on a diet of grains for either their entire lives or the end of their lives ("grain-finished") in order to fatten them up. Beef labeled "grass-fed" has eaten a grass-only diet. As a result, it's lower in saturated fat and contains higher levels of omega-3 fatty acids—important for heart health, brain function, and more—than grain-fed beef.

Pasture-raised: This feel-good phrase connotes that not only were the animals raised without cages and with access to the outdoors, they actually got to live the way we imagine farm animals should live: outside on fresh, green pasture. However, since there's no legal definition of "pasture-raised," it's a good idea to do your own research by calling the company in question and asking them how their animals are raised.

I'll be the first to admit that eating grass-fed beef is more expensive than grain-fed and that eating antibiotic-free chicken is going to cost more than conventional. Not everyone can do it all the time. But that's why we supplement: to help combat the effects of the less-than-ideal diet most of us eat every day.

> **BOTTOM LINE:** Hormones, antibiotics, and pesticides are par for the course when it comes to industrially produced meat, poultry, and dairy products. The animals we're eating are sick or contaminated, and so are we.

ENVIRONMENTAL TOXINS

Currently, there are an astonishing 84,000 synthetic chemicals manufactured or processed in the United States,[39] with about 1,000 new ones introduced each year.[40] Most people just assume these chemicals have undergone extensive safety testing before being released to the market. But unfortunately, that's not the case.

Consider this stunner. There are six internationally agreed upon tests for screening the toxicity of high-produce volume (HPV) chemicals: acute toxicity, chronic toxicity, developmental/reproductive toxicity, mutagenicity, ecotoxicity, and environmental fate. Sadly, according to a 1998 EPA report, only 7 *percent* of the 3,000 HPV chemicals that the United States makes or imports have undergone all six safety tests. And 43 *percent*—nearly half!—have not been subjected to a single, solitary one.[41]

How can this be? Because our laws have it backward. The 1976 Toxic Substances Control Act only requires that a new chemical be tested for toxicity before being introduced to the market if there is evidence that it may be harmful.[42] And once it's on the market, it's very difficult to remove. Talk about a Catch-22! How will evidence surface that a new chemical is toxic if it's not required to be tested?

As a result of our lax laws, American industry releases 4 billion pounds of toxic chemicals into the environment annually—72 million pounds of which are now known to cause cancer.[43] Humans have never been exposed to such a deluge of disease-causing chemicals in our history.

And don't think that just because you live outside of a major city that this isn't your problem. In today's modern environment, toxins are everywhere. From the volatile organic compounds in your painted walls . . . to the formaldehyde in your wrinkle-resistant clothing . . . to the flame retardants in your couch . . . to the pesticides on your food . . . to the dioxins in your coffee filters . . . to the phthalates in your air freshener . . . to the lead in your lipstick . . . to the Teflon in your frying pan . . . to the parabens in your lotion . . . to the BPA in your hard water bottle . . . to the stain-resistant coating on your carpet . . . to the vinyl in your shower curtain . . . to the pharmaceutical drugs tainting your water supply.

The Chemicals Inside You

Sure, you feel healthy, but if you were to take samples of your blood and urine and have them analyzed them for toxin content, you might be surprised at what you'd find.

Without a doubt, DDT, the long-banned pesticide and "probable human carcinogen," would show up. According to a report published in the journal *Environmental Health Perspectives,* the pesticide is so stable that "there is now not a single living organism on the planet that does not contain DDT."[44]

A chemical known as PFOA, used to manufacture Teflon and the coatings lining microwave popcorn bags and pizza boxes, would also very likely be present. This chemical, a "likely human carcinogen" that is linked with heart disease and stroke, is present in the blood of over 98 percent of Americans.[45]

You could also expect to see the toxic chemical BPA in your test results, as a recent study conducted by the Centers for Disease Control (CDC) discovered it in 90 percent of those studied.[46] BPA mimics the effects of human hormones and has been linked to prostate and breast cancer. If you've ever eaten food out of a can, had dental sealants, or drunk water out of a hard plastic bottle, you've been exposed to BPA.

And don't forget BDE-47, the fire retardant that American couches, chairs, and mattresses are regularly doused with. This suspected carcinogen is so widely applied to items we sit and lie down on that it appeared in nearly all of the participants the CDC tested.[47] Animal studies show chemicals in this class have effects on the thyroid gland and liver and may affect the brain and immune system.[48]

Those are just the chemicals you can *count* on being in your system. The truth is, you probably harbor hundreds of the 1,000 toxic chemicals tracked by the EPA Office of Toxic Substances. Even newborn babies— who have never breathed our air, drunk our water, or eaten our food— are contaminated. A benchmark study led by the Environmental Working Group identified 287 different industrial chemicals in the umbilical cord blood of ten babies born in 2004. On average, each infant had been exposed to about 200 different chemicals before even leaving the womb.[49]

BOTTOM LINE: *Even if you make an effort to live a clean lifestyle, your body is still contaminated with hundreds of toxic chemicals because they are so prevalent in common everyday household items.*

Toxins, Oxidative Stress, and Disease

So why is all this toxic exposure bad for you? What exactly do toxins do to your body?

A vast majority of toxic chemicals increase oxidative stress, in other words, the stress that is put on your body from being constantly bombarded by free radicals. Also known as oxidants, free radicals are oxygen compounds that are unstable because they're missing an electron. Since their ultimate goal in life is to become stable, free radicals will use any means necessary to achieve it—including stealing electrons from other molecules. This stripping of electrons can damage healthy cells.

The problem is, free radicals multiply. In fact, they're a lot like vampires. Once a free radical takes an electron from another molecule, that molecule then becomes a free radical. The newly initiated free radical then goes looking for another molecule to pillage, initiating a vicious cycle of cellular damage.

Your body produces some free radicals during normal metabolism, and others come from the environment. Cigarette smoke, pollution, pesticides, and other toxic chemicals are all huge generators of free radicals.

As with a lot of things, it's a case of balance. You want to have a certain level of free radicals in your body, because they destroy viruses and bacteria. But too many, and you're looking at cellular destruction, aging, and disease. In fact, most scientists today agree that nearly all chronic diseases—from cancer to heart disease to Alzheimer's disease to Parkinson's disease—involve oxidative stress.

Let's take lung cancer as an example. When you breathe in cigarette smoke, it stimulates the creation of free radicals in your lungs. Those free radicals go to work attacking the cells in your lungs and creating more free radicals in the process. If they manage to damage your DNA, your lung cells will mutate and grow abnormally. If the mutated cells reproduce, you'll get lung cancer.

The good news is that your body came equipped with its own antioxidant defenses, so it's prepared to quench a certain amount of free radicals and keep your cells healthy. The bad news is that the level of oxidative stress that you and every other American are experiencing from industrial toxin exposure is way higher than nature ever intended. It's overwhelming our defenses and making us sick.

Just consider these troubling statistics. Fewer people smoke now than they have in decades, yet cancer has surpassed heart disease as the number-one killer of people under age eighty-five.[50] In fact, if you're an American woman, you have a one-in-three chance of getting cancer in your lifetime, and a one-in-five risk of dying from it.[51] If you're a man, your prospects are even worse: you have a one-in-two chance of getting cancer, and a one-in-four risk that it will kill you.[52] The incidence of certain cancers is accelerating at breakneck speed: bone marrow, bladder, and liver cancer cases all doubled from 1950 to 2001.[53]

At a conference in Paris in 2004, a group of leading scientists and doctors stated that "Industrial chemicals have been incriminated as a major cause of increasing cancer rates and other chronic diseases."[54] Two years later, the European Union passed REACH (Registration, Evaluation, Authorisation, and Restriction of Chemicals) legislation, which puts the burden on chemical manufacturers to prove their products are safe. It also calls for phasing out toxic chemicals like phthalates and flame-retardants from consumer products. I wish the United States would follow suit!

BOTTOM LINE: *Toxins cause oxidative stress, and oxidative stress is at the heart of most—if not all—chronic, degenerative diseases.*

Minimizing Your Exposure

As a member of this society, you are going to be interacting with a certain amount of toxic chemicals. You can't live in a bubble. But you can take some precautions to limit your exposure.

Go Low-VOC

Volatile organic compounds (VOCs) are carbon-containing chemicals that easily turn into gasses. You can often spot them by smell because the products that contain them stink—like paints and lacquers, glues and adhesives, and solvents. But VOCs are also hidden in the strangest places, like carpet cleaners, disinfectants, and air fresheners (of all things).

- Whenever possible, choose products that contain no or low levels of VOCs. For example, many brands of latex paint now offer no-VOC lines.

- Disinfect surfaces and freshen air naturally with essential oils. (Thyme essential oil, for example, almost completely kills bacteria within one hour of contact.[55])

Choose Safe Plastics

BPA and phthalates are both hormone-disrupting chemicals with opposite functions. BPA makes plastics hard, so it's found in hard plastic water bottles, baby bottles, and food storage containers. It's also used in the resin lining of canned foods and beverages. Phthalates, on the other hand, soften plastics, so they show up in toys, shower curtains, vinyl flooring, and food packaging. Bizarrely, they are also frequently contained in air fresheners, hairsprays, and shampoos, since they make scents last longer.

- Store food in glass containers, or at the very least, in plastic containers labeled BPA-free. Never heat food in plastic containers.

- Limit your use of canned foods and beverages, or buy your canned goods from Eden Organic, which has developed a BPA-free tin can: http://www.edenfoods.com/.

- Swap your plastic shower curtain for a cloth one, and if you're going to put in new kitchen flooring, choose linoleum over vinyl.

- Shop for phthalate-free cosmetics. You can find a listing of drugstore-brand cosmetics that don't contain phthalates by visiting the website of the Environmental Working Group at www.ewg.org/node/21288. Or you can go a step further and look for natural-brand cosmetics that carry the NPA Natural Seal, which strictly disallows harmful synthetic ingredients at www.npainfo.org/NPA/Custom/PersonalCareProducts .aspx.

Eat Organic Produce

Conventional produce is routinely sprayed with pesticides. Make no mistake: pesticides are poisons, meant to kill living things. The idea that humans are somehow immune to their effects is false. And since a recent USDA study found that 64 percent of fresh fruits and vegetables tested had detectable pesticide residues, it just makes sense to choose organic.[56]

- Look for certified organic produce, which is grown without pesticides.

- If you can't afford to buy all your fruits and vegetables organic, at least avoid the "dirty dozen"—those with the highest levels of pesti-

cide residue—apples, celery, sweet bell peppers, peaches, strawberries, nectarines (imported), grapes, spinach, lettuce, cucumbers, blueberries (domestic), and potatoes.[57]

- Wash conventional produce before eating. It turns out that washing
food with plain water is just as effective at getting rid of pesticides as
produce wash solutions are. You can also peel the skins off some
types of produce to lower pesticide levels. (The downside of that is
that the peel contains fiber and important nutrients.)

Say No to Teflon

Non-stick pans are convenient, but they're not worth the price tag of
cancer, heart disease, and stroke. They contain PFOA, and so do other
non-sticky things, like fast food containers, pizza boxes, and microwave
popcorn bags. DuPont, makers of Teflon, has committed to phasing
PFOA out by 2015. Luckily, you don't have to wait until then to limit
your exposure.

- Get rid of your non-stick pans—today! Cook with stainless steel
instead.

- Make your own popcorn at home, sans microwave.

- Don't eat fast food. It's not just the food that's bad for you—it's the
packaging too!

CHRONIC STRESS

Today's twenty-four-hour, information-saturated, digitally connected
way of living is a recipe for chronic stress. There are so many demands
placed on us, all of which have to be addressed "right now." Stress may
seem insignificant. But it's killing us—literally. A landmark study published in the *Journal of the American Medical Association* in 1999 found a
link between chronic stress and a higher risk of mortality in older
adults.[58] In other words, stressed-out folks were more likely to die than
their relaxed peers.

The Stress Response

The human body interprets every demand, small or large, as a stressor.
And it responds to all stressors in the same basic fashion: the stress

response. This complicated set of physiological reactions is brilliant because it keeps you alive during dangerous situations. Here's how it's supposed to work:

1. You experience an acute stressor. Thousands of years ago, this could have been a tiger trying to eat you. Today, maybe it's a child running in front of your car.

2. In response to the stressor, your adrenal glands release cortisol into your bloodstream. Cortisol is the stress hormone that initiates several lifesaving metabolic changes in your body, including an increase in blood sugar.

3. This extra load of blood sugar is used by your brain, heart, and skeletal muscles for immediate energy so you can fight or run or slam on your brakes.

4. Once the stressor is dealt with, cortisol quickly leaves your system and things return to their normal metabolic state.

That's in a perfect (and imaginary) world. Unfortunately, in this imperfect (and real) world, it's more likely that as soon as you've dealt with one stressor, another one is on its heels. For example, you have a tiff with your spouse over breakfast, then you get caught in a traffic jam that makes you late for work, then you're handed an impossible deadline, and then you get a call from your daughter's school that she's sick and you need to come pick her up. From the time you wake up in the morning to the time you finally get to bed at night, you've probably dealt with dozens of low-grade stressful events.

Your stress response system is supposed to be finely tuned for responding to acute events. But if you're like most people, your system is always on, and you're swimming in a constant stream of low- to moderate-grade stress. This causes significant derangements in metabolism, because your body never gets to return to that blissful state of homeostasis.

BOTTOM LINE: *Your body is well adapted to manage acute, occasional stress. But it was never meant to be on stress alert 24/7.*

How Chronic Stress Affects You

When you are chronically stressed, several things get metabolically out of whack.

- Your cortisol level stays elevated, which means your blood sugar does too. And whatever blood sugar isn't burned gets stored as belly fat.

- Your immune system gets suppressed, which lowers your resistance to infection.

- You produce too much adrenaline, which can cause heartburn and ulcers.

- Your blood pressure increases, which puts you at higher risk of stroke, heart attack, and kidney failure.

- And believe it or not, your hippocampus (the part of your brain responsible for memory storage) may shrink, impairing your ability to remember.[59]

But perhaps the most damaging effect chronic stress has on your system is that it interferes with your body's ability to regulate the inflammatory response. This again has to do with increased cortisol levels.

One of cortisol's roles is to keep inflammation under control. Unfortunately, cortisol is like alcohol: your body can develop a tolerance to it. Alcoholics can drink far more liquor than average folks without getting drunk because their bodies no longer respond to it the way they're supposed to. In the same way, stressaholics' bodies stop responding to cortisol the way they're supposed to. As a result, their bodies lose the power to halt inflammation. And inflammation is now known to be at the heart of most chronic diseases.[60]

BOTTOM LINE: *Chronic stress has multiple negative effects on your health that can increase your risk of disease and death.*

PUTTING IT ALL TOGETHER

In this chapter, we've learned that about 90 percent of Americans don't eat enough disease-fighting fruits and vegetables, so it's very unlikely you're getting all the nutrition you need from your diet. And even if you are the rare one in ten, due to poor soil quality, a tomato today is not nearly as nutritious as a tomato from a hundred years ago. That means it's much harder to get all the vitamins, minerals, phytonutrients, and antioxidants from your diet than it used to be.

We've also highlighted the amazing amount of hidden and dangerous "ingredients" in the food you eat, including the hormones, antibiotics, and pesticides tainting your meat, poultry, and dairy products, as well as the preservatives, artificial sweeteners, chemical food dyes, and GMOs contained in the processed foods sitting in your kitchen cabinet.

Finally, we've discussed the great number of environmental toxins inhabiting your home and your body, and how chronic stress has become a staple of modern living.

The common thread among all these factors is that they put undue stress on your body—stress that the average American diet can't fully counteract, as it itself is part of the problem. Poor soil, a sick food chain, environmental toxins, and chronic stress all cause oxidative stress, inflammation, internal toxicity, and hormonal imbalances. And the best way I know to combat these problems is through the prudent, targeted use of dietary supplements. I'll teach you how to do just that, by creating your own personalized Supplement Pyramid, in the following chapters.

CHAPTER 2

The Supplement Pyramid Overview

Once you understand the importance of nutritional supplements, the next question is: "Now what?"

By far the most common questions I am asked have to do with what to take and, equally important, what not to take. After all, there are a staggering amount of choices out there. Anyone who has walked into the supplement section of a natural foods store or conducted a quick online search on a vitamin supersite can attest to that. Making things even more complicated, there are new products coming to market almost daily. It's easy to get lost with all the options to consider.

So how do you know if you're taking the right supplements? Should you add the latest Amazonian herb you just read about to your supplement regimen? What if you want to cut back a little to save money—which supplements should you keep and which ones should you pitch? These are the exact type of questions your Supplement Pyramid can answer for you.

WHAT IS A SUPPLEMENT PYRAMID?

You're familiar with the food pyramid, right? It's an educational graphic tool that helps you design and follow a healthy diet by telling you how many servings you should eat from different food groups. The Supplement Pyramid is like the food pyramid in that it's an educational graphic tool, but that's where the similarities end.

Unlike its food counterpart, the Supplement Pyramid is personalized to meet your specific nutritional needs. After all, with the exception of a few foundational nutrients, there is no such thing as a one-size-fits-all supplement regimen. I think you'd agree with me that my needs are not yours and your needs are not mine.

Why a pyramid? First, because the pyramid structure is symbolic of stability. And second, because as you ascend up the levels of the pyramid, they shrink in size, representing their order of importance to your health. That means you're going to build your Supplement Pyramid from the bottom up, like a real pyramid.

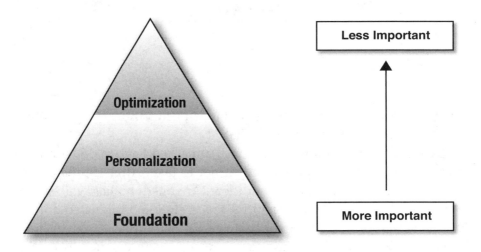

THE THREE LEVELS

Your Supplement Pyramid will have three levels.

The bottom tier is the Foundation Level. It's made up of nutrients essential to life. Because of their vital importance to human biology, we all need to take the same foundational supplements. The middle tier is the Personalization Level. This is the level that's all yours. It's comprised of nutrients specific to your personal medical history and health needs. (You'll establish these needs through medical quizzes and blood testing included in Chapter 4.) The top tier is the Optimization Level. This is where all of the "extra" supplements come in that really take your health to the next or optimal level.

The Foundation Level

The Egyptian pyramids have lasted for over 4,000 years because of one thing—a solid foundation. Your Supplement Pyramid needs a sturdy base too. The supplements comprising this level support basic life processes, such as cellular energy production, growth, repair, and regeneration.

No matter who you are or what you're going through, you need the same foundational supplements as everybody else. Think of them as the essential nutrients for living well as a human. They include four building blocks:

1. An ideally dosed multivitamin/mineral

2. Omega-3 fatty acids

3. Coenzyme Q_{10} (as ubiquinol)

4. Probiotics

The Personalization Level

The middle part of the Supplement Pyramid is all about you. It's about finding the right supplements to help you prevent the diseases most likely to affect you personally. If you're itching to find out which supplements will help you train for a marathon or reverse your cells' biological clocks to prevent aging, we'll get to that. Those types of personal health and wellness goals belong in the Optimization Level. This level is really designed to prevent disease.

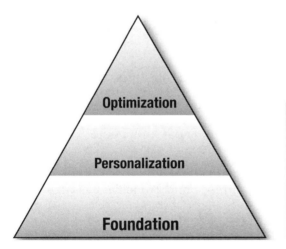

Optimization

Personalization

Foundation

Personal Prevention
Supplements
Probiotics
Ubiquinol CoQ$_{10}$
Omega-3 Fatty Acids
Ideally Dosed
Multivitamin

You'll complete three basic procedures in order to identify the supplements in your Personalization Level:

1. Personal and Family Medical Inventories

2. Medical Quizzes

3. Laboratory Testing

Personal and Family Medical Inventories

We all face different health challenges throughout our lives. Some of these you'll have dealt with directly. You may have a history of heart disease, for example, or perhaps just some of the warning signs, like high blood pressure, elevated triglycerides, or insulin resistance. Other health challenges may not have touched you yet, but have affected members of your family, putting you at greater risk. A father, an aunt, or a grandparent may have had cancer or Alzheimer's disease, for example.

Creating a personal and family medical inventory will help you identify past, ongoing, and potential problem spots for you to protect against. And that's the beauty of the Personalization Level. This is not a one-size-fits-all solution. It's tailored to your own specific medical needs. Accounting for your personal and family health history is the first step in developing it.

Your medical inventory will be comprised of questions pertaining to major organ systems, including:

- The cardiovascular system: heart and blood vessels

- The nervous system: brain and nerves

- The muscular system: muscles

- The digestive system: stomach, liver, and intestines

- The endocrine system: pancreas, glands, and hormones

- The immune system: thymus, spleen, and lymph nodes

- The skeletal system: bones and joints

- The respiratory system: lungs, sinuses, and bronchial passages

- The urinary system: kidneys and bladder

I'll also ask you questions to see how you're doing in the following areas:

- Diabetes/metabolism

- Eyes/ears/nose/throat

- Mental health/mood

You'll note the obvious diseases, as well as the strange symptoms that haven't been diagnosed yet. For example, let's say your older sister suffers from chronic tremors of her hands, but her doctors don't know why. And your mom remembers a great aunt that had similar problems. This information would be included in your inventory as a potential nerve disorder and would require appropriate supplementation.

Once you've identified past problems that you don't want to come back, current problems to address, and potential problems in the future, you can take appropriate steps to protect yourself.

Medical Quizzes

After you finish your personal and family medical inventory, you'll take a series of medical quizzes to assess how you're doing in different areas . . . heart health, cognitive function, immune strength, and more. These quizzes aren't the kind of fluff you'd find in a mainstream health magazine. Each one is based on real clinical risk assessments that doctors use for major organ systems.

The answers you give on each quiz will be used to calculate a risk score for that particular body function. This deeper level of detail will help identify potential problems that weren't picked up in your personal and family medical inventory. Based on your risk scores in different categories, I'll make very specific supplement suggestions to complete your Personalization Level.

Laboratory Testing

The final step in developing your Personalization Level is to learn about the array of laboratory tests that can further help you personalize your Supplement Pyramid. I think this is the most exciting part of the Personalization Level because lab testing can tell you all kinds of things about what's going on inside your body that would be hard to figure out otherwise. I'll recommend tests that will help you identify:

- Which nutrients you may be lacking

- Whether you're part of the 70 percent of Americans deficient in omega-3 fatty acids

- The level of toxic heavy metals in your system

- How much oxidative stress your body is under

- If your levels of various hormone and neurotransmitters are normal

- Whether food allergies are making you sick

I'll even provide a quick cognitive test that you can take right at home to determine if you're showing any signs of age-related cognitive decline.

The Optimization Level

The top part of your Supplement Pyramid is the Optimization Level. Supplements in this level do exactly what the name implies. They don't necessarily meet your medical needs—that's what the personalization level is for. These supplements simply "optimize" your regimen.

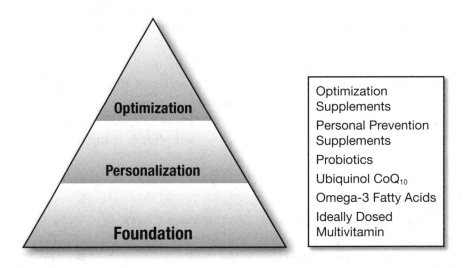

Optimization

Personalization

Foundation

Optimization Supplements

Personal Prevention Supplements

Probiotics

Ubiquinol CoQ$_{10}$

Omega-3 Fatty Acids

Ideally Dosed Multivitamin

This level is where you'll find supplements that help you live a longer, healthier life. You could also think of them as anti-aging supplements. These might include extra antioxidants, proteins, and amino acids, or maybe even the latest longevity herb.

Supplements at this level may not be essential to your overall health. But that's not to say they aren't important. They could help extend your lifespan or make your later years healthier. However, when it's all said and done, you can do without them.

That's why the Supplement Pyramid is structured the way it is—so you always meet your foundational survival needs first, your disease prevention needs second, and your anti-aging goals last. I know that not everyone is always flush with cash. So if you need to cut back on expenses, then the supplements in the Optimization Level should be the first to go. That way, you'll still be providing your body with the core, foundational nutrients for survival and the custom-tailored supplements that will help you prevent disease.

Now that you understand what it is and how it functions, I hope you're getting excited about creating your very own personalized Supplement Pyramid! Once you complete chapters four, five, and six you'll know exactly the right supplements you should be taking for your foundational requirements, your disease prevention needs, and your health optimization. But first . . . how can you identify high-quality supplements?

CHAPTER 3

Choosing High-Quality Supplements

It's almost time to build your own personalized Supplement Pyramid. But before we get into the specifics of what *kinds* of products you'll be taking every day, let's go over how to choose the best *quality* products.

It's a sad but true fact that quality among nutritional supplements varies widely. Therefore, it's a good idea to ask yourself the following questions before making a purchase:

- How do I know that the ingredients inside my supplements match what's advertised on the labels?

- How can I be sure that my supplements contain the full amount they say they do?

- How do I know that my supplements aren't contaminated with pesticides, heavy metals, or microbes?

- How can I tell if my supplements are providing therapeutic dosages of key ingredients versus just a sprinkling?

- How can I keep myself from being hoodwinked by supplement charlatans who care only about lining their pockets at my expense?

The dilemma is real, but the solution is simple: Stick with a company that has an established track record of selling high-quality products. Established companies use only pure, potent raw materials. They follow—and in many cases exceed—all government regulations for processing and manufacturing. They test their products regularly to make sure they contain everything they say they do—and nothing they don't.

And because they are in business for long-term benefit and not short-term gain, they include dosages of key ingredients high enough to impact your health. That way, they'll keep you as a loyal customer.

In this chapter, I'll give you some guidelines to help you distinguish between high-quality supplements you can purchase with confidence and low-quality supplements you should avoid wasting your money on.

SUPPLEMENTS VERSUS INGREDIENTS

So what is a dietary supplement, anyway? And how is it different from a dietary ingredient?

According to the Dietary Supplement Health and Education Act of 1994 (DSHEA), a dietary supplement (also known as a nutritional supplement) is a product that is intended for ingestion (such as capsules, tablets, soft gels, liquids, powders, and so on) and is meant to supplement the diet. A dietary ingredient refers to the raw material used to make the finished dietary supplement, and includes vitamins, minerals, herbs and other botanicals, and amino acids. A dietary ingredient can also be a concentrate, metabolite, constituent, or extract of any of the above ingredients.

DSHEA also established what dietary supplements are *not*. They are not drugs. (So it's not legal to put, say, Viagra, in a men's multivitamin.) They are not conventional foods. (That means it's not allowable to market a soup as a dietary supplement.) And finally, they are not food additives. (As a result, they don't need FDA pre-market approval.)

THE IMPORTANCE OF HIGH-QUALITY RAW MATERIALS

It may seem obvious, but a high-quality supplement begins with high-quality raw materials. If you put garbage in, you get garbage out. It's as simple as that! Many companies try to cut corners and save a few pennies by using inexpensive raw materials. But you can't get a quality end product by starting with junk any more than you can build a sturdy house on a foundation of quicksand.

A note of caution: Cost can often be an indicator of quality. I hate to say it, but you get what you pay for. Products sourced from only the best-validated raw materials and produced by manufacturers following legally established quality procedures cost more than products that don't. Don't skimp on your health!

SHOULD YOU BUY ORGANIC SUPPLEMENTS?

Organically grown raw materials are desirable because they are grown without the use of harmful pesticides, but they are not always cost effective. Don't worry though. If you follow my suggestions for choosing a high-quality product, you can be assured that it's been tested for the absence of contaminants—whether or not it's made from organic raw materials.

THE FOUR BASIC ELEMENTS OF A QUALITY PRODUCT

In drafting quality procedures for dietary supplement manufacturing—known as Good Manufacturing Practices, or GMPs—the FDA came up with a pretty good definition of quality: "Quality means that the dietary supplement consistently meets the established specifications for identity, purity, strength, and composition . . . "[1] That covers the basics pretty well. As you'll see later in this chapter, I have a few additional standards for quality. But every quality nutritional supplement should, at a minimum, have the identity, purity, strength, and composition it purports to. Let's look at each one of these factors individually.

Identity

Imagine you bought a product that said it was ginkgo, but it turned out upon laboratory analysis to be a totally different herb—one that didn't have any of ginkgo's researched properties. Believe it or not, this has happened on occasion. In some cases, the result is simply an ineffective product. In other cases, though, the consequences are much more dire—such as when digitalis, an herb that can cause cardiac arrest, was accidentally substituted for the herb plantain by a raw material supplier in 1997.[2]

Therefore, the first criterion of a high-quality product is that it contains everything that's listed on the label, including both active and inactive ingredients. The active ingredients are those that are listed inside the Supplement Facts box. The inactive ingredients are listed beneath it under "Other Ingredients."

Purity

Just as important that a product contains everything that's listed on the label is that it doesn't contain anything that's *not* listed there, such as contaminants and adulterants. You don't want your herbs to be contaminated with heavy metals or your fish oils to be contaminated with PCBs. And you definitely don't want to purchase a product that has been adulterated.

Some unscrupulous raw materials suppliers secretly and intentionally add illegal substances to their ingredients to make them appear to be higher quality than they actually are. For example, the herb bilberry is frequently adulterated with cheaper berries to artificially inflate the level of active constituents. On rare occasions, raw material suppliers have even been known to adulterate their ingredients with prescription drugs to make them more effective.

Strength

It's also important to know that the label of the supplement you're considering purchasing has accurately represented the strength, or potency, of what's inside. After all, a large part of what makes a supplement effective is dose. If the product says it contains 500 milligrams (mg) of vitamin C per tablet, you want to know it does!

By law, dietary supplement manufacturers have to test their products to make sure they provide at least 100 percent of the stated amount of each ingredient. But too often, their numbers come up short. This is illustrated by a recent analysis of coenzyme Q_{10} (CoQ_{10}) products performed by ConsumerLab.com, an independent company that routinely tests the actual potencies of a whole range of nutritional supplements against the potencies stated on their labels. While the majority of CoQ_{10} products passed ConsumerLab.com's stringent quality tests, one product contained just 4 percent (8 mg) of the stated amount of CoQ_{10} (200 mg) per serving!

On the flip side, sometimes dietary supplements contain more of an ingredient than what's stated on the label. To some extent, that's to be expected. Over time, the potency of supplements diminishes. In order to provide at least 100 percent of the stated amount of each ingredient at the time the consumer buys it, supplement manufacturers include overages. But would you expect your calcium supplement to provide nearly *twice* the amount of vitamin D it says it does? I wouldn't! But that's exactly what ConsumerLab.com found in a recent analysis of calcium products. Two of the twenty-three products the company selected for testing contained 172.5 percent and 182.2 percent of their stated values for vitamin D.

Composition

Composition is sort of an amalgam of the three other quality factors: identity, purity, and strength. It means that the formula as a whole is composed of the same ingredients listed on the label, in the same potencies, without any contaminants.

VETTING SUPPLEMENTS FOR IDENTITY, PURITY, STRENGTH, AND COMPOSITION

Now that you understand the four basic elements that make up a quality product, how do you look for them? Here are some tips.

1. Check for GMP Compliance

As of June 2010, it became mandatory that all nutritional supplements made or sold in the United States be manufactured in accordance with GMPs, a set of manufacturing processes, safety procedures, packaging standards, and laboratory testing protocol that help ensure a quality product.

The requirements include provisions related to:

- The design and construction of physical plants that facilitate maintenance
- Cleaning of work areas
- Proper manufacturing operations with calibrated machines
- Quality-control procedures
- Testing final product or incoming and in-process materials
- Handling consumer complaints
- Maintaining records

According to the FDA's website, "Under FDA regulations at 21 CFT part 111, all domestic and foreign companies that manufacture, package, label, or hold dietary supplements, including those involved with the activities of testing, quality control, packaging and labeling, and distributing them in the U.S., must comply with the Dietary Supplement Current Good Manufacturing Practices (CGMPs) for quality control."[3] That means that even if a supplement sold in the United States is made in Europe, it still has to be manufactured in accordance with GMPs. However, since it's a lot easier for the FDA to monitor facilities in the

United States rather than halfway across the world, I think your best bet is going with supplements made in America.

Unfortunately, being made in America is not an absolute guarantee of quality. The truth is that not all supplement companies have your health and safety in mind. In fact, from June 2008 to June 2012, the FDA inspected 450 supplement firms and found violations among half of them.[4] Therefore, it's important to choose your brand wisely!

So how do you verify that the company you are considering buying from is aboveboard? Call them and ask for verification of their GMP compliance. The good ones will have no problem providing this information to you.

2. Choose Brands That Test and Test Again

The only surefire way to know a product is accurately labeled is to test it. By law, every nutritional supplement manufacturer should be subjecting each raw material they use in a particular product, as well as the finished product itself, to a series of identity and purity tests. For example, sophisticated analytical techniques such as high-performance liquid chromatography (HPLC) and mass spectrometry (MS) can distinguish between true bilberry and a cheap imposter. And purity tests can easily determine if a product has been contaminated or adulterated.

SHOULD YOU AVOID INGREDIENTS FROM CHINA?

In general, the best sources of raw material are the United States, Japan, and Europe. Despite negative headlines, China can also be a good source.

You know the saying, "One bad apple can spoil the whole bunch"? That's what happened in China. You've heard the stories . . . infant formula tainted with melamine, a toxic and illegal additive . . . Chinese toys contaminated with lead, a neurotoxin . . . dietary supplements corrupted with undisclosed prescription drugs.

These are serious incidents. But they are the exception and not the rule. So don't let them scare you from taking supplements that contain raw material manufactured in China. There are numerous reputable Chinese-based companies producing high-quality raw materials. The key is to find nutritional supplement brands you can trust . . . those that test ALL raw materials for quality and safety BEFORE developing a product, as they are required to do by law.

But you'd be surprised that not all companies do this. So you need to pick up the phone and ask. Now, in some cases, the supplement company doesn't perform the actual testing themselves. However, they only purchase ingredients from trusted suppliers that have had their raw materials tested by third-party laboratories, and they freely share the results with the company and with you, the consumer. That's perfectly fine. Ultimately, you just want to know that the testing has been done.

3. Ask for a Certificate of Analysis

I wouldn't just take a company's word for it that they test their raw materials and finished products, though. Ask for proof. To validate the quality of any product, pick up the phone and request that the company send you a Certificate of Analysis, commonly referred to as a C of A. This document is a summary of all the tests that have been done on the product to assure that it contains the ingredients it says it does, that the ingredients are present in the doses listed on the label, and that it is free of contaminants such as heavy metals and microbes.

If the company in question tells you they don't have C of As for their products or don't release them, then that's probably a good reason for you to find another company from which to purchase your supplements.

I have provided a section later in this chapter that teaches you how to evaluate a C of A.

4. Do a Search on ConsumerLab.com

One way to find out if your nutritional supplement makes the grade is to do a search on www.ConsumerLab.com. As I mentioned before, this company routinely tests what's inside a product versus what's stated on the label, and reveals which brands passed and which didn't. Of course, they can't test all the nutritional supplements in the world, but it's a good place to start.

The site is subscription-based, so you'll have to shell out about $33 a year to access their testing results. But it also has a great encyclopedia of natural products, which allows you to look up just about any dietary ingredient and see whether or not it is scientifically supported.

5. Take It from Me

If you don't have the time or inclination to do your own research, check out the companies I have listed in Appendix A. These are companies that I have personally scrutinized for quality and that I recommend as sources from which to purchase your supplements.

Just remember: identity, purity, strength, and composition are the four basic elements of a quality nutritional supplement. But that's just the beginning. The following are some other factors to consider when making your choice.

ARTIFICIAL ADDITIVES

It might be surprising to find out that some supplement brands routinely add things like artificial colors—and, in the case of chewables, artificial flavors—to their products. Just as you want to avoid artificial additives in your food, you also want to steer clear of them in your supplements. That's one reason I prefer health food store brands to drugstore brands: what's *not* in the tablet!

Look at the inactive ingredients of popular drugstore vitamin brands (which are listed below the Supplement Facts box), and you'll find all kinds of things that have no place in a nutritional supplement. In addition to artificial dyes, they also contain hydrogenated oils (in other words, trans fats!), and artificial preservatives.[5] High-quality nutritional supplements won't contain any of this junk.

EVALUATING A CERTIFICATE OF ANALYSIS

Okay, you've done your homework. You've called the company and asked for a C of A, and they've sent it to you. Now what? It's comparison time!

Go back to the store with the C of A in hand and compare it to the

---

IS ALL THIS WORK REALLY NECESSARY?

I know that all of this seems like a lot of work for purchasing supplements. But once you get into the habit of calling companies, it's really not that hard. And it's well worth it. You're taking supplements for your health, right? What's more important than your health?

If you were to judge people's purchasing behavior, you would conclude that cars and cell phones are more important than health. We have no problem investigating those two things thoroughly before making a purchase. Yet we're reticent to do the same with supplements. Value your health by treating your supplement purchases with just as much—if not more—importance.

product you're interested in purchasing. I've included a sample C of A here. Use the steps provided on the following page to navigate the document and verify that it matches the product in question—including everything from color and pill shape to active ingredients and dosages.

LifeExtension®
QUALITY SUPPLEMENTS & VITAMINS, INC.

CERTIFICATE OF ANALYSIS

Product Name: ❶	Calorie Control Weight Management Formula with CoffeeGenic
Item Number: ❷	01694
Description: ❸	Tan speckled powder
Lot Number:	0391j1
Manufacture Date:	November 2011
Best By Date: ❹	November 2013

ASSAYS ◄——— This part confirms the label claims.

TEST ❺	SPECIFICATION	RESULT ❻
LuraLean propolmannan (*Amorphophallus konjac K. Koch, ssp. Amorphophallus japonica*) fiber extract (root)	2000 mg	100 %
Phase 2 Phaseolus vulgaris white kidney (bean) extract	445 mg	100%
CoffeeGenic Green Coffee (*Coffea arabica*) extract (bean)	200 mg	100%
Integra-Lean African mango (*Irvingia gabonensis*) proprietary extract (seed)	150 mg	100%
Tea Slender Green Tea Phytosome decaffeinated extract (leaf) bound to phospholipids (from lecithin)	150 mg	100%
Caffeine	8 mg	103%

MICROBIOLOGICAL TESTS ◄——— This part confirms a pure product without harmful pathogens above accepted standards.

TEST	SPECIFICATION	RESULT ❼
Total Plate Count	< 10,000 cfu/g	50 cfu/g
Yeast & Mold	< 1,000 cfu/g	75 cfu/g
Escherichia coli	Negative/10 g	Negative/10 g
Salmonella	Negative/10 g	Negative/10 g
Staphylococcus aureus	Negative/10 g	Negative/10 g

HEAVY METAL TESTS

TEST	SPECIFICATION	RESULT ❽
Lead (Pb)	< 3.0 mcg/day	0.98 mcg/day

Reviewed and Approved by Life Extension
Quality Assurance/Quality Control ❾

❶ Verify the name on the product matches the name on the C of A.

❷ Verify the product number, usually located right above the Supplement Facts on the back panel.

❸ Verifying the color will have to be at home as most stores won't let you open the product.

❹ Make sure it hasn't expired.

❺ Verify that all active ingredients are included.

❻ Verify that the C of A results show between 95% and 110% of the stated label dose for each ingredient.

❼ Verify that each pathogen is completely negative or well below the accepted standard.

❽ Verify that the listed contaminants are completely negative or well below the accepted standard.

Please note that testing only for lead is a well-accepted practice in the supplement industry.

❾ Verify that the C of A has been approved by a company quality control officer and has their signature.

Avoiding Common Supplement Scams

Several scams are common to the supplement industry. Let's go over several of them so you can be sure to avoid them.

Scam #1: Underdosing

One of the most prevalent scams is to underdose. It goes like this: include a "hot" ingredient in a product, refer to exciting research results on the ingredient in product advertising, but never reveal the amount of the nutrient shown to be effective (much higher than what is actually in the product).

An example of this deceptive practice is found in the prostate formulas now offered by many different companies. One of the key ingredients in these products is the bark of the Pygeum africanum tree, which acts through several mechanisms to alleviate—and in some cases prevent—benign prostatic hyperplasia (enlargement of the prostate that causes difficulty with urination).

Studies performed with this bark clearly show that no less than 100 mg of pygeum is needed to produce the desired biological effect. Yet some companies advertise the benefits of this herb, while only putting 10 mg of it in their formulations—an amount far too small to achieve the desired benefits. The main reason why? To save money. They are counting on you not to do your homework!

Scam #2: Adulteration

Another common scam is to substitute expensive ingredients with cheap, fake ones that are adulterated to make them look like the real thing.

Let's go back to pygeum. This herb is high in phytonutrients known as sterols. Some raw material suppliers try to get around the high cost of pygeum by diluting it with sterols from other plants that don't necessarily have the same effect. Crude analytical testing of this fake raw material, which only searches for sterol content, will not pick up that the pygeum has been diluted. Unless a manufacturer uses advanced testing procedures that can pinpoint the exact identity of the herbs—not just the sterol content—the supplier could easily get away with the scam.

Keep in mind that well-established companies utilize state-of-the-art testing instruments, such as high-pressure liquid chromatography and gas chromatography/mass spectrometry, which reveal the inconsistencies hidden by the melting point procedure. These machines are very expensive but are essential to maintaining quality in the supplement industry.

Scam #3: Bait and Switch

Responsible dietary supplement manufacturers will request that raw material suppliers submit samples of their ingredients so they can test them for quality. This is a great practice, except that sometimes suppliers pull a bait and switch. They send the manufacturer a sample of high-quality material that will easily pass quality testing for identity, purity, and potency. But once the manufacturer has approved the high-quality material for use in their products, the supplier will switch it out for lower-quality material, hoping the manufacturer will assume it's the same stuff. For this reason, good companies have all of the active ingredients in their products lab-analyzed *before* they go into individual capsules or tablets.

Some time ago, a supplier desperately wanted the business of three top supplement companies. This supplier "guaranteed" that the materials it shipped would meet the highest quality standards. They provided an impressive stack of documents showing how their materials met these companies' exacting requirements. But when told that each of its shipments would not be accepted until they passed advanced chemical analyses, the supply company decided that it would rather not work with these top companies. So what's the point? Stick with well-established companies.

HOW TO READ A SUPPLEMENT LABEL

Knowing how to read a supplement label is the last step in helping you choose a high-quality product. Here's what you need to know.

Principal Display Panel

The principal display panel, or the front of the package, tells you some important information:

- The product name

- The brand name

- The number of tablets/capsules/soft gels or the weight of the powder

Supplement Facts Panel

The Supplement Facts panel is where the real meat of the label is. Here, you'll learn:

- The serving size

- The servings per container

- The active ingredients and their potencies (listed inside the Supplement Facts panel)

- Standardizations

- The daily values

- The inactive ingredients (listed underneath the Supplement Facts panel)

- Allergen information

Serving size is important because you want to know how many tablets or capsules or soft gels or teaspoons of powder you have to take to get the potencies listed. Take calcium as an example. One product may look like it has more calcium than another, because it says it provides 1,000 mg per serving, while the other only provides 500 mg. But this is meaningless information if you don't look at serving size. If the serving size of the first product is four capsules and the serving size of second product is two capsules, you actually have to take the same amount of capsules (four) to get to 1,000 mg.

"Servings per container" is also an important consideration, because it helps you evaluate the cost of different supplements against one another. A product that costs $20 but provides 100 servings is more cost effective than one that costs $10 but only provides 40 servings.

Of course, the most crucial information is what the active ingredients are and what kinds of potencies are provided in one serving. Potencies are listed in different measurements depending upon the ingredient. Most vitamins and minerals are listed in milligrams (mg), or thousandths of a gram. However, some are required in such tiny amounts by the body that they are included, and therefore listed, in micrograms (mcg), or thousandths of a milligram. The daily value for calcium, for example, is 1,000 mg (or 1 gram). But the government's recommended daily value for vitamin B_{12} is just 2.4 mcg.

Fat-soluble vitamins, such as vitamins A, D, and E, are measured in international units (IU). Unlike grams, milligrams, and micrograms—which are weight measurements—international units measure biological activity. The reason is that these vitamins come in different forms with different biological activity. Measuring them in IUs allows for meaningful comparisons between different forms.

Finally, probiotics are measured in colony-forming units (CFU). Like IUs, CFUs measure activity rather than weight. That's important, since probiotics are organisms that weigh the same whether they arc alive or dead. You don't want to know how much you're getting by weight—you want to know how many colonies of beneficial bacteria will be able to form in your gut.

Also, many botanical ingredients are standardized to their active constituents. In this case, you may see an herb listed this way:

Saw Palmetto (*Serenoa repens*) (fruit) [std. to 85%–95% total fatty acids and sterols (272 mg)] 320 mg

This means that there is 320 mg of saw palmetto herb per serving, and that it is standardized to contain 85 to 95 percent total fatty acids and sterols, for a minimum of 272 mg of these active constituents.

You'll also notice that some ingredients have daily values while others don't. The reason is that the government has only established daily values for certain essential nutrients, such as vitamins and minerals. Therefore, anything other than a recognized essential nutrient will not have a daily value. (Even if it's essential to your health, like omega-3 fatty acids!)

Finally, underneath the Supplement Facts box, you'll find the inactive or "other" ingredients—such as excipients, binders, fillers, and ingredients used to make capsules—which play a number of critical roles in the manufacturing process, including:

- Achieving uniform density for accurate dosing

- Dispersing the active ingredients evenly throughout a solid tablet, capsule, or soft gel

- Protecting active ingredients from rapid inactivation due to heat and moisture

- Promoting tablet disintegration, as well as capsule and soft gel dissolution, so it doesn't pass right through your system without benefit

- Sustaining the release of active ingredients into the body over time

- Keeping a product from degrading and being susceptible to microbes

You may have noticed that some companies refer to excipients as a threat to your health and advertise that their products are "pure and free of excipients." However, not having excipients can actually be a detriment, since they play so many important roles in delivering a quality product. In fact, this tactic may be used to draw attention away from inferior active ingredients!

Just make sure the product you are considering purchasing uses excipients with GRAS (Generally Regarded As Safe) status and that they are used sparingly.

Directly underneath the Supplement Facts box should be allergen information. By law, a product must disclose if it contains any of the eight major food allergens: milk, eggs, peanuts, tree nuts (almonds, cashews, walnuts, and so on), fish, shellfish, soy, and wheat.

Romance Copy Panel

In marketing, the panel that tells you all about the product benefits is called "romance copy" because its purpose is to romance you into buying the product. This is where you'll find what are called "structure/function" claims. Dietary supplements are legally prohibited from claiming to diagnose, treat, cure, or prevent any disease—even if there is research to support these claims. Instead, manufacturers can only speak about the product in terms of how it affects a structure or function of the body. So, for example, it's illegal for a product to say that it alleviates arthritis pain, because arthritis is a disease. However, it can say that it supports joint health, function, and flexibility, because those are structures and functions of the body. As a result, you sometimes have to read between the lines to understand what a product does.

Other Information

It is also required that product labels list the contact information of the manufacturer so that you can get in touch with them if you have a question or if you have an adverse reaction to the product (which, despite what the media says, is actually quite rare). Other useful information on product labels is the suggested usage, that is, how much you should take and when. Don't overlook the *when*! Some products are fine to take on an empty stomach, but others—such as fish oils, fat-soluble vitamins, and certain herbs—are better absorbed with meals. Finally, somewhere on the label it should tell you how to store it. In general, you want to keep your dietary supplements in a cool, dry place—that is, not your bathroom cabinet! Others, such as probiotics, flax oil, and powdered seeds, need to be refrigerated.

So there you have it: some simple steps you can follow to ensure you're getting the highest quality nutritional supplements available!

BOTTOM LINE: *High-quality supplements—those that are made from high-quality raw materials . . . that have been manufactured according to GMPs . . . that have been tested for identity, purity, strength, and composition . . . that are dosed appropriately . . . that are provided in superior forms . . . and that are free of undesirable ingredients—work in preventing, treating, and, in some cases, curing disease. (Even if they can't say that!) Products that don't meet these standards don't work, may be dangerous, and are a waste of your time and money.*

CHAPTER 4

The Foundation Level

Now that you know how to choose high-quality supplements and read product labels, let's get started building your pyramid. It starts with the Foundation Level, which is comprised of the same four basic supplements for everyone:

1. An ideally dosed multivitamin

2. Omega-3 fatty acids

3. Coenzyme Q_{10} (as ubiquinol)

4. Probiotics

Let's take a look at each one individually.

FOUNDATIONAL MULTIVITAMIN/MINERAL

The very first and most important supplement of your foundation—and thus your whole pyramid—is an ideally dosed daily multivitamin/mineral (which I'll refer to simply as a multivitamin or multiple throughout the rest of this chapter).

I once asked a friend of mine if he took a multivitamin. His response was, "Vitamins and minerals are so passé. I want to take the latest innovations."

Don't be like my friend. Never think of the basic vitamins and minerals as outdated. From vitamin A to the mineral zinc, your body is totally dependent on these nutrients for optimal health. And I promise you this: You can always live without the latest Amazonian herb that claims to cure everything, but you can never live without vitamins and minerals. By the way, a multivitamin is usually a lot cheaper than herbal and plant extracts!

I can't stress enough, though, that not all multivitamins are the same. There are your basic, bare-bones multivitamins that provide minimal doses of some essential nutrients. And then there are your robust multivitamins that deliver ideal doses of a full spectrum of essential nutrients. What is the main difference between these multiples? Dosage. The first type is based on the government's "recommended dietary allowance," or RDA, and the second reflects what I call the "ideal daily intake," or IDI.

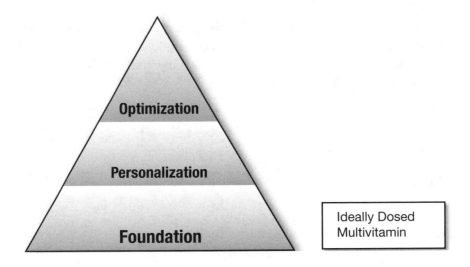

To fully comprehend the difference between these two approaches, we have to go back a little bit in time. Have you ever wondered who established the RDAs for all the vitamins and minerals, and how they got the numbers they did?

During World War II, the U.S. National Academy of Sciences (NAS) had a goal of preventing nutrient deficiency diseases in the armed forces, in civilians being rationed food, and in children enrolled in school lunch programs. The NAS created a committee, later named the Food and Nutrition Board, to answer questions such as: How much vitamin D is necessary to prevent rickets? How much vitamin C is needed to prevent scurvy? How much vitamin B_1 (thiamine) is required to prevent beriberi? The numbers the committee members agreed to in 1941 became the RDAs, which are specific to life stage and gender.

Although they're updated every five to ten years, the RDAs haven't changed significantly over time. Today, most conventional doctors use recommended daily intakes or RDIs, instead of RDAs. These are basically the same thing, but they're broader in scope because they establish the daily dose needed to keep 98 percent of people healthy (or more accurately, free of nutrient deficiency diseases) across every demographic.

Now that you understand the historical background, here's my point: both the RDAs and the RDIs are pretty much useless, because they set the bar very, very low. I believe it's time for our government to stop asking, "What level of a nutrient prevents horrible, disfiguring diseases?" and start asking, "What level of a nutrient will create the most vibrant, optimal health in human beings?"

What if, instead of RDAs and RDIs, we promoted IDIs—science-based ideal daily intakes of vitamins and minerals that far exceed expectations set forth by the U.S. government because they are all about optimizing health. Dosing vitamins and minerals at this level goes way beyond protection against deficiencies. It enters the world of optimizing energy levels, hormonal balance, cardiovascular wellness, bone strength, digestive ease, visual acuity, cognitive agility, emotional stability, and joint integrity.

TABLE 4.1 RECOMMENDED INTAKES OF VITAMINS AND MINERALS		
VITAMINS AND MINERALS	AVERAGES OF RDA AND RDI	IDI
Vitamin A (90% beta-carotene)	900–5,000 IU	5,000 IU
Vitamin B_1 (Thiamine)	1.5 mg	125 mg
Vitamin B_2 (Riboflavin)	1.5 mg	50 mg
Vitamin B_3 (Niacin)	20 mg	190 mg
Vitamin B_5 (Pantothenic acid)	10 mg	600 mg
Vitamin B_6 (Pyridoxine)	2 mg	100 mg
Vitamin B_{12} (Cyanocobalamin)	6 mcg	600 mcg
Vitamin C	100 mg	2,000 mg
Vitamin D_3	400 IU	2,000 IU
Vitamin E	30 IU	100 IU
Biotin	30–300 mcg	3 mg

TABLE 4.1 continued		
VITAMINS AND MINERALS	**AVERAGES OF RDA AND RDI**	**IDI**
Boron	None	3 mg
Calcium	1,000 mg	1,000 mg
Choline	100–500 mg	500 mg
Chromium	25 mcg	500 mcg
Copper	900 mcg	1 mg
Folate	400 mcg	400 mcg
Inositol	None	250 mg
Iodine	200 mcg	1 mg
Lipoic acid	None	100 mg
Lutein	None	15 mg
Lycopene	None	3 mg
Magnesium	400 mg	400 mg
Manganese	1 mg	2 mg
Molybdenum	25 mcg	125 mcg
PABA	30 mg	200 mg
Potassium	35–80mg	35–80 mg
Selenium	25 mcg	200 mcg
Zinc	15 mg	35 mg

Yet given the condition of soil and the sick American food chain, eating healthy is not enough to obtain these higher doses. What you really need is a carefully formulated multivitamin—in addition to a healthy diet—to provide the IDI of key nutrients. (By the way, IDI is not an official dosing system. I made it up. However, it's based on a combination of published scientific research and my own personal experience.)

One of my goals with this book is to educate you on the potential health benefits from higher nutrient dosing. And there are a lot of them—some of which you probably know about and some of which will surprise you! Let's take a look at some commonly recognized benefits of higher vitamin and mineral doses, as well as some lesser-known ones.

TABLE 4.2 HEALTH BENEFITS OF IDEAL DAILY INTAKES (IDI)

Nutrient	Ideal Daily Intake	Commonly Recognized Health Benefits	Lesser Known Health Benefits
Vitamin A (as 90% Beta-carotene)	5,000 mg	Maintains healthy skin and good eyesight; Necessary for growth and development; Essential for immune function	May improve lung function in asthma[1]; Supports mucosal linings[2]
Vitamin B$_{12}$	600 mcg– 1 mg	Helps synthesize red blood cells and prevent anemia	Improves nerve function[3]; Protects from coronary artery disease[4]
Vitamin C	2,000 mg	Manufactures collagen and prevents scurvy; Needed for wound repair and healthy gums; Essential for immune function	Supports heart function[5]; Protects from ulcers[6]
Vitamin D	2,000–5,000 units	Needed for bone strength and prevents rickets; Essential for immune function	Lowers risk of colon cancer[7]; Reduces risk of falls[8]
Vitamin E	400 units	Necessary for reproductive function; Helps synthesize red blood cells; Essential for immune function	Induces breast cancer cell death[9]; Induces prostate cancer cell death[10]
Vitamin K$_2$	1,100 mcg	Needed for healthy blood clotting	Reduces bone fracture risk[11]; Reduces risk of coronary artery disease[12]
Calcium	1,200 mg women; 600 mg men	Necessary for bone and teeth strength and prevents osteoporosis	Inhibits production of body fat[13]
Chromium	450 mcg	Supports optimal blood sugar levels	Increases brain activity in adults with early memory decline[14]
Copper	1 mg	Aids iron absorption; Needed for the crosslinking of collagen and elastin	Protects against osteoporosis[15,16]
Magnesium	400 mg	Relaxes the muscles; Supports bone health	Associated with lower risk of heart disease[17]

TABLE 4.2 continued			
NUTRIENT	**IDEAL DAILY INTAKE**	**COMMONLY RECOGNIZED HEALTH BENEFITS**	**LESSER KNOWN HEALTH BENEFITS**
Selenium	200 mcg	Plays a role in thyroid function; Essential for immune function	Decreases hospitalizations in HIV patients[18]
Zinc	35 mg	Needed for reproductive health; Essential for immune function	Enhances antibody production[19]

As you can see, vitamins and minerals have much more potential than simply eliminating nutrient-deficiency diseases! When dosed appropriately, they can make the difference between surviving and thriving.

As an educated consumer, get into the habit of looking at the back of the label—where the Supplement Facts are—not the front. The front label is nothing more than marketing jargon to grab your attention; the real information is on the back.

BOTTOM LINE: *Vitamins and minerals are absolutely essential to your health, but the RDAs were developed with one purpose only: to prevent nutrient-deficiency diseases. To support vibrant, optimal health, you need to take a higher potency multivitamin.*

BIG NAME MULTIVITAMINS & THE RDI

Big-name multivitamins are dosed at the RDI, sometimes a little more and sometimes even a little less. This is how they keep their products cheap—and pretty much ineffective for anything but preventing deficiencies. As an example, the typical multivitamin provides 60 mg of vitamin C, a little less than the RDI, but enough to protect you from developing scurvy. But what about all the other health benefits attributed to vitamin C—benefits like a stronger immune system, cardiovascular support, and even younger-looking skin?

Even with a healthy diet, taking a bare-bones multiple vitamin will not provide you with these benefits. You might get 200 mg per day . . . maybe. Yet the IDI of vitamin C is closer to 2,000 mg daily.

OMEGA-3 FATTY ACIDS

The second supplement of your foundation is a high-quality omega-3 fatty acid supplement.

Chances are, you've heard of omega-3 fatty acids, because they've had their fair share of media exposure lately. But if you're like most people, you're not exactly sure what they are or what they do.

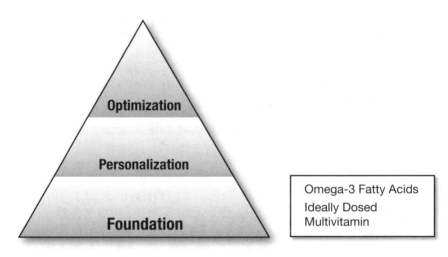

Optimization

Personalization

Foundation

Omega-3 Fatty Acids
Ideally Dosed
Multivitamin

In the simplest terms, omega-3 fatty acids are healthy fats. They're sometimes called "essential fatty acids" because, quite simply, they are essential to health—you can't live without them. Yet your body can't make them. So you either have to get them through your diet or through supplementation. Omega-3 fatty acids are so critical to human health that I'm betting within the next decade or two the U.S. government will assign them an RDI, giving them equal status with vitamins and minerals.

> **BOTTOM LINE:** Omega-3 fatty acids are so critical to human health that I'm betting that within the next decade or two the U.S. government will assign them an RDI, giving them equal status with vitamins and minerals.

An abundance of scientific research substantiates the wide-ranging health benefits of omega-3 fats. Some of these benefits include:

1. Supporting mental health (including very real benefits for patients who are depressed,[20] bipolar,[21] borderline personality,[22,23] or schizophrenic[24])

2. Promoting cognitive agility (from helping overcome learning disabilities in children[25] to slowing cognitive decline in people with Alzheimer's disease and dementia[26,27])

3. Decreased risk of cardiovascular disease (such as lowering triglycerides[28] and blood pressure,[29] and reducing the risk of heart attack,[30] sudden death,[31] stroke,[32] and arrhythmia[33])

4. Lowering systemic inflammation[34] (and thus supporting just about every bodily system imaginable)

The last one on the list, lowering inflammation, is more important than you might realize. I firmly believe—and I'm not alone in this—that inflammation is the common denominator of all age-related diseases, such as cancer, heart disease, and diabetes. Lowering levels of chronic, low-grade inflammation in your body is probably the single most important thing you can do to promote optimal health.

One of the reasons so many of us are walking around with chronic, low-grade inflammation is the standard American diet (SAD), which is high in inflammatory omega-6 fatty acids (found in all vegetable oils,

INFLAMMATION: A DOUBLE-EDGED SWORD

Inflammation is your body's primary defense against a threat. Whether in response to a broken bone, a virus, or even a splinter, inflammation increases blood flow to mobilize white blood cells to the affected area. Redness, heat, swelling, and pain—the four telltale signs of inflammation—are the result. This response is very helpful for acute situations, because it fights off infection.

But once the problem is fixed, your body is supposed to call off the troops and go back to normal. Unfortunately, it doesn't always happen that way—especially as you age. The result is chronic, low-grade inflammation, which can end up damaging the very cells it was supposed to protect.

nuts, seeds, and grains) and sorely lacking in anti-inflammatory omega-3 fatty acids. (An astonishing 70 percent of Americans are estimated to be deficient in omega-3s![35])

Don't get me wrong; you need omega-6 fats to live. But in caveman days, our species consumed a ratio of 2:1 to 3:1 omega-6 to omega-3.[36] These days, that ratio is totally out of whack. In fact, would you believe the average American consumes fifteen to seventeen times more omega-6 than omega 3?[37] No wonder our inflammation levels are through the roof!

The United States hasn't set an RDI for omega-3 fatty acids yet, but several other countries—such as Canada, Sweden, the United Kingdom, Australia, and Japan—have. It usually falls somewhere between 300 and 500 mg per day of EPA plus DHA. But that's a bare minimum. If you have cardiovascular disease, the American Heart Association recommends 1 gram of fish oil daily. And raise that number to 2–4 grams if your triglycerides are elevated.

Also keep in mind that how much omega-3 you need is directly proportional to how much omega-6 you consume. Remember, you're shooting for a 2:1 to 3:1 ratio of omega-6 to omega-3, just like our hunter-gatherer ancestors used to eat. A study in the *American Journal of Clinical Nutrition* estimated that, given how many omega-6 fatty acids Americans consume, we need to ingest a whopping 3.5 grams of omega-3s daily to counteract their inflammatory properties![38]Just to put that in perspective, one 3-ounce serving of wild coho salmon provides a little shy of 1 gram of omega-3.[39]

BOTTOM LINE: *Omega-3 fatty acids are as important to your health as vitamins and minerals—and help prevent a boatload of chronic degenerative diseases—but most Americans are deficient in them. You need to take an omega-3 product every day to help balance the average diet's skewed ratio of omega-6 to omega-3.*

COENZYME Q_{10}: UBIQUINOL

The third supplement of your foundation is coenzyme Q_{10} (CoQ_{10}), in the ubiquinol (not ubiquinone) form.

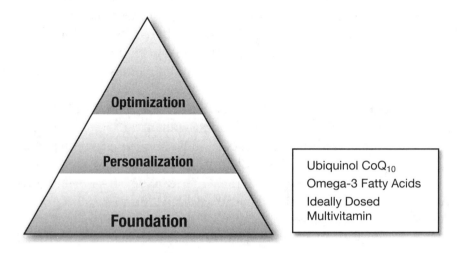

Ubiquinol CoQ_{10}
Omega-3 Fatty Acids
Ideally Dosed
Multivitamin

I'm betting you're fairly familiar with multivitamins and omega-3 fatty acids, but coenzyme Q_{10} may be new to you. I'm hoping to change that! This one supplement can make such a big difference in your health and well-being that I think every single American adult could benefit from taking it.

What the heck is a coenzyme? Well, "co" means "with" or "together." And enzymes catalyze all the chemical reactions in your body that sustain life. So coenzymes work together with enzymes to keep you alive. Sounds important, huh?

HOW TO GET MORE FROM YOUR COQ_{10}

You can amplify the effects of CoQ_{10} by taking it with a vitality-enhancing substance from the Himalayas called shilajit. The latest studies reveal that when shilajit is combined with CoQ_{10}, cellular energy gains substantially increase.

In a breakthrough preliminary study in mice, the combination of CoQ_{10} and shilajit produced a 56 percent increase in cellular energy production in the brain—40 percent better than CoQ_{10} alone. In muscle there was a 144 percent increase, or 27 percent better than CoQ_{10} alone.

Coenzyme Q_{10} specifically works with enzymes inside the mitochondria of your cells to produce energy in the form of ATP—energy your cells need to function. If your CoQ_{10} levels are low, you won't just feel tired and drained. Every cell, tissue, and organ in your body will suffer because they're all powered by ATP.

CoQ_{10} is most well known for promoting cardiovascular health. And that makes sense when you think about it, because your heart demands more energy than almost any other organ in your body. But CoQ_{10} has other benefits too. Scores of human clinical trials have shown that CoQ_{10}:

1. Is helpful in multiple heart conditions (including congestive heart failure,[40] cardiomyopathy,[41] high blood pressure,[42] and recovery from heart attack[43])

2. May slow the progression of Parkinson's disease, a degenerative brain disease[44,45]

3. Helps control blood sugar in diabetics[46,47]

4. Increases feelings of vigor in healthy folks[48]

5. Boosts the amount of fat burned during low-intensity exercise.[49]

CoQ_{10} is naturally produced in the body, but as you get older, you make less of it. Tissue samples have revealed that CoQ_{10} levels tend to peak at around age twenty and then continuously decrease with age.[50] But it's not just aging that diminishes CoQ_{10} levels.

Statin drugs, used for lowering cholesterol, are notorious CoQ_{10} robbers. In fact, just one month of statin treatment can lower your CoQ_{10} levels by 40 percent![51] Finally, people with certain cardiovascular disease states are prone to having low levels of CoQ_{10} in their heart tissues, where they need it most.

BOTTOM LINE: *All of your cells need energy to function—particularly your heart and brain cells—and CoQ$_{10}$ plays a critical role in cellular energy production. Unfortunately, many factors conspire to deplete CoQ$_{10}$ levels, making supplementation advisable. Ubiquinol is absorbed much better than the more common ubiquinone, so it's the preferred form.*

PROBIOTICS

The fourth and final supplement of your foundation is a probiotic product.

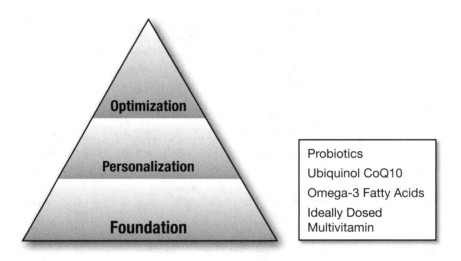

Thanks to the success of the yogurt brand Activia, you've probably heard of probiotics. They're the good-for-you bacteria that inhabit your gastrointestinal (GI) tract—and occur in fermented foods such as yogurt and raw sauerkraut—where they play a key role in maintaining gut health. And let me be frank: You are only as healthy as your gut.

Think about it: Your survival is dependent on your gut's ability to extract protein, carbohydrates, fats, vitamins, and minerals from your food. When your gut health is compromised, it doesn't matter how healthy a diet you eat—you won't be able to access all the nutrition it provides. Not only that, a good portion of your immune system—about 70 percent—is actually located within your GI tract.[52] And the makeup of bacteria in your gut influences how well your immune system works.

Importantly, good bacteria (also known as "friendly flora") aren't the only ones who take up residence in your GI tract. Bad bacteria live there too. Now, as long as you have a healthy balance of good to bad—most experts agree 80 percent to 20 percent is ideal—it's okay and even normal to host some of the bad guys. But if too many bad bacteria are living in your gut, your digestive and immune function can get really out of whack. In fact, I believe a lot of the rampant problems of the digestive system we're seeing today—from simple indigestion to inflammatory bowel disease—are due to a lack of beneficial bacteria.

A large body of scientific evidence points to the multiple benefits of probiotics, including:

1. Supporting digestive health (providing relief from indigestion,[53] diarrhea,[54] constipation,[55] gastritis caused by the bacterium *Helicobacter pylori*,[56] inflammatory bowel disease,[57] and irritable bowel syndrome[58]).

2. Promoting increased immune function (including crowding out pathogenic bacteria,[59] strengthening the mucosal barrier to protect against infection,[60] secreting chemicals that break down toxins produced by bad bacteria,[61] and increasing levels of antibodies[62] and infection-fighting cells[63]).

3. Supporting women's health, by helping fight urinary tract infections,[64] yeast infections,[65] and bacterial vaginosis[66,67].

4. Manufacturing key nutrients (such as B vitamins,[68] short-chain fatty acids,[69] and certain amino acids[70]).

5. Combating metabolic syndrome (including lowering blood pressure[71] and bad cholesterol[72] and improving insulin sensitivity[73]).

6. Preventing cancer (specifically of the colon,[74] liver,[75] and bladder[76]).

So why are so many of us lacking in these friendly flora? For starters, antibiotics. As I stated in Chapter 1, antibiotics are life-saving drugs, and many times they're necessary to combat bacterial infections. But they don't just kill harmful bacteria—they wipe out *all* bacteria, including the good guys that keep you healthy. If you've ever taken antibiotics, you've disrupted your bacterial balance.

Other factors that can lower your levels of beneficial bacteria—and make room for the bad guys to multiply—include alcohol consumption, smoking, stress, and eating a typical, enzyme-deficient American diet. Fortunately, you can control those factors by making better lifestyle choices. But one thing you can't control is aging. Researchers have documented that as we get older, our populations of probiotic bacteria decline.[77] This sets the stage for disease-causing bacteria to flourish.

If you suffer from any kind of digestive complaint, you will almost certainly benefit from probiotic supplementation. If you frequently find yourself getting sick, probiotics could keep you on your feet when the next cold and flu season hits. And if you are overweight, prediabetic, and/or have elevated blood pressure and blood lipids, a probiotic product could help normalize your metabolism. But since these beneficial bugs are so vital to human health and well-being—and few of us live a totally "clean" lifestyle—I recommend that everyone take them as a matter of course.

BOTTOM LINE: *You are only as healthy as your gut, and your gut is only as healthy as the microbes that inhabit it. Since so many factors diminish levels of beneficial bacteria in the GI tract, it's essential to replenish their numbers with daily probiotic supplementation.*

INGREDIENT FORM OF FOUNDATIONAL SUPPLEMENTS

Is there really a difference between supplements you buy at the drugstore versus the ones you find in a health food store? In a word, yes. Just as important as getting the proper dosage of a certain ingredient is getting the best form. And as a rule, health food store brands tend to include superior forms of ingredients in their products. I'll take you through the most popular types of supplements and tell you which forms are best.

Vitamins and Minerals

Assuming that all vitamins and minerals are the same is like assuming that all cars are the same. Much the same way the model of a car can dramatically affect how well it performs, the form of a vitamin or mineral can dramatically affect how well it is absorbed and utilized. For example, organic minerals (such as those chelated, or bound, with amino acids) are much better absorbed than inorganic minerals. But since inorganic minerals are cheap, that's the kind you'll see in most drugstore supplements.

Now you might think that it's always better to buy "natural" vitamins. But the truth is, the human body does not distinguish between vitamins that are naturally derived and those that are synthetically manufactured, with two exceptions. In the case of beta-carotene (a precursor to vitamin A) and vitamin E, the natural forms are absorbed better because the synthetic forms are not identical to what is found in nature. But for everything else, synthetics are not only just fine—they're preferable, since they do not contain impurities and allergens that natural forms can.

Most vitamins aren't even available as "natural," because the resources and energy it would take to extract them from foods is prohibitive. The real issue is not whether an ingredient is natural or synthetic, but whether it is pure and identical to what is found in nature.

TABLE 4.3. PREFERABLE FORMS OF VITAMINS AND MINERALS

	PREFERABLE FORM	WHY IT'S BETTER
Vitamin A	90% beta-carotene (natural, not synthetic)	Beta-carotene is a precursor to vitamin A, meaning your body uses it to make vitamin A. The benefit of beta-carotene is that it is water-soluble, unlike preformed vitamin A (retinol), which is fat-soluble. As a result, it cannot build up to toxic levels in the body. At the same time, it's a good idea to take some preformed vitamin A, just in case your body has difficulty converting beta-carotene into vitamin A. Natural beta-carotene is absorbed better than synthetic.
B vitamins	Coenzyme form, when available	Before B vitamins can be utilized by the body, they must be converted into their active coenzyme form. You can skip this process by buying B vitamins already in their coenzyme form.
Vitamin C	Buffered form (Mineral ascorbates, Ester C)	Some people experience stomach upset or acid reflux from taking vitamin C as ascorbic acid. For these individuals, buffered forms (which neutralize the acidity of vitamin C with alkaline minerals) are recommended. If you have no stomach issues, ascorbic acid is fine.
Vitamin D	Vitamin D_3	A recent systematic review and meta-analysis has concluded that vitamin D_3 is significantly better absorbed than vitamin D_2.[78] One of the studies reviewed found D_3 is 87% more potent than D_2.[79] However, D_2 is a good choice for vegans as D_3 is derived from wool.

TABLE 4.3 continued		
	PREFERABLE FORM	**WHY IT'S BETTER**
Vitamin E	If taking alpha-tocopherol, choose the natural form (d-alpha tocopherol), not the synthetic form (dl-alpha tocopherol). However, I recommend taking mixed tocopherols.	Vitamin E consists of eight different compounds: four tocopherols and four tocotrienols.[80] At the very least, you should take natural alpha-tocopherol rather than synthetic because it is absorbed better. However, I prefer mixed tocopherols (providing gamma, delta, alpha, and beta tocopherols) because taking alpha tocopherol alone can displace gamma tocopherol and both are important. The very best products will include mixed tocopherols and tocotrienols.
Minerals	Choose organic mineral forms (minerals bound to amino acids or Krebs Cycle intermediates, such as citrate, malate, etc.) over inorganic forms if you do not produce adequate stomach acid.	Organic minerals are generally better absorbed than inorganic. That's because in order for the body to absorb a mineral, it has to be in its ionic state, which means separated into its charged particles. Organic minerals readily ionize regardless of pH; however, inorganic minerals need to be in the presence of stomach acid to be ionized, and not everyone produces sufficient stomach acid to efficiently accomplish this. As a result, calcium citrate is about 22–27% better absorbed than calcium carbonate.[81] However, if you have no problem producing stomach acid (in other words, if your digestion is strong), then inorganic mineral forms are probably fine.

Omega-3 Fatty Acids

Omega-3 fatty acids can be either derived from animals or plants. Cold-water fatty fish—such as tuna, mackerel, salmon, herring, Arctic cod, and sardines—are the most common animal source of omega-3s. However, these healthy fats are also present in krill and shark liver. Omega-3s are harder to come by in plants. The best sources of vegetarian omega-3s are flax and chia seeds.

Importantly, the omega-3 fatty acids found in animals are not the same as those found in plants. Fish, krill, and shark all contain omega-3 as eicosapentaenoic acid (EPA) and docosahexaenoic acid (DHA). Flax and chia seeds both contain omega-3 as alpha-linolenic acid (ALA).

HOW TO CHOOSE A QUALITY FISH OIL PRODUCT

Choosing a quality fish oil product involves several factors. First, it's absolutely imperative that your fish oil be fresh (as measured by oxidation levels). Taking rancid fish oil can be worse for your health than taking nothing at all! Second, you want to make sure your fish oil contains only negligible levels of contaminants such as heavy metals (including mercury), PCBs, and dioxins.

When choosing a fish oil, check to see how it was graded by the International Fish Oil Standards program, a third-party validation system that has a 5-star ranking system of fish oil quality. A fish oil supplement is given 5 Stars if it meets criteria in five specific areas:

Star 1—Product complies with all CRN/GOED/WHO testing categories

CRN = Council for Responsible Nutrition

GOED = Global Organization for EPA and DHA Omega-3

WHO = World Health Organization

All three of these organizations have set strict standards for fish oil quality

Star 2—Contains the same quantity of active ingredients that is listed on the product label

Star 3—Has an oxidation level less than 75% of the CRN/GOED standard

Star 4—Has PCB levels less than 50% of CRN/GOED Standard

Star 5—Has dioxin levels less than 50% of the WHO Standard

You can interpret the 5-Star Rating the following way:

5 Star: Exceptional Product Batch

4 Star: Very Good Batch

3 Star: Good Batch

2 Star: Fair Batch

1 Star: Poor Batch

What's the difference? EPA and DHA are the exact forms the human body is designed to use, so these are perfectly compatible with your natural biochemistry. ALA is a shorter-chain fat that needs to be converted before it can be used. While in theory your body can convert ALA into EPA and DHA, in reality this conversion is pretty inefficient. As a result, it's very difficult to meet your need for omega-3 fatty acids just through flax or borage oil. For that reason, I recommend an animal-derived omega-3 supplement for most people.

If you're a vegetarian, then flax and chia seeds represent your best options for omega-3 supplementation. In fact, it's *especially* important that vegetarians take an essential fatty acid product because their diet provides little, if any, omega-3.

Coenzyme Q_{10}

There are two forms of CoQ_{10} available in supplements: ubiquinol and the more common ubiquinone. (Both of these names are variations on the word "ubiquitous," since CoQ_{10} exists in almost every cell of the body.) The form you want to take is ubiquinol, because it's absorbed significantly better than ubiquinone. Just compare the numbers.

In one study, when subjects were administered 1,200 mg per day of ubiquinone, they achieved blood CoQ_{10} levels of 3.96 mcg/mL[82] (considered an ideal concentration for people with cardiovascular disease[83]). Yet in another study, a much smaller dose of ubiquinol—just 150 mg—resulted in blood levels of CoQ_{10} nearly as high: 3.84 mcg/mL.[84] Comparing the results of these studies suggests that ubiquinol is absorbed up to eight times better than ubiquinone!

Bonus: ubiquinol is the active antioxidant form of CoQ_{10}, so it also protects your cells from free-radical damage.

Another method for confirming the quality, and in this case, the efficacy, of your CoQ_{10} product is to see if it's actually affecting your blood levels of the nutrient. Before starting on the product, take a CoQ_{10} blood test. This establishes your baseline level of CoQ_{10}. After three to six months of taking your CoQ_{10} product of choice, recheck your status. A high-quality product should increase your blood level significantly over your baseline reading. (Some people, however—those with congestive heart failure, for instance—may require higher amounts of supplemental CoQ_{10} to see a rise in blood levels.) You'll learn more about blood tests in Chapter 5.

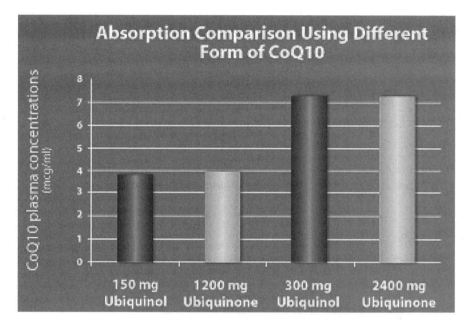

Probiotics

There are many different strains of probiotics to choose from. Below is a table showing some of the most studied strains and what they're good for. As you can see, different probiotic strains have different benefits. Therefore, it makes sense to choose a probiotic supplement that has a variety of strains to get the biggest array of benefits.

HOW TO GET MORE FROM YOUR PROBIOTICS

You can increase the efficacy of probiotics by taking them with prebiotics—complex sugars that act as food for beneficial bacteria. That way, once the probiotics reach your GI tract, they'll have fuel to spur their growth and proliferation. Some examples of prebiotics include fructooligosaccharides (FOS), inulin, oligofructose, galactooligosaccharides (GOS), xylooligosaccharides, and pectin. Other ingredients to look for are sodium alginate and grape seed extract. These ingredients help protect the live bacteria as they travel throughout the GI tract.

TABLE 4.4. SPECIFIC BENEFITS OF INIDCATED PROBIOTICS

BENEFIT*	INDICATED PROBIOTIC
Reduce infection risk during and after antibiotic treatment	*S. cerevisiae boulardii; Lactobacillus rhamnosus* GG; *Bacillus coagulans* GBI-30; *Bifidobacterium longum* BB536
Treat yeast infections, bacterial vaginosis, and urinary infections	*L. rhamnosus* GR-1; *L. reuteri* RC-14; *L. fermentum* RC
Reduce frequency and severity of colds, flu, and other infections	*L. casei* DN-114001; *L. rhamnosus* GG; *L. acidophilus* NCFM; *Bifidobacterium longum* BB536
Alleviate symptoms of irritable bowel syndrome	*Bifidobacterium infantis* 35624; *L. plantarum* DSM9843
Soothe eczema	*L. rhamnosus* HN001; *L. rhamnosus* GG
Avoid traveler's diarrhea	*S. cerevisiae boulardii; L. rhamnosus* GG
Alleviate diarrhea from rotavirus infection (stomach flu) and use of antibiotics	*L. rhamnosus* GG; *L. reuteri* MM53
Improve lactose intolerance	*L. acidophilus*
Boost immune function	*L. casei* Shirota; *L. casei* CRL431
Alleviate constipation	*Bifidobacterium longum* BB536
Improves symptoms of inflammatory bowel disease	*Bifidobacterium longum* BB536
Relieve allergy symptoms	*Bifidobacterium longum* BB536

*Sources

1. Reid G. The scientific basis for probiotic strains of Lactobacillus. Appl Environ Microbiol. 1999 Sep;65(9):3763–3766.
2. Sachs, Jessica Synder. Best cure for stomach troubles—which probiotics work and why. CNN. March 10, 2009.
http://www.cnn.com/2009/HEALTH/03/10/healthmag.probiotics.stomach/index.html
3. BB536 Clinical Studies. HumanClinicals.org. http://www.humanclinicals.org/BB536.html

Also beware that since probiotics are alive, they can die. Therefore, you should make sure that the manufacturer has taken steps to preserve the potency of its product. Some methods of achieving this are:

- Packaging the product in amber glass bottles, which protect the bacteria from degradation by light

- Keeping the product refrigerated

- Using shelf-stable varieties of probiotics, such as *Bifidobacterium longum* BB536, which maintain their potency at room temperature

- Formulating in such a way as to protect probiotic bacteria from being destroyed by stomach acid, such as enteric coating or a patented gel formulation utilizing sodium alginate from seaweed and grape skin. Some manufacturers are using a new capsule-within-a-capsule probiotic delivery system that protects the bacteria as it moves from the stomach into the small intestine.

DOSAGE OF FOUNDATIONAL SUPPLEMENTS

It's a commonsense proposition: Your supplements are only going to work if they are provided in the right dosages. After all, if most of the research on coenzyme Q_{10} used a dosage of at least 100 mg, and your product only provides 25 mg, you're probably not going to get much benefit from it. The question is, how do you figure out which products contain effective potencies—without getting a degree in nutritional and herbal science?

Here are some basic tips for getting the right dosages for your foundational supplements:

1. **For vitamins and minerals,** aim for potencies of vitamins and minerals comparable to the ideal daily intakes (IDIs) I presented in the table on page 53. If the dosing of the product you're looking at is too low, keep searching. (One caveat: because calcium is a bulky mineral that takes up a lot of room in a tablet, it's very difficult to find the full IDI in a multivitamin. Therefore, you may need to take an additional calcium supplement.)

2. **For omega-3 fish oil,** a good product will provide at least 1 gram of fish oil in one soft gel. The IDI is between 2 and 4 grams daily—especially if you have elevated triglycerides or blood pressure, cardiovascular disease, mental illness, or neurodegenerative diseases such as Alzheimer's disease or dementia.

3. **For omega-3 flax products,** take at least 1 gram of ALA daily, preferably more. I like to recommend flaxseed oil in the liquid form because it provides a nice dosage of 6 grams of ALA per tablespoon.

4. **For coenzyme Q_{10},** I recommend at least 100–200 mg of ubiquinol (not ubiquinone, which is not as well absorbed) daily for preventive purposes and 200–400 mg daily if you have cardiovascular disease, Parkinson's disease (or other neurodegenerative diseases), or diabetes. For the average healthy person, 100 mg per day is a good starting dose.

5. **For probiotics,** keep in mind that these good bacteria are living organisms. Therefore, quality products aren't measured in milligrams but in colony-forming units, or CFUs. Look for products that provide at least 1 billion CFUs per strain per day, and keep in mind that some studies have used as much as 10 billion CFUs per strain daily to achieve results in specific disease states.

CHAPTER 5

The Personalization Level

Everyone's health challenges are different. Some of them you may already be experiencing. Perhaps you have diabetes, for example, or your doctor may have warned you that your blood sugar indicates you are prediabetic. Or there could be other health challenges—such as cancer or heart disease— that haven't touched you yet, but have struck members of your family, signalling that you are at greater risk.

I've created two lists of bodily systems on the following pages. For the first list, place a mark next to each health problem affecting you or an immediate family member (father, mother, sisters, and brothers). Record the obvious diseases, as well as any symptoms your immediate family members have, whether or not there's an official diagnosis. For example, if your mother suffers from frequent colds, but her doctors don't know why, just place a mark next to "immune problems." Or maybe you've suffered a heart attack. So you would place a mark next to "heart and lungs." For the second list, place a mark next to each health problem you have experienced directly.

Keep in mind, this initial inventory is not meant to be very specific. It's simply identifying general problem areas based on your—and your immediate family's—past medical history. In the following sections of this chapter, you'll take medical quizzes and learn about blood, hormone, nutrient, and oxidative stress tests for collecting more detailed information.

FAMILY MEDICAL INVENTORY

Do you, or does anyone in your family, suffer from problems related to any of the following?

- **Heart:** Arrhythmia, elevated cholesterol and/or triglycerides, angina, heart attack, heart failure, stroke

- **Lungs:** Shortness of breath, asthma, bronchitis, emphysema

- **Blood Pressure & Blood Vessels:** Hypertension, aneurisms, varicose veins, spider veins, arteriosclerosis (hardening of the arteries), poor circulation

- **Cancer & Precancerous Lesions:** All forms

- **Diabetes & Metabolic Disorders:** Diabetes, insulin resistance, metabolic syndrome (marked by large waist size, high triglycerides, high blood pressure, low HDL cholesterol, and/or high blood sugar)

- **Brain & Nerves:** Normal age-related cognitive decline, tremors, dementia, Alzheimer's disease, Parkinson's disease, diabetic neuropathy, Huntington's disease

- **Bones & Joints:** Osteopenia (low bone-mineral density), osteoporosis, joint pain and stiffness, osteoarthritis, rheumatoid arthritis

- **Immune Problems:** Frequent colds/flu/illness, autoimmune diseases

- **Kidneys:** Chronic kidney disease, renal failure

- **Eyes, Ears, Nose & Throat:** Allergies, sinus disorders, glaucoma, age-related macular degeneration, hearing loss, tonsillitis

PERSONAL MEDICAL INVENTORY

Do you personally suffer from problems related to the following?

- Inflammatory & Pain Syndromes
- Low Energy/Fatigue
- Overweight & Obesity
- Muscles & Skin
- Gastrointestinal System
- Low Thyroid
- Urinary Tract & Bladder Infections
- Depression
- Anxiety

On page 236, you'll find a worksheet with an empty pyramid. Once you've completed your medical inventories, find the recommended supplements on the following page for each body system you've marked off and add them to the Personalization Level of your pyramid. (They are listed in order of most to least important. At a minimum, I would suggest adding the first supplement listed within each group.) Remember, these are in addition to the supplements in your Foundation Level: an optimally dosed multivitamin, omega-3 fatty acids, CoQ_{10}, and probiotics.

RECOMMENDED SUPPLEMENTS FOR SPECIFIC BODY SYSTEMS

❏ **Heart**

Pomegranate extract

Stand-alone vitamin D_3

Aged garlic extract

❏ **Lungs**

Natural vitamin E

N-acetyl-cysteine

Panax ginseng

❏ **Blood Pressure & Blood Vessels**

Pomegranate extract

Grape seed extract

Olive leaf extract

❏ **Cancer**

Cruciferous vegetable extract

Stand-alone vitamin D_3

Reishi mushroom or curcumin extract

❏ **Diabetes & Metabolic Disorders**

Chromium and/or cinnamon extract

Green coffee bean extract

R-lipoic acid

❏ **Brain & Nerves**

Benfotiamine (fat-soluble vitamin B_1) and Methyl cobalaimine (active form of B_{12})

Blueberry extract

Magnesium-L-threonate

❏ **Bones & Joints**

Stand-alone vitamin D_3 (bones)

Dedicated bone formula (bones)

MSM (joints)

Glucosamine (joints)

❏ **Immune Problems**

Stand-alone vitamin D_3

Thymus extract

Selenium

❏ **Kidneys & Urinary Tract**

Cranberry extract

Horsetail

Grape seed extract

❑ **Eyes, Ears, Nose & Throat**
Lutein & Zeaxanthin
Astaxanthin
Natural vitamin E

❑ **Inflammatory & Pain Syndromes**
Curcumin
Boswellia extract
Tart cherry extract

❑ **Low Energy/Fatigue**
Rhodiola
Glutathione
Magnesium citrate

❑ **Overweight & Obesity**
Irvingia extract
Fucoxanthin
Green coffee bean extract

❑ **Muscles & Skin**
D-ribose
Propionyl-L-Carnitine
Diosmin

❑ **Gastrointestinal System**
Zinc-carnosine
Artichoke extract
Picrorhiza extract

❑ **Low Thyroid**
L-tyrosine
Iodine
Selenium

❑ **Urinary Tract & Bladder Infections**
Cranberry extract
Hibiscus extract
D-mannose

❑ **Depression**
Tryptophan or 5-HTP
SAMe
Saffron extract

❑ **Anxiety**
GABA
Lemon balm
Valerian

Let's use me as an example. First, I started taking the foundational supplements everyone should be taking. Soon after, I took a medical inventory and placed marks by the following body systems:

- Blood Pressure & Blood Vessels

- Cancer

My dad suffered from high blood pressure, and my mom died of lung cancer. Unfortunately, she was a smoker. I was exposed to secondhand smoke most of my life, so I wanted to protect myself against its effects.

Based on my medical inventory, I added grape seed extract and crucifer-ous vegetable extract to my pyramid. I decided that since heart disease is the number-one killer of men, I would prioritize grape seed extract (for heart disease prevention) over cruciferous vegetable extract (for cancer prevention). My pyramid now looked like this:

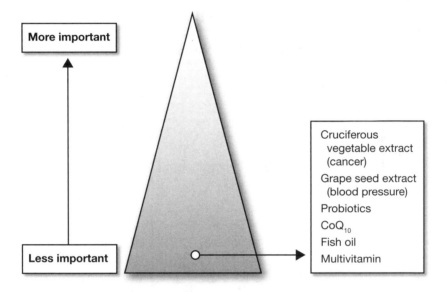

So take your inventories and fill in your pyramid on page 236.

You can get more specific. That's what the remaining sections in this chapter are for. Let's start with some medical quizzes to get more detailed with the Personalization Level of your pyramid. There is an empty pyra-mid at the end of Chapter 10 that you can use as a worksheet. (Tip: use pencil! Your pyramid may go through several incarnations.)

MEDICAL QUIZZES

Now that you have a basic idea of some supplements you might need based on your medical inventory, let's dig a little deeper. I've developed seventeen medical quizzes on various body systems to provide another layer of detail beyond your inventory. By completing these quizzes, we'll be able to pinpoint with more accuracy which supplements you really need.

Let's go back to my pyramid. If you remember, after taking my medical inventory, I decided it was more important to protect myself against heart disease than cancer. However, after completing the heart and cancer quizzes, my responses showed just the opposite. It turns out I have no heart disease risk factors except a family history of high blood pressure, but I do have some cancer risks because of secondhand smoke and my exposure to radiation as a radiology resident.

Based on my quiz results, my pyramid changed. Cancer prevention supplements are more important for me than heart disease supplements. So here is how my pyramid looks now:

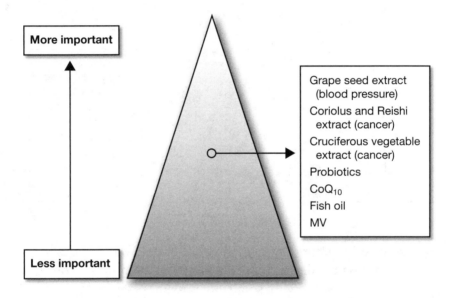

Can you see how your Supplement Pyramid will help you prioritize your supplements? By completing the medical quizzes, I now have a better understanding of what's important for my health. My pyramid identifies my needs and helps organize and prioritize all of my supplements based on those needs.

Let's say in the far-off future, my financial situation changes and I can no longer afford the full suite of supplements. My pyramid not only tells me how to build my regimen, but also how to make changes and eliminate products. In this case, assuming my medical history and quiz answers don't change, I'll stop taking grape seed extract first, and move down the pyramid, eliminating less important supplements before I ax more important supplements.

Take as many quizzes as you need to take. I recommend taking them all. But you can start off with the ones covering the parts of the body that most concern you today. There's no rush. Take your time and build your pyramid slowly. Or go fast and take all of the quizzes. It's totally up to you.

Here's how I would approach the quizzes:

1. Identify the most important quizzes for you, using your inventory as a guide.

2. Take the quizzes and record your results, as well as the suggested supplements based on those results.

3. Continue reading Chapter 5 for laboratory tests you might want to get to further refine the Personalization Level of your pyramid.

4. Speak with your doctor or call Life Extension health advisors (see Appendix A). They will help you decide which lab tests to get and then help you develop the Personalization Level of your pyramid.

Each quiz comes with its own set of instructions, as well as directions on how to tally and interpret your scores. Specific supplements are suggested based on your score. A detailed explanation of each supplement is provided in the Appendix B.

Now, if this all seems too much for you, and you don't have the patience to fill out a bunch of quizzes or complete the laboratory tests I suggest later in this chapter, then you can just use the recommendations from your personal and family medical inventories to build the Personalization Level of your pyramid.

Please note: These quizzes, although developed from clinical risk assessment questions, do not replace the advice of your doctor. They are simply meant to help you identify possible risk factors or symptoms of various diseases so you can protect yourself against those diseases.

BUILD YOUR SUPPLEMENT PYRAMID ONLINE

Build your personalized supplement pyramid online at www.mysupplement pyramid.com. You can complete your inventories and take all of the quizzes by creating a FREE online account. All of your supplement suggestions, quizzes, and inventories are stored digitally in place for easy access.

MEDICAL QUIZ 1 Heart & Circulation

*If you have known heart disease, have suffered a heart attack, or have had heart or vascular procedures, skip to Quiz Results and Suggestions.

Do you have circulation problems (such as cold, blue extremities)?	Yes – 1 point	No – 0 points	
Is your bad (LDL) cholesterol high (over 130 mg/dL)?	Yes – 1 point	No – 0 points	Don't know – 0.5 points
Do you have high fasting blood sugar (over 101 mg/dL) or have diagnosed diabetes?	Yes – 2 points	No – 0 points	Don't know – 0.5 points
Do you have high triglycerides (equal to or greater than 150 mg/dL)?	Yes – 1 point	No – 0 points	Don't know – 0.5 points
Is your good (HDL) cholesterol low (under 40 mg/dL for men and under 50 mg/dl for women)?	Yes – 1 point	No – 0 points	Don't know – 0.5 points
Is your CRP level (a marker of inflammation) high (greater than 3.0 mg/dL), or do you have an inflammatory condition such as psoriasis, bowel inflammation, rheumatoid arthritis, or other autoimmune disorders?	Yes – 2 points	No – 0 points	Don't know – 0.5 points
Is your homocysteine level high?	Yes – 1 point	No – 0 points	Don't know – 0.5 points
Is your fibrinogen level high (greater than 300 mg/dL)?	Yes – 1 point	No – 0 points	Don't know – 0.5 points
Is your testosterone level low (less than 300 ng/dL for men and less than 15 ng/dL for women)?	Yes – 1 point	No – 0 points	Don't know – 0.5 points
Do you smoke?	Yes – 3 points	No – 0 points	
Do you eat fish at least twice a week?	Yes – 0 points	No – 1 point	
Do you eat whole grains and dark fruits and vegetables every day?	Yes – 0 points	No – 1 point	

Note: If your score ends in 0.5, round down to get your point total. **Point Total:** _____

Quiz 1: Results and Suggestions

Below are some lifestyle and supplement suggestions for you to follow. You do not have to implement every lifestyle suggestion or take every supplement recommended for your point score. However, I would recommend at a minimum adding the first supplement listed for your score to the Personalization Level of your Supplement Pyramid. (They are listed in order of importance.)

Lifestyle Suggestions

❑ Complete a cardiac blood panel that identifies heart disease factors to help personalize suggestions.
❑ Eat a diet high in protein, vegetables, and fiber (especially soluble fiber)—and low in refined carbohydrates, especially soda and desserts.
❑ Aim to get thirty to sixty minutes of exercise most days of the week.

Supplement Suggestions

In addition to the supplements in your Foundation Level, consider adding these to your Personalization Level:

0–1 points: You're doing great! Stick to the lifestyle suggestions above.

2–3 points: 1) pomegranate extract, 2) stand-alone vitamin D_3

4–6 points: 1) pomegranate extract, 2) stand-alone vitamin D_3, 3) aged garlic

7–9 points: 1) pomegranate extract, 2) stand-alone vitamin D_3, 3) aged garlic, 4) niacin

10 points or more: 1) pomegranate extract, 2) stand-alone vitamin D_3, 3) aged garlic, 4) niacin, 5) resveratrol

If you have . . .

❑ A past history of heart disease—pomegranate extract, stand-alone vitamin D, aged garlic, niacin, resveratrol
❑ Had a heart attack—The supplements listed above, plus EDTA chelation therapy
❑ High bad (LDL) cholesterol—Red yeast rice, sytrinol, polycosanol
❑ High triglycerides (TG)—Increase foundational fish oil dose to 3–4 grams EPA + DHA
❑ Low good (HDL) cholesterol—Niacin (not niacinamide), Indian gooseberry
❑ High CRP—Increase foundational fish oil dose to 3–4 grams EPA + DHA, curcumin, boswellia
❑ High fibrinogen—Nattokinase
❑ High homocysteine—Complete B complex, trimethylglycine, SAMe

---

All suggestions are based on general risk. Once you complete a cardiac blood panel, more specific supplements can be suggested based on your actual risk factors. For instance, you might need cholesterol-lowering supplements if your "bad" (LDL) cholesterol level is too high. But without knowing your cholesterol level, I cannot make specific suggestions.

MEDICAL QUIZ 2 | Cancer

*If you have cancer of any kind, skip to Quiz Results and Suggestions.

Do you have a family history of cancer?	Yes – 2 points	No – 0 points	Don't know – 0.5 points
Do you have any genetic markers for cancers (i.e., BRCA gene for breast cancer)?	Yes – 2 points	No = 0 points	Don't know = 0.5 points
Do you smoke?	Yes = 2 points	No = 0 points	
Do you work with chemicals, dyes, or paints?	Yes = 2 points	No – 0 points	
Have you had more than ten X-ray procedures in your life or been exposed to radiation?	Yes – 2 points	No – 0 points	
Do you have, or have you had removed, any suspicious skin lesions?	Yes – 1 point	No – 0 points	
Do you suffer from chronic viral infections, such as hepatitis, Epstein Barr, herpes, etc.?	Yes – 1 point	No – 0 points	
Are you overweight (body mass index of 25–29.9) or obese (body mass index of 30 or above)?*	Yes – 1 point	No – 0 points	
Do you eat red meat more days a week than not?	Yes – 1 point	No – 0 points	
Do you eat at least 25 grams (women) or 35 grams (men) of fiber a day?	Yes – 0 points	No – 1 point	

Note: If your score ends in 0.5, round down to get your point total.   **Point Total:** _____

Medical Quiz 2 (continued)

Quiz 2: Results and Suggestions

Below are some lifestyle and supplement suggestions for you to follow. You do not have to implement every lifestyle suggestion or take every supplement recommended for your point score. However, I would recommend at a minimum adding the first supplement listed for your score to the Personalization Level of your Supplement Pyramid. (They are listed in order of importance.)

Lifestyle Suggestions

❏ Eat a diet high in fruits and vegetables, particularly cruciferous vegetables such as broccoli and kale.

❏ Lose weight if you are overweight or obese: According to the American Cancer Society, 20 percent of all cancer deaths among women and 14 percent among men can be attributed to excess pounds.

❏ Get thirty minutes of exercise per day.

Supplement Suggestions

In addition to the supplements in your Foundation Level, consider adding these to your Personalization Level:

0–1 points: You're doing great! Stick to the lifestyle suggestions above.

2-3 points: 1) cruciferous vegetable extract, 2) stand-alone vitamin D_3

4-5 points: 1) cruciferous vegetable extract, 2) stand-alone vitamin D_3, 3) curcumin

6-7 points: 1) cruciferous vegetable extract, 2) stand-alone vitamin D_3, 3) curcumin, 4) reishi

8–9 points: 1) cruciferous vegetable extract, 2) stand-alone vitamin D_3, 3) curcumin, 4) reishi, 5) coriolus

If you have . . .

10 points or more or have cancer: 1) cruciferous vegetable extract, 2) stand-alone vitamin D_3, 3) curcumin, 4) reishi, 5) coriolus, 6) lignans

---

* **Don't know your body mass index? You can use the CDC's Adult BMI Calculator:**
http://www.cdc.gov/healthyweight/assessing/bmi/adult_bmi/
english_bmi_calculator/bmi_calculator.html.

MEDICAL QUIZ 3　Diabetes & Metabolic Disorders

*If you have diabetes, skip to Quiz Results and Suggestions.

Have you been diagnosed with prediabetes, or is your blood sugar consistently between 101–125 mg/dL? Yes – 3 points　No – 2 points　Don't know – 0.5 points

Do you drink more than one sugary drink a day and/or eat dessert every day? Yes – 2 points　No – 0 points

Are you forty-five years old or older? Yes – 1 point　No – 0 points

Do you carry your extra weight around your waist? Yes – 1 point　No – 0 points

Is your good (HDL) cholesterol low (under 40 mg/dL for men and under 50 mg/dl for women)? Yes – 2 point　No – 0 points　Don't know – 0.5 points

Do you have high triglycerides (equal to or greater than 150 mg/dL)? Yes – 2 points　No – 0 points　Don't know – 0.5 points

Is your blood pressure consistently high (equal to or greater than 130/80)? Yes – 2 points　No – 0 points　Don't know – 0.5 points

Do you exercise more days a week than not? Yes – 0 points　No – 1 points

Do you have darker, thicker skin around the armpits and/or neck region (acanthosis nigricans)? Yes – 1 point　No – 0 point

Note: If your score ends in 0.5, round down to get your point total.　**Point Total:** _____

Medical Quiz 3 (continued)

Quiz 3: Results and Suggestions

Below are some lifestyle and supplement suggestions for you to follow. You do not have to implement every lifestyle suggestion or take every supplement recommended for your point score. However, I would recommend at a minimum adding the first supplement listed for your score to the Personalization Level of your Supplement Pyramid. (They are listed in order of importance.)

Lifestyle Suggestions

❑ Lose weight if you are overweight or obese. You can lower your blood pressure, blood sugar, and cholesterol levels simply by losing 10 percent of your body weight, or 15 pounds for a 150-pound woman.

❑ Eat a diet high in protein, vegetables, and fiber (especially soluble fiber)—and low in refined carbohydrates, especially soda and desserts.

❑ Aim to get thirty to sixty minutes of exercise most days of the week.

Supplement Suggestions

In addition to the supplements in your Foundation Level, consider adding these to your Personalization Level:

0–1 points: You're doing great! Stick to the lifestyle suggestions above.

2–3 points: 1) chromium and/or cinnamon extract

4–6 points: 1) chromium and/or cinnamon extract, 2) green coffee bean extract

7–9 points: 1) chromium and/or cinnamon extract, 2) green coffee bean extract, 3) R-lipoic acid

If you have . . .

10 points or more or have diabetes: 1) chromium and/or cinnamon extract, 2) green coffee bean extract, 3) R-lipoic acid, 4) green tea extract

MEDICAL QUIZ 4 | Brain and Nerves

*If you have Alzheimer's disease (or any type of dementia), Parkinson's disease, or tremors, or any kind of neuropathy, skip to Quiz Results and Suggestions.

Do you have sharp or burning pain in your extremities?	Yes – 3 points	No – 0 points
Do you work with chemicals, dyes, or paints?	Yes – 2 points	No – 0 points
Have you suffered from head trauma?	Yes – 2 points	No – 0 points
Are you over age fifty?	Yes – 1 point	No – 0 points
Do you have joint stiffness or rigid limbs?	Yes – 1 point	No – 0 points
Do you have trouble keeping your balance while walking?	Yes – 1 point	No – 0 points
Do you have sleep disturbances?	Yes – 1 point	No – 0 points
Do you have trouble swallowing?	Yes – 1 point	No – 0 points
Do you have difficulty concentrating?	Yes – 1 point	No – 0 points
Do you lose your train of thought easily?	Yes – 1 point	No – 0 points

Point Total: _____

Quiz 4: Results and Suggestions

Below are some lifestyle and supplement suggestions for you to follow. You do not have to implement every lifestyle suggestion or take every supplement recommended for your point score. However, I would recommend at a minimum adding the first supplement listed for your score to the Personalization Level of your Supplement Pyramid. (They are listed in order of importance.)

Lifestyle Suggestions

❏ Stay physically active to ensure proper blood supply to the brain.
❏ Keep your brain challenged: learn a new language, do crossword puzzles, play video games.
❏ Eat a diet high in fruits and vegetables, particularly blueberries, and omega-3 fats.

Supplement Suggestions

In addition to the supplements in your Foundation Level, consider adding these to your Personalization Level:

Medical Quiz 4 (continued)

0–1 points: You're doing great! Stick to the lifestyle suggestions above.

2–3 points: 1) Benfotiamine (fat-soluble vitamin B_1) and Methylcobalamine B_{12}* (active form B_{12})

4–6 points: 1) Benfotiamine (fat-soluble vitamin B_1) and Methylcobalamine B_{12} (active form B_{12}), 2) blueberry extract

7 points or more: 1) Benfotiamine (fat-soluble vitamin B_1) and Methylcobalamine B_{12} (active form B_{12}), 2) blueberry extract, 3) magnesium threonate

If you have . . .

Alzheimer's disease: 1) pregnenolone, 2) curcumin, 3) R-lipoic acid, 4) quercetin, 5) resveratrol

Parkinson's disease/tremors: 1) creatine, 2) mucuna pruriens, 3) acetyl-L-carnitine, 4) green tea, 5) resveratrol

MEDICAL QUIZ 5 | Memory

This test is different. It's a simple short-term memory quiz. Slowly read each line once (and only once!). Then look away and try to recall the numbers in that line, in the exact order. Each line comes with a numbered score. The last line that you can recall is your score.

4 8 6	10 points
2 5 7 8	9 points
5 8 2 5 7	8 points
9 1 3 4 0 6	7 points
6 7 2 8 4 3 8	6 points
1 3 8 9 0 7 5 2	5 points
0 9 3 7 0 4 6 9 1	4 points
6 6 9 4 6 2 7 8 1 0	3 points
9 6 2 4 3 7 2 0 1 9 5	2 points
6 3 1 0 9 9 7 1 4 2 6 5	1 point

Point Total: _____

Medical Quiz 5 (continued)

Quiz 5: Results and Suggestions

The average short-term memory can only hold around seven pieces of information. However, with age, ongoing stress, chronic diseases, drug use, nutritional deficiencies, and poor lifestyle habits, the amount of information we can hold can drop off.

Below are some lifestyle and supplement suggestions for you to follow. You do not have to implement every lifestyle suggestion or take every supplement recommended for your point score. However, I would recommend at a minimum adding the first supplement listed for your score to the Personalization Level of your Supplement Pyramid. (They are listed in order of importance.)

Lifestyle Suggestions

❑ Play memory games. A good website to check out is www.lumosity.com, which offers more than forty games based on the latest scientific research to help improve your ability to pay attention, remember information, and perform cognitive tasks.

❑ Eat a diet rich in antioxidants, including plenty of fruits and vegetables in a range of colors, and omega-3 fatty acids, such as cold-water fatty fish like salmon and tuna.

❑ Maintain an active social life, which has been shown to delay age-related memory loss.

Supplement Suggestions

In addition to the supplements in your Foundation Level, consider adding these to your Personalization Level:

0–3 points: Excellent! Stick to the lifestyle suggestions above.

4–6 points: Good. Consider 1) blueberry extract.

7–9 points: Needs work. Consider 1) blueberry extract, 2) magnesium threonate

10 points: Poor. Consider 1) blueberry extract, 2) magnesium threonate, 3) phosphatidyl serine (PS)

MEDICAL QUIZ 6 — Blood Pressure and Blood Vessels

Is your blood pressure consistently high (equal to or greater than 130/80)?	Yes – 4 points	No – 0 points	Don't know – 0.5 points
Do you have abdominal or brain aneurisms?	Yes – 3 points	No – 0 points	
Do you smoke?	Yes – 2 points	No – 0 points	
Do you have varicose veins?	Yes – 1 point	No – 0 points	
Do you have spider veins?	Yes – 1 point	No – 0 points	
Do you have dark skin?	Yes – 1 point	No – 0 points	
Are you overweight (body mass index of 25–29.9) or obese (body mass index of 30 or above)?*	Yes – 1 point	No – 0 points	
Do you drink more than two alcoholic drinks every day?	Yes – 1 point	No – 0 points	
Do you limit your salt intake?	Yes – 0 points	No – 1 point	
Do you have sleep apnea?	Yes – 1 point	No – 0 points	

Point Total: _____

Quiz 6: Results and Suggestions

Below are some lifestyle and supplement suggestions for you to follow. You do not have to implement every lifestyle suggestion or take every supplement recommended for your point score. However, I would recommend at a minimum adding the first supplement listed for your score to the Personalization Level of your Supplement Pyramid. (They are listed in order of importance.)

Lifestyle Suggestions

❏ Lose weight if you are overweight or obese.
❏ Eat more fruits and vegetables.
❏ Get regular aerobic exercise (minimum thirty minutes per day, three days per week).

* **Don't know your body mass index? You can use the CDC's Adult BMI Calculator: http://www.cdc.gov/healthyweight/assessing/bmi/adult_bmi/ english_bmi_calculator/bmi_calculator.html.**

Medical Quiz 6 (continued)

Supplement Suggestions

In addition to the supplements in your Foundation Level, consider adding these to your Personalization Level:

0–1 points: You're doing great! Stick to the lifestyle suggestions above.

2–3 points: 1) pomegranate extract

4–6 points: 1) pomegranate extract, 2) grape seed extract

7–9 points: 1) pomegranate extract, 2) grape seed extract, 3) olive leaf extract

10 points or more: 1) pomegranate extract, 2) grape seed extract, 3) olive leaf extract, 4) hawthorn extract

If you have only . . .

Varicose or spider veins, try diosmin (derived from the citrus bioflavonoid hesperidin).

Aneurysms, try hawthorn extract.

MEDICAL QUIZ 7　Hormone Imbalances in Men

This test does not use points. Simply circle the appropriate answer.

Are you easily tired?	Yes	No
Are you constipated two or more days a week?	Yes	No
Do you have cold extremities (hands and feet)?	Yes	No
Are you depressed or do you feel like you have the "blues"?	Yes	No
Have you lost muscle mass and gained fat?	Yes	No
Do you have a low sex drive?	Yes	No
Have you gained weight around your midsection?	Yes	No
Do you experience erectile dysfunction?	Yes	No
Do your feet and ankles swell?	Yes	No
Do you crave sweets?	Yes	No

Total Yes Answers: _____

Medical Quiz 7 (continued)

Quiz 7: Results and Suggestions

Answering "yes" to any of the above questions indicates that you should get your hormone levels tested. Additional sections later in this chapter cover the tests in more detail. Below are some lifestyle and supplement suggestions for you to follow.

Lifestyle Suggestions

❏ Get a complete thyroid panel—TSH, total T4, free T4, and free T3.

❏ Get a complete hormone panel—Testosterone, estradiol (a form of estrogen), DHT, SHBG, DHEA, progesterone, pregnenolone, PSA (prostate specific antigen) and vitamin D*.

Supplement and Hormone Suggestions

Once you receive your lab results, follow these suggestions:

Low testosterone—prescription testosterone via gels or creams, DHEA, and pregnenolone supplements

High estrogen—zinc, chrysin, calcium-d-glucarate and grape seed extract, DIM

Low DHEA—DHEA supplement

Low pregnenolone—pregnenolone supplement

High DHT—natural 5-alpha reductase inhibitors like saw palmetto and sesame lignin supplements

High SHBG—cruciferous vegetable extract supplement

Low thyroid—prescription bioidentical thyroid hormones or tyrosine and iodine supplements

* While it is called "vitamin" D, this nutrient is actually a hormone.

MEDICAL QUIZ 8   Hormone Imbalances in Women

This test does not use points. Simply circle the appropriate answer.

Are you easily tired?	Yes	No
Are you constipated two or more days a week?	Yes	No
Do you have cold extremities (hands and feet)?	Yes	No
Are you depressed or do you feel like you have the "blues"?	Yes	No
Are you menopausal?	Yes	No
Do you have hot flashes?	Yes	No
Do you experience vaginal dryness?	Yes	No
Are you more anxious and irritable than usual?	Yes	No
Are your periods irregular or heavy?	Yes	No
Do you have fibroids?	Yes	No
Do you have ovarian cysts?	Yes	No
Do you have endometriosis?	Yes	No
Do your feet and ankles swell?	Yes	No
Do your breasts swell?	Yes	No
Do you crave sweets?	Yes	No
Have you lost muscle mass and gained fat?	Yes	No
Do you have a low sex drive?	Yes	No

Total Yes Answers: _____

Medical Quiz 8 (continued)

Quiz 8: Results and Suggestions

Answering "yes" to any of the above questions indicates that you should get your hormone levels tested. Additional sections later in this chapter cover the tests in more detail. Below are some lifestyle and supplement suggestions for you to follow.

Lifestyle Suggestions

❏ Get a complete thyroid panel—TSH, total T4, free T4, and free T3.

❏ Get a complete hormone panel—Testosterone, total estrogen, estradiol (a form of estrogen), DHT, SHBG, DHEA, progesterone, pregnenolone, and vitamin D*.

Supplement and Hormone Suggestions

Once you receive your lab results, follow these suggestions:

Low estrogen—prescription bioidentical hormone therapy or supplements of lignans, hops, black cohosh, DIM

Low DHEA—DHEA supplement

Low progesterone—over-the-counter progesterone cream

Low pregnenolone—pregnenolone supplement

Low testosterone—prescription testosterone via gels or creams, DHEA, and pregnenolone supplements

Low thyroid—prescription bioidentical hormone therapy or tyrosine and iodine supplements

---

* While it is called "vitamin" D, this nutrient is actually a hormone.

MEDICAL QUIZ 9 Inflammatory Conditions

This test does not use points. Simply circle the appropriate answer.

Are you over age fifty?	Yes	No
Do you have rheumatoid arthritis?	Yes	No
Do you have lupus?	Yes	No
Do you have psoriasis?	Yes	No
Do you have eczema?	Yes	No
Do you have inflammatory bowel disease?	Yes	No
Do you have Alzheimer's disease?	Yes	No
Do you have any form of heart disease?	Yes	No
Do you have cancer or are you a cancer survivor?	Yes	No
Do you have age-related or exercise-induced arthritis?	Yes	No
Are you prediabetic or diabetic?	Yes	No
Do you suffer from migraines?	Yes	No
Are you obese (body mass index of 30 or higher)?	Yes	No
Do you have occasional undiagnosed rashes?	Yes	No
Do you have chronic sinusitis?	Yes	No

Total Yes Answers: _____

Medical Quiz 9 (continued)

Quiz 9: Results and Suggestions

Answering "yes" to any of these questions may indicate that you have chronic inflammation.

Below are some lifestyle and supplement suggestions for you to follow. You do not have to implement every lifestyle suggestion or take every supplement recommended for your number of yeses. However, I would recommend at a minimum adding the first supplement listed to the Personalization Level of your Supplement Pyramid. (They are listed in order of importance.)

Lifestyle Suggestions

❏ Get your vitamin D levels tested and, if less than 30–40 ng/mL, take a vitamin D_3 supplement to optimize your levels.

❏ Eat an anti-inflammatory diet. (Stress cold-water fatty fish, such as salmon and tuna, and plenty of fruits and vegetables. Avoid meat, processed foods, wheat, sugar, alcohol, and so on.)

❏ Engage in gentle exercise every day. If you are inactive, start with simple range-of-motion and stretching exercises.

Supplement Suggestions

Omega-3 fatty acids are naturally anti-inflammatory, so remember to take your foundational supplements, which include an omega-3 fatty acid product. In addition, here are recommendations if you said yes to:

One question: 1) curcumin

Two or three questions: 1) curcumin, 2) boswellia

Four or five questions: 1) curcumin, 2) boswellia, 3) black cumin seed oil

Six or more questions: 1) curcumin, 2) boswellia, 3) black cumin seed oil, 4) black tea theaflavin

MEDICAL QUIZ 10 Bones

*If you have diagnosed osteoporosis, skip to Quiz Results and Suggestions.

Have you ever been told you have osteopenia (low bone density)?	Yes – 3 points	No – 0 points	
Do you have hyperparathyroidism (overactivity of the parathyroid glands)?	Yes – 3 points	No – 0 points	
Do you take steroids regularly or have you used them three or more times in the past two years?	Yes – 2 points	No – 0 points	
Do you engage in weight-bearing exercise two or more times per week?	Yes – 0 points	No – 2 points	
Are you of Caucasian or Asian descent?	Yes – 1 point	No – 0 points	
Are you a woman?	Yes – 1 point	No – 0 points	
Do you have low levels of estrogen (ovaries removed, postmenopausal)?	Yes – 1 point	No – 0 points	Don't know – 0.5 points
Do you have low levels of testosterone?	Yes – 1 point	No – 0 points	Don't know – 0.5 points
Are you over age fifty?	Yes – 1 point	No – 0 points	
Do you have a small body type or frame?	Yes – 1 point	No – 0 points	
Are you physically active more days a week than not?	Yes – 0 points	No – 1 point	

Note: If your score ends in 0.5, round down to get your point total.   **Point Total:** _____

Medical Quiz 10 (continued)

Quiz 10: Results and Suggestions

Below are some lifestyle and supplement suggestions for you to follow. You do not have to implement every lifestyle suggestion or take every supplement recommended for your point score. However, I would recommend at a minimum adding the first supplement listed for your score to the Personalization Level of your Supplement Pyramid. (They are listed in order of importance.)

Lifestyle Suggestions

❏ Start performing weight-bearing exercises, which force you to work against gravity.

❏ Eat foods rich in calcium and vitamin D, such as dairy products, green vegetables, and salmon.

❏ Get your estrogen and testosterone levels checked. If low, replenish with an appropriate bioidentical hormone prescription.

Supplement Suggestions

In addition to the supplements in your Foundation Level, consider adding these to your Personalization Level:

0–1 points: You're doing great! Stick to the lifestyle suggestions above.

2 points: Stand-alone vitamin D_3

3–5 points: Complete bone formula that contains: calcium, vitamin D_3, boron, magnesium, zinc, manganese, silicon, and vitamin K_2

If you have. . .

6 points or more or osteoporosis: 1) complete bone formula that contains: calcium, vitamin D_3, boron, magnesium, zinc, manganese, silicon, and vitamin K_2, 2) strontium

MEDICAL QUIZ 11 Respiratory

*If you're a current smoker or have asthma, skip to Quiz Results and Suggestions

Did you quit smoking within the last two years?	Yes – 2 points	No – 0 points
Are you over age forty?	Yes – 1 point	No – 0 points
Have you worked with chemicals, paints and/or dyes?	Yes – 1 point	No – 0 points
Have you worked in construction?	Yes – 1 point	No – 0 points
Do you have a chronic cough?	Yes – 1 point	No – 0 points
Do you have chronic allergies?	Yes – 1 point	No – 0 points
Do you eat cured meats two times a week or more?	Yes – 1 point	No – 0 points
Do you have HIV?	Yes – 2 points	No – 0 points

Point Total: _____

Quiz 11: Results and Suggestions

Below are some lifestyle and supplement suggestions for you to follow. You do not have to implement every lifestyle suggestion or take every supplement recommended for your point score. However, I would recommend at a minimum adding the first supplement listed for your score to the Personalization Level of your Supplement Pyramid. (They are listed in order of importance.)

Lifestyle Suggestions

❏ Improve the air quality in your home by switching to all-natural cleaning products and air fresheners in your household; choosing low-VOC paints, solvents, and glues; and adding houseplants to every room.

❏ Avoid cigarette smoke, smog, and eating cured meats.

❏ Eat a diet rich in antioxidants, including plenty of fruits and vegetables in a range of colors.

Medical Quiz 11 (continued)

Supplement Suggestions

In addition to the supplements in your Foundation Level, consider adding these to your Personalization Level:

0–1 points: You're doing great! Stick to the lifestyle suggestions above.

2–3 points: 1) vitamin E*

4–6 points: 1) vitamin E*, 2) N-acetyl cysteine (NAC)

7–9 points: 1) vitamin E*, 2) NAC, 3) Panax ginseng

If you have. . .

Scored 10 points or are a smoker: 1) vitamin E*, 2) NAC, 3) Panax ginseng, 4) broccoli extract

Asthma: 1) green tea, 2) butterbur, 3) rosmarinic acid, 4) vitamin E*

* Look for the natural "d" form rather than the synthetic "dl" form.

MEDICAL QUIZ 12 Eyes

*If you have macular degeneration, cataracts, or glaucoma, skip to Quiz Results and Suggestions.

Are you between fifty-five and sixty-nine years old?	Yes – 1 point	No – 0 points
Are you seventy years old or older?	Yes – 2 points	No – 0 points
Do you smoke?	Yes – 2 points	No – 0 points
Do you eat a diet high in fat?	Yes – 1 point	No – 0 points
Are you a woman?	Yes – 1 point	No – 0 points
Are you obese (body mass index of 30 or above)?*	Yes – 2 point	No – 0 points

Point Total: _____

* Don't know your body mass index? You can use the CDC's Adult BMI Calculator: http://www.cdc.gov/healthyweight/assessing/bmi/adult_bmi/ english_bmi_calculator/bmi_calculator.html.

Medical Quiz 12 (continued)

Quiz 12: Results and Suggestions

Below are some lifestyle and supplement suggestions for you to follow. You do not have to implement every lifestyle suggestion or take every supplement recommended for your point score. However, I would recommend at a minimum adding the first supplement listed for your score to the Personalization Level of your Supplement Pyramid. (They are listed in order of importance.)

Lifestyle Suggestions

❏ Wear UV-blocking sunglasses whenever you go outside, especially in the summer months and in southern latitudes, even if it is cloudy.

❏ Eat a low-glycemic diet (stress foods that will not cause spikes in your blood sugar) high in fruits and vegetables. High-glycemic diets can contribute to diabetes, and diabetes can lead to vision loss.

❏ Get regular eye exams.

Supplement Suggestions

In addition to the supplements in your Foundation Level, consider adding these to your Personalization Level:

0–1 points: You're doing great! Stick to the lifestyle suggestions above.

2–3 points: 1) lutein

4–6 points: 1) lutein, 2) zeaxanthin

7–9 points: 1) lutein, 2) zeaxanthin, 3) beta-carotene (in addition to what's in your multivitamin)

If you have . . .

Macular degeneration: 1) lutein, 2) zeaxanthin, 3) bilberry, 4) beta-carotene

Cataracts: 1) Eyedrops containing N-acetyl-Carnosine

Glaucoma: 1) pine bark extract, 2) bilberry extract, 3) lutein

MEDICAL QUIZ 13 | Joints

*If you have diagnosed osteoarthritis, skip to Quiz Results and Suggestions.

Do you have pain in your joints?	Yes – 1 point	No – 0 points
Do you have joint stiffness?	Yes – 1 point	No – 0 points
Do you have joint swelling?	Yes – 1 point	No – 0 points
Are you over age fifty?	Yes – 1 point	No – 0 points
Are you a woman?	Yes – 1 point	No – 0 points

Point Total: _____

Quiz 13: Results and Suggestions

Below are some lifestyle and supplement suggestions for you to follow. You do not have to implement every lifestyle suggestion or take every supplement recommended for your point score. However, I would recommend at a minimum adding the first supplement listed for your score to the Personalization Level of your Supplement Pyramid. (They are listed in order of importance.)

Lifestyle Suggestions

❑ Lose weight if you are overweight. Extra pounds mean extra stress on your joints.

❑ Get regular, low-impact exercise, such as walking, bicycling, or swimming. Moderate exercise can ease joint pain and help you lose weight.

❑ Eat an anti-inflammatory diet. (Stress cold-water fatty fish, such as salmon and tuna, and plenty of fruits and vegetables. Avoid meat, processed foods, wheat, sugar, alcohol, and so on.)

Supplement Suggestions

In addition to the supplements in your Foundation Level, consider adding these to your Personalization Level:

0 points: You're doing great! Stick to the lifestyle suggestions above.

1–2 points: 1) MSM, 2) glucosamine

3–4 points: 1) MSM, 2) glucosamine, 3) hyaluronic acid

If you have . . .

5 points or arthritis: 1) MSM, 2) glucosamine, 3) hyaluronic acid, 4) SAMe and/or type II collagen

If you have only . . .

Pain—try MSM and Korean angelica.

MEDICAL QUIZ 14　Kidneys and Urinary Tract

If you have chronic kidney or urinary disease, do not take any supplements before consulting your doctor.

Are you diabetic?	Yes – 2 points	No – 0 points
Do you have high blood pressure?	Yes – 2 points	No – 0 points
Are you over age sixty-five?	Yes – 1 point	No – 0 points
Have you had protein in a urine sample within the past year?	Yes – 1 point	No – 0 points
Have you had blood in a urine sample within the past year?	Yes – 1 point	No – 0 points
Do you take prescription pain medications?	Yes – 1 point	No – 0 points
Do you have urinary retention?	Yes – 1 point	No – 0 points

Point Total: _____

Quiz 14: Results and Suggestions

Below are some lifestyle and supplement suggestions for you to follow. You do not have to implement every lifestyle suggestion or take every supplement recommended for your point score. However, I would recommend at a minimum adding the first supplement listed for your score to the Personalization Level of your Supplement Pyramid. (They are listed in order of importance.)

Lifestyle Suggestions

❏ Drink plenty of fluids.

❏ Avoid alcohol, caffeine, and carbonated beverages.

❏ Eat a diet low in refined carbohydrates (especially soda and desserts) and high in fiber (especially soluble fiber).

Supplement Suggestions

In addition to the supplements in your Foundation Level, consider adding these to your Personalization Level:

0–1 points: You're doing great! Stick to the lifestyle suggestions above.

2–3 points: 1) cranberry extract, 2) horsetail

4–6 points: 1) cranberry extract, 2) horsetail, 3) grape seed extract

7–9 points: 1) cranberry extract, 2) horsetail, 3) grape seed extract, 4) N-acetyl-cysteine

MEDICAL QUIZ 15 | Chronic Infections

This test does not use points. Simply circle the appropriate answer.

Do you suffer from any chronic viral infection?	Yes	No
Do you suffer from any chronic bacterial infection?	Yes	No
Do you have HIV/AIDS?	Yes	No
Do you have chronic viral hepatitis?	Yes	No

Total Yes Answers: _____

Quiz 15: Results and Suggestions

Answering "yes" to any of these questions requires targeted supplementation for that particular infection.

Below are some lifestyle and supplement suggestions for you to follow. You do not have to implement every lifestyle suggestion or take every supplement recommended for your point score. However, I would recommend at a minimum adding the first supplement listed for your score to the Personalization Level of your Supplement Pyramid. (They are listed in order of importance.)

Lifestyle Suggestions

❏ Get your vitamin D levels tested and, if less than 30–40 ng/mL, take a vitamin D_3 supplement to optimize your levels.

❏ Eat an anti-inflammatory diet. (Stress cold-water fatty fish, such as salmon and tuna, and plenty of fruits and vegetables. Avoid meat, processed foods, wheat, sugar, alcohol, and so on.)

❏ Engage in gentle exercise every day. If you are inactive, start with simple range-of-motion and stretching exercises.

Supplement Suggestions
If you have . . .

Chronic viral infection: 1) andrographis, 2) aronia, 3) bitter melon, 4) Japanese honeysuckle

Chronic bacterial infection: 1) aged garlic, 2) oregano oil, 3) beta-glucan, 4) andrographis

HIV/AIDS: 1) selenium, 2) R-lipoic acid, 3) magnesium, 4) lactoferrin, 5) astragalus, 6) DHEA

Chronic viral hepatitis: 1) silymarin (from milk thistle), 2) N-acetyl cysteine, 3) R-lipoic acid, 4) Polyenylphosphatidyl choline, 5) Schisandra chinensis

MEDICAL QUIZ 16　Chronic Fatigue

If you have chronic fatigue syndrome, skip to "Results and Suggestions."

Are you between the ages of forty and fifty?	Yes – 1 point	No – 0 points	
Are you a woman?	Yes – 1 point	No – 0 points	
How do you rate your stress level?	High – 2 points	Moderate – 1 point	Low – 0 points
Do you suffer from depression?	Yes – 1 point	No – 0 points	
Do you have a sore throat or tender lymph nodes?	Yes – 1 point	No – 0 points	
Do you experience unrefreshing sleep?	Yes – 1 point	No – 0 points	
Do you experience extreme exhaustion lasting more than twenty-four hours after physical or mental exercise?	Yes – 1 point	No – 0 points	
Do you have muscle or joint pain?	Yes – 1 point	No – 0 points	
Are you sensitive to chemicals, dyes, and perfumes?	Yes – 1 point	No – 0 points	
Do you suffer from food sensitivities?	Yes – 1 point	No – 0 points	
Do you have any one of the following: eating disorders, Fibromyalgia, chronic cystitis (interstitial), irritable bowel syndrome, chronic headaches, or temporo-mandibular disorders?	Yes, I have 1 – 1 point Yes, I have 2 – 2 points Yes, I have 3 or more – 3 points No – 0 points		

Point Total: _____

Medical Quiz 16 (continued)

Quiz 16: Results and Suggestions

Below are some lifestyle and supplement suggestions for you to follow. You do not have to implement every lifestyle suggestion or take every supplement recommended for your point score. However, I would recommend at a minimum adding the first supplement listed for your score to the Personalization Level of your Supplement Pyramid. (They are listed in order of importance.)

Lifestyle Suggestions

❑ Engage in gentle exercise every day. If you are inactive, start with simple range-of-motion and stretching exercises.

❑ Start a meditation practice: Begin by sitting quietly for just five minutes a day, increasing to thirty minutes daily over time.

❑ Get better sleep, by keeping a consistent sleeping schedule, avoiding alcohol and caffeine before bed, and keeping your bedroom a dark, restful haven with no light or sound disturbances.

Supplement Suggestions

In addition to the supplements in your Foundation Level, consider adding these to your Personalization Level:

0–1 points: You're doing great! Stick to the lifestyle suggestions above.

2–3 points: 1) rhodiola, 2) glutathione

4–6 points: 1) rhodiola, 2) glutathione, 3) magnesium citrate

If you have . . .

7 points or more or chronic fatigue syndrome: 1) rhodiola, 2) glutathione, 3) magnesium citrate, 4) NADH (the coenzyme form of vitamin B_3 or niacin) and/or N-acetyl-cysteine

MEDICAL QUIZ 17 | Fibromyalgia and Pain Syndromes

*If you have fibromyalgia or a chronic pain syndrome, skip to Quiz Results and Suggestions.

Have you experienced trauma to your extremities (hands and feet), including surgeries?	Yes – 1 point	No – 0 points
Have you suffered head or neck trauma, including surgeries?	Yes – 1 point	No – 0 points
Are you a woman?	Yes – 1 point	No – 0 points
How would you rate your stress level?	High – 2 points	Moderate – 1 point	Low – 0 points
Are you between the ages of twenty and forty?	Yes – 1 point	No – 0 points
Have you recently suffered a sudden illness (such as heart attack, stroke, or infection)?	Yes – 1 point	No – 0 points

Point Total: _____

Quiz 17: Results and Suggestions

Below are some lifestyle and supplement suggestions for you to follow. You do not have to implement every lifestyle suggestion or take every supplement recommended for your point score. However, I would recommend at a minimum adding the first supplement listed for your score to the Personalization Level of your Supplement Pyramid. (They are listed in order of importance.)

Lifestyle Suggestions

❑ Get your vitamin D levels tested and, if less than 30–40 ng/mL, take a vitamin D_3 supplement to optimize your levels.

❑ Eat a diet high in protein, vegetables, and fiber (especially soluble fiber)— and low in refined carbohydrates, especially soda and desserts.

❑ Aim to get thirty to sixty minutes of exercise most days of the week.

Supplement Suggestions

In addition to the supplements in your Foundation Level, consider adding these to your Personalization Level:

Medical Quiz 17 (continued)

0 points: You're doing great! Stick to the lifestyle suggestions above.

1–2 points: 1) magnesium citrate

3–4 points: 1) magnesium citrate, 2) tart cherry extract

5–6 points: 1) magnesium citrate, 2) tart cherry extract, 3) boswellia

7–8 points: 1) magnesium citrate, 2) tart cherry extract, 3) boswellia, 4) MSM

If you have . . .

Fibromyalgia or chronic pain syndrome: 1) magnesium citrate, 2) tart cherry extract, 3) boswellia, 4) MSM, 5) Korean angelica

---

My Pyramid

Now that you have completed the medical quizzes of concern to you, it's time to make adjustments to the Personalization Level of your pyramid. Return to page 236 and add in suggestions from your quiz results. Add the recommended supplements (or at the very least, the top-recommended supplement) for your point score.

BLOOD TESTS

So far, you've identified your four Foundation Supplements—an ideally dosed multivitamin, omega-3 fatty acids, coenzyme Q_{10} (as ubiquinol), and probiotics. You've also made good headway into determining which supplements make up your Personalization Level by completing your personal and family medical inventories, as well as medical quizzes relevant to you. We're not done yet, though. After all, this is a book about building your own personalized nutritional regimen, and the best way to do that is to see exactly what's going on inside of you. How do we do that? Blood tests!

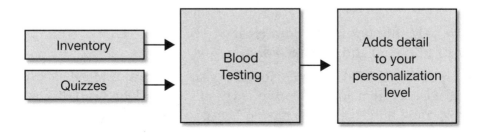

Every year, your doctor probably orders a standard blood panel that checks very basic markers of your health. And that's good. But to create a solid, health-promoting pyramid beyond what the basic tests provide, we need more information.

In this section, I'll outline different blood tests you can undergo that will help pinpoint the exact supplements you need. Now, I can't cover all of the myriad blood tests that are available, so I'm just going to focus on the ones most relevant to people in this country: those that assess the health of your heart, the strength of your bones, your levels of inflammation and oxidation, and your ability to metabolize sugar. (For additional blood tests, you can visit the Life Extension lab page at www.lef.org/Vitamins-Supplements/Blood-Tests/index.htm.)

Cover Your Bases with a Comprehensive Metabolic Panel (Chemistry/CBC)

This blood test is a comprehensive metabolic evaluation and includes all of the basics: fasting blood sugar level, liver and kidney function tests, cholesterol and triglyceride levels, a complete blood count, electrolyte measurements, and more. It's a general test that everybody should get.

Who Should Get This Test
The general population

Why This Test Is Important
A great place to start: identifies areas where you may need further testing

How to Make Sense of the Results
Your doctor or Life Extension doctors (see Appendix A) will review the tests with you and make supplement suggestions, helping fill in the Personalization Level of your pyramid.

Get a Deeper Look into Your Heart with a Specialized Cardiac Panel

Despite the fact that you go in for your yearly checkup and get a clean bill of health from your doctor, you may still be at risk for heart disease. How could this be? Because the risk factors doctors typically use to test for coronary artery disease—such as LDL cholesterol, HDL cholesterol, high blood pressure, and triglycerides—are important, but they don't tell the whole story. In fact, would it shock you to find out that nearly 75 percent of heart attacks that put people in the hospital occur in those with normal cholesterol levels?[1]

The truth is, there are many additional risk factors for cardiovascular disease that the conventional tests miss, such as homocysteine, vitamin D, C-reactive protein, and fibrinogen. Let's look at each one individually.

Homocysteine

Homocysteine is a sulfur-containing amino acid that typically winds up in the blood from eating meat. Unlike most amino acids, which are beneficial, homocysteine is considered an independent risk factor for heart disease. Studies have shown that just a 25 percent increase in homocysteine is associated with a 49 percent higher risk of ischemic heart disease.[2] It's theorized that high blood levels of homocysteine may directly damage the delicate endothelial cells lining the insides of the arteries—resulting in vascular inflammation, blood clot formation, and arterial plaque rupture.

Fibrinogen

Fibrinogen, another independent risk factor for heart disease, is a protein that encourages blood to clot. While some blood clotting is necessary to prevent blood loss after an injury, excessive clotting can cause serious damage to the body. If a clot ruptures and blocks an artery leading to the heart, for example, it becomes starved of oxygen and causes a heart attack. If a ruptured clot blocks an artery leading to the brain, the result is a stroke.

C-Reactive Protein

C-reactive protein (CRP) is a measure of systemic inflammation. As opposed to acute inflammation, which happens in response to illness or injury and is short lived and specific, systemic inflammation is a state of low-level inflammation that is ongoing and body wide. Scientists are realizing how important inflammation really is; it is now understood to be the common denominator among all chronic age-related diseases. Uncontrolled systemic inflammation puts you at risk for many degenerative diseases, including heart disease.[3]

Vitamin D (Vitamin D 25-OH)

"What does vitamin D have to do with heart disease?" you may be thinking. A lot! This vitamin, which is actually a hormone, is important to every cell and tissue throughout the body—including the entire cardiovascular system. Not only are people who are deficient in vitamin D more likely to have high blood pressure[4] and arterial stiffness[5] than those with normal levels, they're also 60 percent more likely to experience a cardiovascular event—such as heart attack, heart failure, or stroke.[6]

Who Should Get This Test
The general population, but especially people with a personal or family history of heart disease

Why This Test Is Important
Identifies additional heart disease risk factors missed by conventional tests

How to Make Sense of the Results
Your doctor or Life Extension doctors (see Appendix A) will review the tests with you and make supplement suggestions, helping fill in the Personalization Level of your pyramid.

Assess Risk Accurately with Advanced Cholesterol Measurements: VAP Test

There's more to cholesterol than just "good" and "bad." Researchers are realizing that not all LDL ("bad") cholesterol is the same. When it comes to LDL, size matters: Smaller, denser LDL particles are more "atherogenic"—meaning they're more likely to harden your arteries—than larger, fluffier ones. Likewise, not all HDL ("good") cholesterol is alike either. In this case, the smaller particles are more protective because they appear to be better at removing cholesterol from the endothelium (the lining of the blood vessels).[7] Unfortunately, a conventional cholesterol test will only estimate your LDL and HDL levels; it won't tell you anything about the size of your particles.

Who Should Get This Test
The general population, but especially people with a personal or family history of heart disease; people being treated for high cholesterol

Why This Test Is Important
To get a more comprehensive and reliable assessment of your risk of heart disease

How to Make Sense of the Results
Your doctor or Life Extension doctors (see Appendix A) will review the tests with you and make supplement suggestions, helping fill in the Personalization Level of your pyramid.

A much more accurate test is the VAP test, which provides a more comprehensive cholesterol risk assessment by directly measuring—not estimating—total cholesterol, HDL ("good") cholesterol, LDL ("bad") cholesterol, VLDL ("extra bad") cholesterol, and several clinically relevant cholesterol subclasses. As a result, this test allows your doctor to fully assess your risk of coronary heart disease and more effectively tailor follow-up assessments and treatment strategies.

The VAP test covers things like:

- Total cholesterol and all subtype measurements
- Atherogenic (plaque-forming) particles like LP(a) & APO-B100
- LDL-cholesterol density patterns and particle size
- Measurements of the most protective to least protective forms of HDL cholesterol

Fine-Tune Cholesterol Measurements with Apolipoprotein Testing

Here's a shocker for you: despite what you've been told, there are not two kinds of cholesterol. All cholesterol is, in fact, the same. What makes it either "good" or "bad" is not the cholesterol itself, but the kind of lipoprotein to which it's attached.

Who Should Get This Test
People who have had a heart attack in the past or who have peripheral vascular disease

Why This Test Is Important
To measure more sensitive cholesterol risk factors called apolipoproteins that your doctor isn't checking

How to Make Sense of the Results

Your doctor or Life Extension doctors (see Appendix A) will review the tests with you and make supplement suggestions, helping fill in the Personalization Level of your pyramid.

As the name implies, lipoproteins are combinations of fat and protein. They act as cholesterol taxis, carrying cholesterol around the body. HDL, which stands for high-density lipoprotein, is thought of as good because it protects against cardiovascular disease. LDL, which stands for low-density lipoprotein, is considered bad because it contributes to cardiovascular disease.

Apolipoproteins make up the protein portion of lipoproteins. They determine whether the lipoproteins are "good" or "bad." For example, APO A-1 acts as an arterial street cleaner, picking up excess cholesterol from the tissues and bringing it to the liver for processing. Therefore, it slows arterial plaque buildup (also known as atherosclerosis) and protects the heart. On the other hand, APO-B is like a litterer, depositing cholesterol in the tissues willy-nilly. As a result, it speeds up plaque buildup and damages the heart.

Since it's really lipoproteins that are the problem and not cholesterol, it makes sense to see which kinds of lipoproteins are shuttling cholesterol around your body. In fact, exciting new research indicates that APO A-1 is a better indicator of arterial plaque formation than the traditional test for HDL cholesterol. Likewise, APO-B appears to be a more accurate way to assess your risk of atherosclerosis than the traditional test for LDL cholesterol. It can also be helpful to measure your APO A-1 to APO-B ratio: A high ratio is cardio-protective while a low ratio indicates increased risk for heart disease.[8,9]

Evaluate Heart Failure Severity with BNP and Galectin-3 Testing

When your heart muscle cells stretch too much, the ventricles in your heart secrete a small protein called B-type natriuretic peptide (BNP). High levels of BNP tell you that your heart is working too hard.

Who Should Get This Test

People with a personal history of heart failure

Why This Test Is Important

To measure two proteins associated with heart failure and assess the severity of heart failure and the effectiveness of treatment

How to Make Sense of the Results

Your doctor or Life Extension doctors (see Appendix A) will review the tests with you and make supplement suggestions, helping fill in the Personalization Level of your pyramid.

BNP levels are elevated in people with congestive heart failure, a condition in which the heart cannot pump adequate blood to meet the body's needs. In fact, how much BNP is in the blood is directly correlated with both the severity and prognosis of this disease.

Even if you have no clinical evidence of cardiovascular disease, this test is a useful marker of risk. High blood levels of BNP predict your risk for first cardiovascular events (so they could, conceivably, forecast a heart attack before you have one), atrial fibrillation, stroke, and heart failure.

Another test that helps identify the development and progression of congestive heart failure measures galectin-3, a protein that plays a role in cardiac fibrosis—the formation of too much fibrous tissue in the heart.[10] The galectin-3 test is used in conjunction with clinical evaluation to determine the prognosis of people diagnosed with heart failure.

Because galectin-3 and BNP measure separate and distinct biological processes, these tests should not substitute for one another but instead complement each other.

Measure Arterial Plaque Stability with Phospholipase A-2 Testing

Arterial plaque is sort of like a game of Jenga. While that stack of blocks may appear stable on the outside, if just one piece comes loose, disaster can strike. Plaque can build up on the walls of the arteries with no symptoms for decades. But should one plaque rupture, it can enter the bloodstream and block an artery, leading to a heart attack or stroke.

Who Should Get This Test

People with a history of bypass surgery or stents and/or unstable angina (chest pain)

Why This Test Is Important

A high level indicates a risk for stent or bypass reocclusion and/or plaque rupture

How to Make Sense of the Results

Your doctor or Life Extension doctors (see Appendix A) will review the tests with you and make supplement suggestions, helping fill in the Personalization Level of your pyramid.

Phospholipase A-2 (Lp-PLA2) is an enzyme that promotes inflammation inside the arteries, leading to the formation of unstable, rupture-prone plaques. Measuring your level of Lp-PLA2 can predict your risk of coronary heart disease and ischemic stroke associated with atherosclerosis. The Lp-PLA2 test is different than conventional cholesterol and inflammation tests because it is so specific. Lp-PLA2 is the only test that provides unique information about how stable your arterial plaques are.

Check Your Inflammation Levels with a Specialized Inflammatory Panel

Who Should Get This Test

The general population; people with inflammatory disorders such as inflammatory bowel disease or autoimmune disorders like rheumatoid arthritis and lupus

Why This Test Is Important

Controlling inflammation is critical to optimal health. Conventional tests are not comprehensive enough for a full evaluation of your inflammation level.

How to Make Sense of the Results

Your doctor or Life Extension doctors (see Appendix A) will review the tests with you and make supplement suggestions, helping fill in the Personalization Level of your pyramid.

Most of us are familiar with inflammation as an acute response of the immune system to injury, such as when we stub our toe or pull a muscle in our back. When inflammation has done its job, it should go away. But that doesn't always happen. In fact, many people in this country are living with chronic, low-grade, systemic inflammation—and researchers now recognize this inflammatory state is the common denominator among age-related diseases such as heart disease and cancer. People with autoimmune disorders—in which the immune defenses of the body turn against itself—also have heightened levels of inflammation.

Now, I'm not saying that inflammation *causes* these diseases. It may simply be that inflammation is a result of our bodies fighting disease. But we do know this: if you have low-grade systemic inflammation, something is wrong. When your inflammation levels are consistently high, your heart, brain, and whole body are at risk.[11]

A specialized inflammatory panel should include:

- Chemistry Profile (electrolytes, liver and kidney function, cholesterol)

- Complete Blood Count (CBC)

- C-Reactive Protein (high sensitivity)

- Sedimentation Rate

- Rheumatoid Factor (RF)

- Antinuclear Antibodies (ANA) Screen

Measure Your Level of Oxidative Stress with Isoprostane Testing

Are you interested in seeing how much your body is aging? The isoprostane test will give you some interesting information. It measures your level of isoprostanes—inflammatory compounds that are produced when essential fatty acids are oxidized—in other words, damaged by highly reactive oxygen compounds known as free radical molecules.

Free radicals are unavoidable in modern living. They come from environmental toxins (such as cigarette smoke, air pollution, and UV radiation), the foods we eat (particularly trans fats, sugar, and animal foods), the water we drink (especially if it's chlorinated), the medications we take, and even our body's own metabolic processes.

The more isoprostanes in your system, the higher your level of oxidative stress.[12] And that's a problem, because oxidative stress—the strain on your body's tissues when the number of free radicals in your system outnumbers the number of antioxidants—is widely believed to be a key contributor the aging process.

While it's good to avoid as many sources of free radicals as possible, the best way to stop them in their tracks is to make sure your body is stocked with plenty of antioxidants, which defuse these highly reactive compounds. Fruits and vegetables are loaded with antioxidants, and certain nutritional supplements are also excellent at combating oxidative stress.

How many antioxidants you need varies from person to person. If you've living in a polluted city, you might need more antioxidants than someone living in the pristine countryside. If you're an industrial worker who is continually exposed to chemicals, you likely need more than a doctor like me who works in a relatively clean office environment.

Isoprostane tests are available at a modest price. Another way to check your level of oxidative stress is through blood or urine panels, which measure things like:

- **Glutathione:** Your body's premier antioxidant

- **N-acetyl-cysteine:** An amino acid needed for the formation of glutathione

- **Other antioxidant amino acids:** Cysteine, methionine, taurine, tryptophan, and tyrosine also act as antioxidants in the body

- **Vitamin and mineral antioxidants:** Beta-carotene (the precursor to vitamin A), vitamins C and E, zinc, and selenium all have significant antioxidant activity

Unfortunately, many of the antioxidants listed above are water-soluble. That means they are very short lived in the blood and urine, so it's difficult to get an accurate reading. And considering these tests are quite expensive, your best bet may be to stick with just measuring isoprostanes.

Who Should Get This Test

Anyone at high risk of oxidative stress, including smokers, people with chronic diseases, those taking prescription medications, and industrial workers

Why This Test Is Important

Although we all need to supplement with antioxidants, some of us need more based on our lifestyles and medical history

How to Make Sense of the Results

Your doctor or Life Extension doctors (see Appendix A) will review the tests with you and make supplement suggestions, helping fill in the Personalization Level of your pyramid.

Two Blood Sugar Tests to Consider

Diabetes has reached epidemic proportions in the United States. Nearly 10 percent of the American population has diabetes,[13] and the U.S. Centers for Disease Control has estimated that if current trends continue, one in three adults will have diabetes by 2050.[14] That's a problem, because adult diabetics are two to four times more likely to suffer from heart disease or a stroke than adults without the disease.[15]

Basic panels will check your fasting blood sugar level, but there are two additional tests you might consider if you're at high risk for diabetes (including having prediabetes) or are currently being treated for the disease.

Measure Insulin Resistance with Glucose Tolerance Testing

Insulin is a hormone secreted by the pancreas in response to eating carbohydrates. It facilitates the transport of blood sugar (known as blood glucose) from the bloodstream into the cells. Once inside, the sugar is used by the cells to make energy.

Unfortunately, your body can become resistant to insulin the same way an alcoholic's body can become resistant to (or tolerant of) alcohol. When your pancreas is constantly pumping out insulin in response to a high-carbohydrate diet (particularly simple carbohydrates such as white flour products and sugary foods and drinks), your body doesn't respond to it in the same way. As a result, sugar is not efficiently removed from the bloodstream and blood glucose levels remain high.

Insulin resistance is the hallmark of type 2 diabetes. The glucose tolerance test measures how quickly your body clears glucose from your blood. It can help determine if your body has become resistant to insulin or if you already have type 2 diabetes.

Check Glycation with Hemoglobin A1C Testing

Another test to consider if you think you might have prediabetes or diabetes is the hemoglobin A1C test. As opposed to a single fasting blood sugar test, which is subject to daily variation, this test evaluates your long-term blood sugar control by measuring your levels of hemoglobin A1C.

Sometimes the sugar in your blood reacts with important proteins in your body through a process called glycation. This is bad news, because it makes the protein-based fibers stiff and malformed, leading to connective tissue damage. Hemoglobin A1C is a reflection of this detrimental reaction: it measures how much of your hemoglobin (that oxygen-carrying protein in red blood cells) is glycated. Therefore, if your hemoglobin A1C level is elevated, it indicates that your blood sugar levels have been high enough for long enough to create alarming numbers of these mutant proteins.

Doctors often prescribe this blood test for their diabetic patients to monitor the progression of the disease and the efficacy of its treatment. However, because glycation is thought to be one of the major contributors to the aging process, I believe everyone should get their hemoglobin A1C level checked.

Who Should Get These Tests
People who are prediabetic, diabetic, or at risk of becoming so

Why These Tests Are Important
To identify insulin resistance and glycation early on so you can make appropriate changes before too much damage has occurred

How to Make Sense of the Results
Your doctor or Life Extension doctors (see Appendix A) will review the tests with you and make supplement suggestions, helping fill in the Personalization Level of your pyramid.

Two Bone Health Tests to Consider

Osteoporosis is a frightening disease. Not only does it threaten your mobility by degrading your bones, it can actually shorten your lifespan. According to a recent study, for a full ten years after a hip fracture, older women are two and a half times more likely to die than the general population, and older men are three times more likely![16] In addition to the standard DEXA scan, which measures bone density, certain blood tests can also help evaluate the health of your bones.

Measure Bone Formation with Alkaline Phosphatase Testing

You may think of bones as hard, lifeless structures, but the truth is, bones are active, living tissue that is constantly being remodeled. Cells called osteoclasts are busy tearing down old, weak bone tissue through a process called bone resorption. Meanwhile, cells called osteoblasts are hard at work building new, strong bone tissue in a process known as bone formation. In an ideal world, these two activities are perfectly balanced. Bone loss typically occurs when bone resorption outpaces bone formation. The result is reduced bone mass and increased susceptibility to fractures.

Bone-specific alkaline phosphatase (bone ALP) is a biomarker of active bone formation. It actually measures your total osteoblast activity, so you can see if you are building new bone quickly enough.

Evaluate Bone Loss with C-Telopeptide Testing and Urine DPD

Bone is made up of two basic substances: protein, mainly type 1 collagen (which gives bone its structure) and minerals, mainly calcium phosphate (which hardens the bone). When type 1 collagen is broken down by osteoclasts, C-telopeptide is released. Therefore, it is a good biomarker of bone resorption. The C-telopeptide test measures the amount of this biomarker in your blood. If your level is high, that means you are breaking down old bone too quickly.

Who Should Get These Tests
People with osteoporosis or low bone density

Why These Tests Are Important
To better evaluate bone breakdown and buildup

How to Make Sense of the Results
Your doctor or Life Extension doctors (see Appendix A) will review the tests with you and make supplement suggestions, helping fill in the Personalization Level of your pyramid.

Another test that measures bone resorption is the deoxypyridinoline (DPD) cross-link urine test. DPD is a crosslink of type 1 collagen. When bones are broken down, DPD is released into the bloodstream and secreted unmetabolized into the urine. Just like C-telopeptide, a high level indicates your rate of bone resorption is too high.

Evaluate Cellular Health with Lactate Dehydrogenase (LD) Isoenzyme Testing

The enzyme lactate dehydrogenase (LD) is found in virtually all of the body's cells, but only a small amount is usually detectable in the blood. It's released from cells into the bloodstream when cells are damaged or destroyed. Therefore, the LD test can be used to get a picture of cellular health. (The higher the level you have, the more cellular damage your body has endured.)

Although there is some overlap, each of the five LD isoenzymes tends to be concentrated in specific body tissues. In general, the isoenzyme locations are as follows:

- LD-1: heart, red blood cells, kidney
- LD-2: heart, red blood cells, kidney (lesser amounts than LD-1)
- LD-3: lungs and other soft tissues
- LD-4: white blood cells, lymph nodes, muscle, liver (lesser amounts than LD-5)
- LD-5: liver, skeletal muscle

This is wonderfully convenient, because it allows you to pinpoint the cellular health of very specific parts of your body.

Who Should Get This Test
The general population

Why This Test Is Important
To identify general problem areas early and begin specific supplements to maintain your health and well-being

How to Make Sense of the Results
Your doctor or Life Extension doctors (see Appendix A) will review the tests with you and make supplement suggestions, helping fill in the Personalization Level of your pyramid.

This has just been a sampling of the many blood tests available to you. As I mentioned earlier, I chose to discuss the ones of interest to the greatest amount of people, but there are dozens more you can take that may be more specific to your personal or family history. For details, check out Appendix A.

HORMONE TESTS

I teach that hormones are the messengers between your brain and your body. When your brain commands an action, it sends the instructions through your hormones to the target tissue, which produces the desired action.

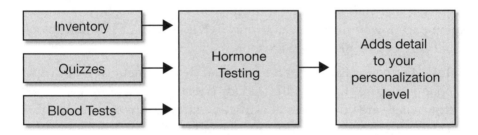

Those actions include everything from decreasing your heart rate and your blood pressure to activating your digestion and urine production. So as you can see, these "messengers" are pretty important to your health.

But what happens to your hormones as you age? They decrease in production. I believe that the steady loss of hormones is one reason we age. Hormone testing will identify hormonal deficiencies and imbalances, helping you personalize your Personalization Level beyond your medical inventory, quizzes, and blood tests.

There are several available methods for testing your hormones. The conventional method is by blood. It produces reliable results that doctors are familiar with and can understand.

The second method is saliva. It's my opinion that saliva results are not as reliable as blood measurements, for a variety of reasons. For instance, if even trace amounts of blood mix with saliva, the results will be inaccurate. Additionally, doctors are still learning how to interpret the results and understand changes from one test to the next.

If you decide to go with saliva testing, just make sure your doctor is experienced at reading the results. When you take the exam, be very careful how you or your doctor collects the saliva, and if you have sores or infections wait until they clear up before taking the test.

A third method of hormone testing is urine. This works well for hormones that are heavily metabolized, like estrogen and cortisol. But collecting urine can be cumbersome as it is best to collect several samples over a twenty-four-hour period.

The last method is hair analysis. This is not reliable for hormones and should be reserved for mineral and micronutrient analysis only.

Discover Hormonal Imbalances with a Female Hormone Blood Panel

As a woman, you probably know how important estrogen is to your overall health and well-being. But did you know that other hormones can impact how you feel just as strongly? A good female hormone blood panel will test for *all* of these hormones:

- **Total Estrogen:** Estrogen affects sexual development, reproduction, bone structure, liver health, mood, cognitive function, and blood flow. There are three types of estrogen: estrone, estradiol, and estriol. The total estrogen test measures the sum total of all three types of estrogen circulating in your bloodstream.

- **Estradiol:** It is the predominant circulating estrogen during a woman's reproductive years.

- **Progesterone:** Progesterone is often thought of as the pregnancy hormone, because it helps prepare your body for conception and pregnancy. Beginning in perimenopause and continuing through menopause, your levels of progesterone drop rapidly.

Who Should Get This Test
Aging women, especially in the perimenopausal, menopausal, and postmenopausal stages

Why This Test Is Important
Low estrogen, as well as an imbalanced estrogen-to-progesterone ratio, is associated with many age-related diseases

How to Make Sense of the Results
Your doctor or Life Extension doctors (see Appendix A) will review the tests with you and make supplement and/or bio-identical hormone suggestions, helping fill in the Personalization Level of your pyramid.

- **Total and Free Testosterone:** While testosterone is thought of as a male hormone, it's important for women too. Low testosterone levels in women can suppress libido and cause sexual dysfunction, while testosterone replacement therapy can improve sexual desire and function, mood, and general well-being.

- **Sex Hormone Binding Globulin (SHBG):** Not technically a hormone, SHBG binds to sex hormones, rendering them biologically inactive. This test can be helpful for detecting excess testosterone levels and polycystic ovarian syndrome in women.

- **Pregnenolone:** This hormone is the "mother hormone" of other steroidal hormones, giving rise to DHEA, progesterone, testosterone, estrogen, and cortisol. If you are low in pregnenolone, chances are you'll be low in all of these important hormones as well.

THE DANGERS OF CONVENTIONAL HORMONE REPLACEMENT THERAPY

Until 2002, mainstream physicians routinely prescribed conventional hormone replacement therapy (HRT) in order to alleviate menopausal symptoms such as hot flashes, mood swings, decreased sexual desire, vaginal dryness, and difficulty sleeping, as well as to prevent heart disease and osteoporosis.

In 2002, however, the results of a landmark study, the Women's Health Initiative (WHI), identified dangers associated with conventional hormone replacement therapy in women, which include nonhuman and nonbioidentical hormones —in other words, hormones that do not look or act like your natural hormones.

After observing 160,000 women, it was determined that conventional HRT side effects included a 26 percent increased risk of breast cancer, 29 percent increased risk of heart attack, 41 percent increased risk of stroke, and a doubling in risk of blood clots relative to the untreated group. Moreover, women receiving conjugated equine (horse-derived) estrogen experienced a sixfold increased risk of uterine cancer.[17–23]

Bioidentical HRT, which prescribes hormones that are biologically identical to those that your body produces, is associated with far fewer side effects than conventional HRT, and there is intriguing evidence that it may even reduce the risk of certain cancers.[24,25]

- **Dehydroepiandrosterone sulfate (DHEA-S):** A metabolite of the hormone DHEA, sometimes called the "youth hormone," DHEA-S is used as a biomarker of adrenal function.

- **Thyroid stimulating hormone (TSH):** Your thyroid gland has several important functions, including regulating your metabolism. Women frequently suffer from an underactive thyroid, which can cause symptoms such as fatigue, weight gain, depression, low libido, and more. TSH stimulates the thyroid to produce hormones that regulate metabolism.

Discover Hormonal Imbalances with a Male Hormone Blood Panel

Just as women tend to think of estrogen as being solely responsible for their hormonal well-being, men tend to concentrate on testosterone. However, each of the following hormones is critical to supporting men's optimal health. A good male hormone blood panel will test for *all* of these hormones:

- **Total and Free Testosterone:** There's no denying testosterone's importance to men's health. Not only is it responsible for sexual development, reproduction, and desire, it also stimulates metabolism, promotes fat-burning, and fuels muscle growth. It even plays a role in maintaining youthful neurological structure and alleviating depression. Unfortunately, after the age of forty, testosterone levels drop 1 percent every year, or 10 percent each decade![26]

- **Dihydrotestosterone (DHT):** Importantly, not all testosterone is good. When testosterone converts to DHT, it not only causes male pattern baldness—it also contributes to the development of an enlarged prostate (which causes urinary problems by squeezing the urethra) and prostate cancer.[27,28,29,30]

- **Pregnenolone:** This hormone is the "mother hormone" of other steroidal hormones, giving rise to DHEA, progesterone, testosterone, estrogen, and cortisol. If you are low in pregnenolone, chances are you'll be low in all of these important hormones as well.

- **Estradiol:** Why would a man check his level of estradiol—the most potent type of estrogen? Because men with elevated estradiol levels are at increased risk of stroke,[31] coronary artery disease,[32,33,34,35] enlarged prostate,[36,37,38] and prostate cancer.[39,40] On the other hand, insufficient estrogen puts men at risk for osteoporosis and bone fracture.[41,42] The key is balance.

- **Sex Hormone Binding Globulin (SHBG):** Not technically a hormone, SHBG binds to sex hormones, rendering them biologically inactive. You can have all the testosterone in the world, but if it's bound to SHBG, it won't do you any good. This test will tell you what percentage of your testosterone is bound up.

- **Prostate-Specific Antigen (PSA):** PSA isn't a hormone either, but is frequently included in a men's hormone panel because it is widely used to screen men for prostate cancer, a hormonally related cancer. High levels of PSA are associated with an increased risk for prostate cancer.

TESTOSTERONE: IMPORTANT FOR MORE THAN JUST SEX

Recent studies have demonstrated that low testosterone in men is strongly associated with metabolic syndrome, type 2 diabetes, cardiovascular disease, and an almost 50 percent increase in mortality over a seven-year period.[44–48]

Restoring testosterone to youthful ranges in middle-aged, obese men resulted in an increase in insulin sensitivity, as well as a reduction in total cholesterol, fat mass, waist circumference, and pro-inflammatory proteins—risk factors for atherosclerosis, diabetes, and metabolic syndrome.[49–51]

Testosterone therapy also significantly improved erectile function and functional capacity, or the ability to perform physical activity without severe duress, in men with heart failure.[52–54]

Why does testosterone decrease in aging men? Two reasons:

1. Less production from the testicles

2. More conversion into estrogen—specifically a form called estradiol

With less testosterone being made and more of it turning into estrogen, a significant decrease in the testosterone to estrogen ratio occurs. This decrease is associated with many age-related diseases.

- **Thyroid stimulating hormone (TSH):** Your thyroid gland has several important functions, including regulating your metabolism. While women are more likely to have an underactive thyroid than men, as many as 10 percent of men over age sixty may suffer from thyroid issues.[43] TSH stimulates the thyroid to produce hormones that regulate metabolism.

Who Should Get This Test
Aging men

Why This Test Is Important
Low testosterone, as well as a low testosterone-to-estrogen ratio, is linked to many age-related diseases

How to Make Sense of the Results
Your doctor or Life Extension doctors (see Appendix A) will review the tests with you and make supplement and/or bio-identical hormone suggestions, helping fill in the Personalization Level of your pyramid.

Find Out if *That's* Why You're So Tired, with a Complete Thyroid Panel

Your thyroid gland is your metabolic throttle. By secreting thyroid hormones, it regulates your metabolism. When you have healthy thyroid hormone levels, your metabolism runs like a well-oiled Indy 500 racing engine. But if you have low levels of thyroid hormones, it putters and sputters like an old lawn mower engine.

Who Should Get This Test
Aging men and women, especially those with low energy, dry skin, and constipation

Why This Test Is Important
Low thyroid activity affects all metabolically active cells and tissues

How to Make Sense of the Results
Your doctor or Life Extension doctors (see Appendix A) will review the tests with you and make supplement and/or bio-identical hormone suggestions, helping fill in the Personalization Level of your pyramid.

Fatigue is probably the number one indicator that something is amiss with your thyroid gland, but having low thyroid function has greater consequences than simply feeling tired all the time. It can actually increase your mortality risk.[55,56,57]

If you suspect you have an underactive thyroid gland, it's a good idea to get a complete thyroid panel. This test should include:

- **Thyroid-Stimulating Hormone (TSH):** TSH, produced by the pituitary gland, stimulates the thyroid gland to produce hormones that regulate metabolism. Therefore, this test evaluates your overall thyroid function.

- **Free Triiodothyronine (T3):** T3 is the biologically active form of thyroid hormone, regulating the rate of metabolism in every cell of your body. This test tells you how much circulating, biologically active thyroid hormone you have.

- **Total Thyroxine (T4):** T4 acts as backup to T3. It is not a biologically active thyroid hormone, but can be converted by the liver into T3 if needed. This test measures the total amount of T4 in your system, both bound (inactive) and free (active).

A SIMPLE HOME TEST TO CHECK YOUR THYROID FUNCTION

If you suspect your thyroid is underactive, and you want to check yourself out at home, there is a simple test you can do called the basal temperature test. Here are the steps:

- Get a basal thermometer (the kind you can use under your tongue). Leave it overnight on your bedside table.

- First thing in the morning, before you get out of bed, tuck the thermometer under your armpit and lay completely still for ten minutes. Set a timer before you begin so that you don't have to move around to look at the clock.

- Record your temperature for three to five days. If your temperature is consistently below 97.8°F, you may have a thyroid problem, and you should have yourself evaluated by a health professional.

- **Free Thyroxine (T4):** Most of the T4 circulating in your body is bound and inactive. This test specifically evaluates the amount of free (active) T4 that is available to your cells and tissues.

Based on the results of your thyroid panel, your doctor can identify whether or not you're running at full throttle—or out of gas. If your thyroid hormone levels are low, you can start bioidentical thyroid replacement therapy or take nutritional supplements that help boost your natural production of thyroid hormones.

NUTRIENT TESTS

I don't have to convince you of the importance of having the proper levels of essential nutrients in your system, or you wouldn't be reading this book. Identifying both outright deficiencies and less-than-ideal levels of specific nutrients in your system will further help to personalize your Personalization Level beyond your medical inventory, quizzes, and blood and hormone tests, some of which may not be reliable or well accepted.

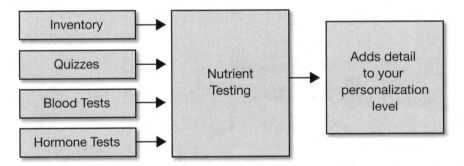

Who Should Get This Test

The general population, especially people with chronic diseases and/or those taking prescription drugs

Why This Test Is Important

Correcting micronutrient deficiencies caused by poor diet, chronic disease, or medications can improve your health outcome.

How to Make Sense of the Results

Your doctor or Life Extension doctors (see Appendix A) will review the tests with you and make supplement suggestions, helping fill in the Personalization Level of your pyramid.

Discover Proper Dosing of CoQ_{10} with CoQ_{10} Blood Testing

I consider CoQ_{10} a foundational nutrient because it is required by your cells to make energy—and without enough energy, all metabolic processes would slow down and eventually cease. CoQ_{10} is also a very powerful antioxidant that protects your cells and tissues from free radical damage. As you can imagine, taking the right dose of this key nutrient is critical.

Without any knowledge of your CoQ_{10} status, I would suggest supplementing with 100 mg per day. But that's just a guess. And I'd rather not guess. I would much prefer to suggest the perfect CoQ_{10} dose for you based on your current blood level of the nutrient. That's because supplemental CoQ_{10} needs vary dramatically from person to person.

Anyone who is taking statin drugs will want to take a CoQ_{10} test because statins may reduce blood CoQ_{10} levels by nearly 40 percent.[58] Even more alarming, the aging process could reduce CoQ_{10} levels in the heart muscle wall by 72 percent.[59] Certain disease states can also compromise your CoQ_{10} status, including heart disease, muscular dystrophy, Parkinson's disease, cancer, diabetes, and HIV/AIDS.

A CoQ_{10} test will measure your blood levels of the nutrient. Once you know your CoQ_{10} status, you will know precisely how much to take to achieve and maintain proper levels of this critical energy-producer and antioxidant.

And here's a bonus. Taking a CoQ_{10} test before and then six to eight weeks after starting a CoQ_{10} supplement will give you hard and fast data as to how well your supplement is working. You should see a noticeable rise in CoQ_{10} levels from your starting point.

Who Should Get This Test

People wanting their perfect CoQ_{10} dosage, and/or aging people, those diagnosed with chronic illnesses, and those taking statin medications

Why This Test Is Important

Measuring your baseline CoQ_{10} blood level helps you identify the right dose for you. Repeating the test after supplementing for six to eight weeks will help you see if your CoQ_{10} supplement is working.

How to Make Sense of the Results

Your doctor or Life Extension doctors (see Appendix A) will review the tests with you and make dosing suggestions.

See if Your Omega-3 Supplement Is Working with Omega Score Testing

The Omega Score test is a great way to find out if your omega-3 supplement is working.

You should be taking between 2 and 4 grams of fish oil daily, or at least 1 gram of ALA from flax oil daily, as one of your foundational supplements. Some people might choose to take more, but most of us will fall within this range.

Without a doubt, the best way to evaluate the quality of your omega-3 supplement is to measure the level of omega-3 fats in your blood at baseline and then again six to eight weeks after taking a supplement, using the Omega Score test. If it's a good-quality product with reasonable bioavailability, your omega-3 blood levels should increase substantially. By how much is difficult to pinpoint. I don't have a scientific answer to this question because there are so many factors involved, including the health of your gastrointestinal tract.

Who Should Get This Test

People wanting their perfect omega-3 fat dose and people who want to verify the quality of the product they are taking

Why This Test Is Important

Not all omega-3 fat supplements are high quality. In addition to checking a product's IFOS rank, checking your blood level is a simple verification of quality.

How to Make Sense of the Results

Your doctor or Life Extension doctors (see Appendix A) will review the tests with you and make dosing suggestions.

FOOD SENSITIVITY TESTS

Food sensitivities are a little-appreciated contributing factor to unwanted weight gain, fatigue, fluid retention, headache, and certain skin conditions. I call these "mystery symptoms." Why? Because if you have any of these symptoms, you've probably been to your doctor (or doctors) several times, and he or she can't figure out why you feel the way you do. Well, maybe the answer to your mystery symptoms is the food you're eating.

As I mentioned before, you are only as healthy as your gut. When you are sensitive to a particular food—or multiple foods—you can't fully digest what you eat, absorb the nutrients from it, or properly eliminate waste. And your health will suffer for it. That's why getting food sensitivity testing is so important.

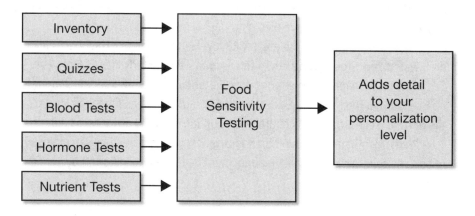

Food Sensitivities versus Food Allergies

Food sensitivities are not the same as food allergies. A classic food allergy occurs when your body mistakes a benign food—say peanuts—for a harmful substance that needs to be attacked. As a result, allergens trigger the immune system to go into overdrive, activating white blood cells and releasing large amounts of the chemical histamine.

Food allergies can be mild, creating symptoms such as itchy, watery eyes; sneezing; itchy, runny nose; rashes; and hives. Or, they can be severe, resulting in a condition called anaphylaxis, in which blood pressure drops and throat swelling becomes so severe it restricts breathing. Anaphylaxis is a serious condition that can be life threatening and requires immediate medical attention. This type of reaction is most frequently mediated by a fast-acting antibody called immunoglobulin E (IgE).

As opposed to the immediate and dramatic surge in histamine release created by a classic food allergy, a food sensitivity can cause a chronic, low-level activation of the immune system. This type of reaction is mediated by a slow-acting antibody called immunoglobulin G (IgG).

The problem with IgG is that it causes the gut wall to release inflammatory substances. These substances generate free radicals that damage the integrity of the gastrointestinal lining, making it more permeable (commonly known as "leaky gut"). Once that happens, bacteria and large, undigested food particles can enter the gut wall and wind up in

FOOD SENSITIVITIES AND WEIGHT MANAGEMENT

Scientific research shows that food sensitivities play an underappreciated but important role in weight management. For example, a clinical study compared levels of IgG antibodies and C-reactive protein (a measure of inflammation) in obese and normal weight juveniles.[64]

Researchers found that the mean CRP level in the bodies of the obese children was **three times** *greater* than the normal weight study kids: 3.6 mg/l vs. 1.2 mg/l, respectively. Furthermore, IgG antibodies were also higher among obese children. Their mean IgG level was 1451 mg/l, whereas the mean level of the normal weight (control) children was 600 mg/l—a **2.4-fold** increase!

Clearly, identifying and avoiding foods that trigger sensitivities can play an important role in your weight management plan and in lowering systemic chronic inflammation.

the bloodstream. Then the immune system sees them as foreign invaders, so it launches yet another attack!

Unfortunately, most people eat the foods they are sensitive to several times daily, so their immune systems are constantly activated. A chronically overworked immune system can cause weight gain, irritable bowel syndrome, and even arthritis.[60,61,62,63] In fact, difficulty losing weight despite dieting is an often-overlooked sign of chronic, low-level immune system activation and the associated inflammation due to undiagnosed food sensitivity.

> **BOTTOM LINE:** *Chronic, low-grade inflammation caused by food sensitivities disrupts normal gastrointestinal function. If your gut is inflamed, you won't absorb all the nutrients from your supplements. So if you're serious about taking supplements, and I hope you are, then avoiding food sensitivities is very important.*

Identify Problem Foods with Food Safe Allergy Testing

I suggest that everyone get a Food Safe Allergy Test—but particularly those who are experiencing discomfort after meals, difficulty losing weight, or have confirmed gut inflammation. Dangerous food allergies are mediated by rapid-acting IgE. Food sensitivities are mediated by slow-acting IgG. Even though it's called the Food Safe Allergy Test, it is actually measuring IgG, not IgE.

The Food Safe Allergy test comes conveniently packaged as a kit. It requires a "finger stick" blood spot to be collected and shipped directly to the laboratory in a prepaid envelope. All of the necessary components for the "finger stick" are included in the kit, along with a complete set of instructions for easy collection.

The Food Safe Allergy Test will analyze your sensitivity to the following ninety-five foods:

FISH

- Cod
- Halibut
- Orange Roughy
- Red Snapper
- Salmon
- Sardine
- Sole
- Trout
- Tuna

MEATS

- Beef
- Chicken
- Egg White
- Egg Yolk
- Lamb
- Pork
- Turkey

FRUIT

- Apple mix
- Apricot
- Avocado
- Banana
- Blueberry
- Cranberry
- Grapefruit
- Lemon
- Nectarine
- Orange
- Papaya
- Peach
- Pear
- Pineapple
- Plum
- Raspberry
- Red Grape
- Strawberry
- Watermelon

DAIRY

- American cheese
- Casein
- Cheddar cheese
- Cottage cheese
- Cow's milk
- Goat's milk
- Lactalbumin
- Mozzarella cheese
- Swiss cheese

VEGETABLES

- Asparagus
- Beet
- Black Olive
- Broccoli
- Cabbage
- Carrot
- Cauliflower
- Celery
- Cucumber
- Garlic
- Green Bean
- Green Pepper
- Kidney Bean
- Lentil
- Lettuce
- Lima Bean
- Onion
- Pea
- Potato
- Soybean
- Spinach
- Squash Mix
- Tomato

NUTS

- Almond
- Peanut
- Pecan
- Sesame Seed
- Sunflower Seed
- Walnut

GRAINS

- Barley
- Buckwheat
- Corn
- Gliadin
- Gluten
- Malt
- Oat
- Rice
- Rye
- Wheat

SHELLFISH

- Clam
- Crab
- Lobster
- Oyster
- Shrimp

MISCELLANEOUS

- Baker's Yeast
- Brewer's Yeast
- Cane Sugar
- Chocolate
- Coffee
- Honey
- Mushroom

Please note: some medications, including but not limited to asthma medications, acid reducers, anti-inflammatory/analgesic drugs, antihistamines, and immune suppressants may influence the results of this test.

Your Food Sensitivity Action Plan

The results from the Food Safe Allergy Test will highlight each individual food tested in one of three colors: red, yellow, or green. Foods appearing in a red bar tested high for IgG antibodies, foods appearing in a yellow bar tested moderate, and foods appearing in a green bar tested low. Here's what to do with your results:

1. Eliminate red and yellow foods from your diet for two weeks. Consider taking anti-inflammatory supplements for your gut, such as:

   - Carnosine
   - Licorice
   - Picrorhiza
   - Omega-3 fish oils (a foundational supplement)
   - Turmeric extract standardized to curcumin

2. One at a time, add back a specific food, starting with the red category. If your mystery symptoms come back, that's a food you need to avoid. Not all foods that create high or moderate IgG antibody levels will cause symptoms.

3. Repeat this process until you've tried adding back all red and yellow foods.

Who Should Get This Test
The general public, people with after-meal discomfort, and those with difficulty losing weight and known gut inflammation

Why This Test Is Important
Food sensitivities increase gut inflammation and decrease the absorption of nutrients from food and supplements.

How to Make Sense of the Results
Your doctor or Life Extension doctors (see Appendix A) will review the tests with you and make supplement suggestions, helping you fill in the Personalization Level of your pyramid.

PUTTING IT ALL TOGETHER

I've presented a lot of information to you in this chapter, and I don't want you to get overwhelmed. So let's recap what to do with everything we've gathered:

Personal and Family Medical Inventories

The personal and family medical inventories are a launching pad for you to start building the Personalization Level of your pyramid. The idea is to identify general problem areas based on your—and your immediate family's—past medical history. After completing these inventories, you should have checked off any health problems affecting you or someone in your family. Add the three top recommended supplements for that body system, listed on page 75–76, to the Personalization Level on your pyramid on page 236.

Shortcut: At a minimum, just add the top recommended supplement for each health problem you've checked off to your Personalization Level.

Medical Quizzes

The medical quizzes let us dive into your personal health history a little deeper and create a supplement program more tailored to your individual needs. Complete and score each quiz. Write down the recommended supplements that correlate with your score. Then rank each of your quiz scores from highest to lowest. The supplements recommended by the quizzes with the highest scores take first priority in the Personalization Level of your pyramid.

Here's an example. Jenny takes all seventeen quizzes and records the following scores:

- Cancer: 6 points (Cruciferous vegetable extract, stand-alone vitamin D_3, curcumin, reishi)

- Heart: 4 points (Pomegranate extract, vitamin D_3, aged garlic)

- Bones: 3 points (Complete bone formula)

- Remaining quizzes: 0–1 point

Therefore, she arranges her pyramid to reflect her greatest needs. Here's her pyramid so far:

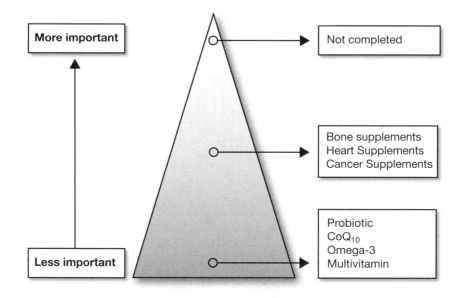

More important

Not completed

Bone supplements
Heart Supplements
Cancer Supplements

Probiotic
CoQ_{10}
Omega-3
Multivitamin

Less important

What happens if you score the same number on two different quizzes? The quizzes are presented in order of importance, so you'll want to prioritize the supplements in whichever quiz came first.

Shortcut: Only take the quizzes you feel pertain to you and skip the rest. At a minimum, just add the top recommended supplement for quiz in which you scored higher than 1 point to your Personalization Level. In Jenny's example, she would only add cruciferous vegetable extract for cancer, pomegranate for heart, and a complete bone formula for bones.

Laboratory Tests

Laboratory tests—including blood tests, hormone tests, nutrient tests, and food sensitivity tests—give you the highest level of detail as to which supplements to add to your Personalization Level. Once you get your test results back, Life Extension doctors will review them with you and make hormone and supplement suggestions.

Shortcut: Unless you have already been diagnosed with a disease, skip the specialized testing and stick to the basics: A complete metabolic panel test, an oxidative stress (isoprostane) test, female/male hormone testing, thyroid hormone testing, and a complete nutritional panel.

CHAPTER 6

The Optimization Level

As we've established, your Foundation Level is made up of nutrients essential to life. These are your "must-take" supplements. Your Personalization Level is about personalizing your nutritional supplement regimen to help prevent and manage disease states that affect you personally. Now, you're ready to move on to the Optimization Level, where you take your regimen to new heights.

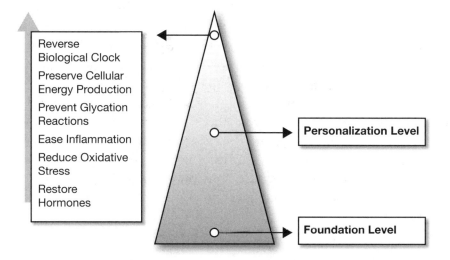

I could have also named the Optimization Level the Anti-Aging Level, because this level includes supplements that help you live healthier, longer. These might include extra antioxidants, proteins, and amino acids, or maybe even the latest longevity herb. Just remember: The supplements in the top level of your pyramid are the icing on the cake. You should only consider taking them after you've established your Foundation and Personalization Levels—not the other way around.

The answer to the question, "Why do we age?" is far from resolved. But researchers have developed some compelling theories. I'd like to share the top theories with you in this chapter, and then offer nutrients that can counter each aging mechanism. I will discuss them in the order I believe to be the most important to the least important.

RESTORE HORMONES

As I stated in Chapter 5, hormones are the messengers between your brain and your body. Without them, many biological reactions would stop or become dangerously deregulated.

The older we get, the fewer hormones we produce. It's just a fact of life. Prominent doctors have long believed that this decline in hormone levels is a major reason why the human body ages—from the cellular level on up.

When I talk about hormones, I am not referring to steroid hormones that are popular among athletes. They often take superhuman doses of steroid hormones to achieve levels that would never naturally occur in the body. Plus, they usually take those hormones in a synthetic form. High doses of synthetic hormones are dangerous, and I do not advocate taking any hormone that your body doesn't make naturally.

What I am talking about is using bioidentical hormones—hormones identical in chemical makeup to those naturally produced by your body—to achieve more youthful levels, similar to those you had when you were in your twenties or thirties. I believe restoring hormones to youthful levels is key to helping your brain "talk" to your body and manage the thousands of biological processes required to live a healthier, longer life.

Here's how to get started:

1. Complete a hormonal blood panel test. This can be ordered from a doctor who specializes in BHRT—bioidentical hormone replacement therapy—or from Life Extension (see Appendix A for information on Life Extension).

2. Speak with a BHRT doctor or if your ordered your blood test from Life Extension, you can speak with one of Life Extension's doctors,

who will review your blood work with you and help you design a hormone restoration program. These doctors cannot write a prescription for you, but they can help you decide what's best for you and help you find a doctor in the area.

3. Begin bioidentical hormone replacement therapy.

4. Obtain follow-up tests to evaluate how your regimen is working.

REDUCE OXIDATIVE STRESS

You might recall from Chapter 5 that oxidative stress is the strain on your body's tissues when the amount of free radicals in your system outnumbers the amount of antioxidants. It is widely believed to be a key contributor to the aging process.

You might also remember that free radicals are unavoidable. While you can reduce your exposure by refusing to smoke, living in an unpolluted area, wearing sunscreen, avoiding processed foods, and filtering your water, one of the key sources of free radicals is your own metabolism.

Yep, every time you breathe in air and breathe out carbon dioxide, you are creating free radicals. (And that process only accelerates with exercise.) Every time you digest food, you are creating free radicals. Every time your body fights an infection or a wound, you are creating free radicals. Therefore, the best approach to fighting free radicals is to make sure your body has the defenses to neutralize them: antioxidants.

To understand how antioxidants work, you first have to understand what free radicals are and why they are so dangerous. A free radical is an atom or group of atoms that is missing an electron from its outer shell. Now, electrons are very codependent. They love to occur in pairs. So an atom or molecule with an unpaired electron becomes extremely unstable—and highly reactive. In fact, it will do anything to get another electron, including stealing one from a healthy cell, which causes the cell to become damaged.

Then guess what happens? That damaged cell is now a free radical, and so it goes about attacking another cell to replace its missing electron. Thus, a whole cycle of cellular damage is set into motion—cellular damage that has been implicated in the development of everything from cardiovascular disease to cancer to arthritis to Alzheimer's disease.[1]

Your body is equipped with its own naturally occurring team of antioxidants, including superoxide dismutase, catalase, glutathione peroxidase, and glutathione reductase. But in our modern world, it's not unusual for free radicals to outnumber the antioxidants in the body. That's where supplemental antioxidants come in. Your foundational supplements do offer some protection from free radicals. But here's a list of some of my favorite additional antioxidant supplements for reducing oxidative stress.

- Pomegranate extract
- Blueberry extract
- Elderberry extract
- Acai extract
- N-acetyl-cysteine
- Superoxide dismutase
- Glutathione

- R-lipoic acid
- Green tea extract
- Black tea extract
- Dark chocolate extract
- Tart cherry extract
- Aronia extract
- Honeysuckle extract

EASE INFLAMMATION

If you're like most people, you're familiar with inflammation as something that occurs on the outside of your body, say, when you get a splinter or stub your toe. The area becomes red, hot, swollen, and painful. But inflammation can happen on the inside of your body, too. Now normally, that's a good thing. When you have a cold or flu, your inflammation levels temporarily go through the roof because inflammatory chemicals are fighting the bacteria or virus. Trouble occurs when your body doesn't turn off the inflammatory response. Then, instead of fighting a foreign invader, it's actually fighting your own cells and tissues.

Ongoing low-level systemic inflammation is now understood to be the common denominator among all chronic age-related diseases. It can cause your cells to mutate. It can wear away your joint cartilage. It can contribute to plaque accumulate in your artery walls. It can destroy the macula of your eye, robbing you of your sight. It can create the development of plaques and tangles in your brain, setting the stage for Alzheimer's disease. It can make you resistant to insulin, leading to diabetes.

The pathological consequences of systemic inflammation are well documented in medical literature. Regrettably, the dangers continue to be ignored, even though proven ways exist to reverse it.

Fortunately, one of the most powerful natural anti-inflammatories is omega-3 fats—one of your foundational supplements. Even if you scored low on the inflammation medical quiz, though, you might consider the following additional anti-inflammatory supplements:

- Boswellia extract
- Bromelain
- Curcumin extract
- Black tea theaflavin extract

PREVENT GLYCATION REACTIONS

Glycation is a process whereby sugars bond to proteins without the benefit of an enzyme to control the reaction. When this happens during cooking, we call it "browning." (That lovely glaze on the outside of a fried steak and that perfectly browned top of a chocolate chip cookie are both, unfortunately, the result of glycation.) When this happens inside the body, we call it "aging."

Either way, it's the same process. Proteins that have been glycated are known as advanced glycation end products (or AGEs). These stiff and malformed mutant proteins have been linked with the development of a number of age-related diseases, such as Alzheimer's disease,[2] cardiovascular disease,[3] and stroke.[4]

To understand what's going on, you have to know a little bit about collagen—a long, strong fiber that gives connective tissue its structure. About a third of the protein in your body is collagen. Sometimes called the "glue" that holds your body together, collagen is found in large amounts in the tendons, ligaments, bones, skin, blood vessels, and cornea.

Glycation causes the collagen in your connective tissue to cross-link, and this leads to some of the undesirable characteristics of aging, such as sagging skin, stiff arteries, deteriorating bones, and cloudy eyes (cataracts). Unfortunately, glycation happens every second throughout your body! While it is a natural consequence of aging, it is far from desirable.

The alarming phenomenon of our aging bodies slowly being cooked to death has motivated scientists to develop ways to block pathological glycation reactions. And the results of their work have pointed toward dietary supplements as one possible answer.

There are three supplements I suggest for preventing glycation:

- Benfotiamine (fat-soluble B_1)

- Pyridoxal-5-phosphate (the coenzyme form of B_6)

- Carnosine (an amino acid compound)

PRESERVE CELLULAR ENERGY PRODUCTION

If the cells in your body fail to make enough energy, they cannot function properly. Unfortunately, that's exactly what happens as you age. Cellular energy production drops and your cells and tissues break down and eventually die.

Why? The answer has to do with tiny little organelles that are present inside most of your cells and are called mitochondria. (The number of mitochondria inside each cell varies; liver and muscle cells may contain hundreds or thousands, while red blood cells contain none.)

Mitochondria generate adenosine triphosphate (ATP), which is your body's main source of energy. As you age, two things happen to your mitochondria. First, they start to die off, so you have fewer energy-producing factories.[5] Second, the existing ones become damaged by free radicals, so they stop working as efficiently, which means they produce less energy than they once did.[6]

In order to preserve your cellular energy production, then, you need to accomplish the following three things:

1. Protect your mitochondria from damage.

In this chapter I've discussed how oxidative stress and glycation reactions hasten the aging process. What I didn't mention is that a high degree of these harmful processes happen—you guessed it—inside the mitochondria. And that's a problem, because in what appears to be a design flaw of nature, mitochondrial DNA (mtDNA) is not encased in a protective coating the way regular nuclear DNA (nDNA) is. As a result, it suffers 10 to 100 times the damage of nDNA![7] Therefore, protecting your existing mitochondria means reducing oxidative stress and glycation reactions by increasing your intake of the antioxidant and anti-glycation supplements mentioned previously.

2. Enhance your mitochondrial function.

Enhancing how well your mitochondria function means helping them make more energy in the form of ATP. CoQ_{10}, one of your four foundational supplements, resides in the inner membranes of the mitochondria, where it transports electrons to help create ATP. You might also consider taking L-carnitine (which helps transport fatty acids into the mitochondria where they can be burned as fuel) for an additional mitochondrial boost.

3. Make new mitochondria.

The final way to preserve your cellular energy production as you age is to make brand-new mitochondria. There are several ways to achieve this. One is vigorous exercise. Research has shown that working out generates more mitochondria throughout your body.[8,9] A second way is to increase your intake of a nutrient called pyrroloquinoline quinine (PQQ) through taking a PQQ supplement. Animal research has shown that PQQ can actually activate the genes that promote the formation of new mitochondria and beneficially interact with genes directly involved in mitochondrial health.[10] Bonus: these same genes also support healthy body weight, normal fat and sugar metabolism, and youthful cellular proliferation.

REVERSE YOUR BIOLOGICAL CLOCK

One of the best ways to see how fast your biological clock is ticking is to look at the length of your telomeres. "My what?" you may be asking. Yes, your telomeres. You may not have heard of them, but telomeres are the bits of DNA at the ends of your chromosomes. Think of them like the plastic caps at the ends of shoelaces: they're supposed to keep your DNA from unraveling.

Every time one of your cells divides, your telomeres shorten. At a certain point, telomeres get too short to allow the cell to divide anymore, and the cell dies. Telomere length has been suggested to be a marker for biological aging. In other words, the shorter your telomeres, the higher your biological age (regardless of your chronological age).

Indeed, shortened telomeres have been associated with shortened lives. In fact, one alarming study found that among people over age sixty, having shortened telomeres put folks at three times higher risk of dying from heart disease and eight times higher risk of dying from infectious disease![11] Shortened telomere length has also been found in many cases of cancer.[12,13]

Which factors contribute to telomere shortening? Not surprisingly, the usual suspects: oxidative stress and inflammation. Diet also plays a role. A recent study found that a high intake of fat, such as butter, and a reduced intake of fruit in elderly men was associated with a decrease in telomere length.[14] For women, a high intake of vegetables was protective against telomere shortening.[15]

If you want to keep your telomeres long, I suggest limiting your butter consumption and eating more fruits and vegetables. However, there are also some supplements that have been shown to increase telomere length. One of these is fish oil, which, if you are not a vegetarian, will make up one of your foundational supplements.[16,17]

Here are some others to consider:

• Resveratrol

• Red reishi mushroom extract

• Astragalus extract

In all likelihood, there is no one cause of aging. Hormonal deficiencies, oxidative stress, inflammation, glycation, mitochondrial damage, and telomere length all likely play a role in why our bodies age. I personally believe that along with a healthy diet and regular exercise, bioidentical hormone replacement therapy and the prudent use of dietary supplements can go a long way to counter these aging mechanisms in our bodies and help us achieve not just the absence of disease—but thriving, optimal health!

CHAPTER 7

Disease Supplement Pyramids

Most of this book has been geared toward making sure you're meeting your nutritional needs, helping you prevent disease, and assisting you in aging as well as possible. But what if you or someone you love already has a disease? Then this chapter is for you. Here, I outline some of the most common chronic diseases and the supplements that can help slow their progression—and even improve their symptoms and outcome. You do not have to take every supplement recommended for your particular health challenge. However, I would recommend at a minimum adding the first supplement listed to the Personalization Level of your Supplement Pyramid. (They are numbered in order of importance.)

■ BOWEL AND GUT DISEASES

Inflammatory Bowel Disease

Given all the reasons outlined in Chapter 1—inadequate fruit and vegetable intake, poor soil quality, a sick food chain, environmental toxins, and chronic stress—it's no wonder that digestive disorders are on the rise. In fact, it's been estimated that up to 70 million Americans suffer from digestive issues.[1] That's one in four! In particular, inflammatory bowel disease (IBD), once rare, is becoming increasingly common.

There are two main kinds of IBD: ulcerative colitis and Crohn's disease. They are grouped together because they have many features in common, namely inflammation of the digestive tract. Whereas ulcerative colitis is usually limited to inflammation of the innermost lining of the large intestine and colon, Crohn's disease can cause inflammation anywhere along the digestive tract and can penetrate into the deep layers of the intestinal wall.

IBD affects as many as 1.4 million people in the United States.[2] Recently, researchers performed a systematic review on IBD to ascertain whether it was increasing in incidence and prevalence. They concluded that "Although there are few epidemiologic data from developing countries, the incidence and prevalence of IBD are increasing with time and in different regions around the world, indicating its emergence as a global disease."[3] It's not limited to adults either—the incidence of Crohn's disease among children more than doubled from 1991 to 2002![4]

As with many chronic diseases, researchers aren't sure what causes IBD. Because it is a disease of ongoing inflammation though, infection is a prime culprit. It's also possible that IBD is an autoimmune disorder, meaning that your body reacts as if it is fighting a pathogen when in fact no threat is present.

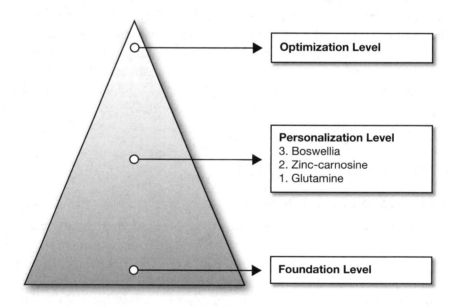

Primary Recommended Supplements

1. **Glutamine:** Food gets absorbed in your small intestine through cells called enterocytes. These cells rely on glutamine, a conditionally essential amino acid, as their major fuel. Levels of glutamine are low in people with moderate-to-severe Crohn's disease, which could

mean it's used at a faster rate by Crohn's patients. Large doses of glutamine have been found to decrease intestinal permeability in patients with Crohn's disease—which is a good thing, because you don't want undigested food particles and bacteria leaking out of your gut into your bloodstream.[5]

2. **Zinc-carnosine:** The gastrointestinal lining, composed of a thick mucous membrane, protects the stomach and intestines from caustic gastric acid. Sometimes though, as in ulcerative colitis, a break in the lining occurs, and we call it an ulcer. Zinc-carnosine (zinc that's chelated, or bonded, to the amino acid L-carnosine) has been shown in numerous human studies to have antiulcer activity by bolstering the ability of the gastric lining to repair itself. [6,7]

3. **Boswellia:** Since IBD is an inflammatory disease, it's essential to tamp down inflammation as a first course of treatment. Boswellia is a powerful anti-inflammatory agent and one of the few herbs that has been the subject of multiple human clinical trials in the treatment of IBD. In fact, boswellia has been found as effective as the drug mesalamine at improving symptoms of Crohn's disease[8] and works as well as the drug sulfasalazine at inducing remission from ulcerative colitis.[9]

Secondary Recommended Supplements

- Saccharomyces boulardii
- Wormwood
- Melatonin

Irritable Bowel Syndrome

An even more common digestive disorder than IBD is irritable bowel syndrome, or IBS. Unlike IBD, IBS doesn't cause permanent damage to the colon—but with its characteristic cramping, abdominal pain, bloating, gas, and alternating bouts of diarrhea and constipation, it is uncomfortable and can seriously impact your quality of life.

Normally, when you eat food, the muscles of your gastrointestinal tract contract and relax rhythmically, moving food through your digestive system until it exits your body. It's thought that in IBS, the contractions are sometimes stronger and longer lasting than normal. As a result, food is hurried along the GI tract without being properly digested—causing gas, bloating, and diarrhea. But sometimes, the contractions may be weak and short lived, causing constipation.

IBS is estimated to affect 11 percent of the global population.[10] Since there are no biological markers to test for it clinically, it's thought to be largely undiagnosed. The cause of IBS isn't clear, but stress, altered gut bacteria, genetics, and food sensitivities may all be involved.

Whatever the cause, multiple factors can exacerbate IBS symptoms. These include certain foods, stress, hormonal changes, and mood issues (such as anxiety and depression).

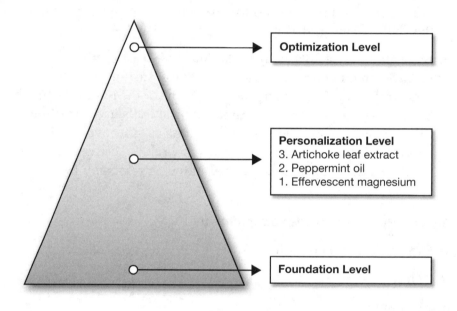

Primary Recommended Supplements

1. **Effervescent magnesium ascorbate crystals:** If your colon isn't contracting enough to enable a bowel movement, your stool can dry up, causing constipation. Effervescent magnesium ascorbate offers quick relief from IBS-associated constipation. Taking 1–2 tablespoons of effervescent magnesium ascorbate crystals (a buffered form of vitamin C) on an empty stomach with several glasses of water will evacuate the bowels within thirty to ninety minutes. You may need to adjust the dose to avoid daylong diarrhea.

2. **Peppermint oil:** If your IBS tends to be diarrhea-dominant, peppermint oil is a great choice. Peppermint is a natural antispasmodic, and this property is concentrated in the oil. Several human clinical studies have shown that peppermint oil that is enteric-coated (which protects the oil from being broken down by stomach acid) can significantly relieve IBS symptoms.[11,12,13,14]

3. **Artichoke leaf extract:** More than just a vegetable, artichoke leaves are a wonderful digestive aid, which is why they are frequently featured in digestive bitters formulas popular in Europe. Artichoke leaf extract (ALE) is particularly good for digesting fats, since it's been shown to increase the production of bile. (Fatty foods are a common trigger for IBS symptoms.) Several human clinical trials have shown that a moderate dosage of ALE can effectively alleviate a range of IBS symptoms.[15,16,17]

Secondary Recommended Supplements

- Saccharomyces boulardii

- Melatonin

- Holy basil

Gastroesophageal Reflux Disease (GERD)

Anyone who has suffered from GERD is all too familiar with the uncomfortable burning sensation that occurs when stomach acid flows back, or refluxes, into the esophagus. But heartburn is only the start. Chronic reflux can cause injury to the delicate tissue of the esophagus, creating ulcerations in the lining of the esophagus and putting its sufferers at higher risk for esophageal cancer.[18]

It's not unusual to experience acid reflux and heartburn every once in a while. But when it happens at least twice a week, a diagnosis of GERD is usually made. The disease is surprisingly common. In fact, 20 percent of Americans experience heartburn twice weekly.[19]

GERD is not, as you may have heard, a disease of excess acid production. It is a dysfunction of the valve that separates the esophagus from the stomach. Therefore, the best way to treat it is not to take antacids, which only mask the problem, but to address the underlying problem that is causing the valve to malfunction: intra-abdominal pressure.

When pressure causes your stomach to bloat, the contents of the stomach, including acid, push against the valve and enter the esophagus. So the key to alleviating GERD symptoms is to lower intra-abdominal pressure by preventing stomach bloating.

Some lifestyle factors that may contribute to stomach bloating include overeating, bending over or lying down after eating, and consuming foods that don't agree with you, such as spicy or fatty foods. But an interesting theory holds that these aren't the primary triggers. Dr. Norm Robillard, author of *Heartburn Cured*, argues that GERD is caused by carbohydrate malabsorption. Improper digestion of carbohydrates causes them to ferment, the theory goes, which creates gas, which causes the stomach to bloat, which results in intra-abdominal pressure, which leads to acid reflux. Supporting this theory are two small studies showing that adopting a low-carb diet improves or eliminates symptoms of GERD.[20,21]

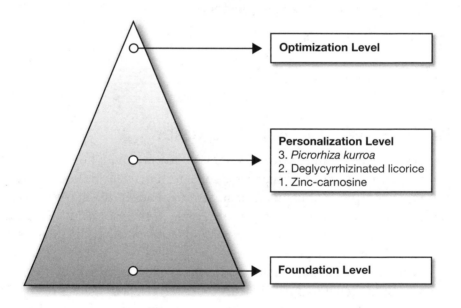

Primary Recommended Supplements

1. **Zinc-carnosine:** Gastric acid is very caustic. It can easily damage the delicate mucosal membrane of the esophagus, creating ulcerations. As I mentioned previously, Zinc-carnosine helps heal the mucosal lining. While it hasn't been tested specifically for esophageal ulcers, the

fact that it can help heal gastric ulcers makes me believe it is probably helpful for all types of ulcerations.

2. **Deglycyrrhizinated Licorice:** Licorice is one of the most prized herbs in traditional Chinese medicine. The deglycyrrhizinated version has the constituent glycyrrhizin, which can elevate blood pressure, removed. Like zinc-carnosine, deglycyrrhizinated licorice also has powerful antiulcer activity. Human clinical studies have shown it can promote ulcer healing and prevent ulcer recurrence.[22,23,24,25]

3. **Picrorhiza kurroa:** Found growing high in the Himalayas, picrorhiza is yet another herb that has been shown to heal stomach ulcers, at least in animals. Rather than increasing the secretion of mucous, however, picrorhiza appears to work by stimulating new tissue growth, nerve cell recovery, and blood vessel formation that may promote recovery from tissue damage.[26,27,28]

Secondary Recommended Supplements

- Melatonin
- Apple polyphenols
- Raft forming alginate

■ BRAIN DISEASES

Age-Related Cognitive Decline and Dementia

As you get older, you inevitably lose some of your cognitive capacity. In fact, new research indicates that cognitive decline—particularly in the areas of abstract reasoning, brain speed, and puzzle-solving—begins at around age twenty-seven.[29] About ten years later, declines in memory can be detected.

Age-related cognitive decline (ARCD) is not technically considered the same thing as dementia; however the line between the two is fuzzy. Both involve loss of mental function, including thinking, memory, and reasoning. And while health officials have tried to portray ARCD as part of normal brain aging and dementia as a disease state, some researchers are now advocating that the two are not distinct conditions so much as different points on the same continuum.[30] The main factor influencing diagnosis tends to be how badly cognitive decline affects a person's ability to function. Therefore, ARCD can easily progress to dementia.

The total number of people living with cognitive impairment in the United States—including ARCD, Alzheimer's disease, and other dementias—exceeds 16 million.[31] That number is expected to surge as the baby-boomer population ages.

The important thing to keep in mind with ARCD is that while it can't necessarily be prevented, it can be attenuated. But first, it's important to understand the various factors that can contribute to mental decline.

- **Oxidative Stress** The brain is particularly susceptible to damage from oxidative stress for two reasons. First, it consumes more than its fair share of oxygen—about one-fifth of that used by the entire body. Second, it contains high concentrations of a type of fat known as phospholipids, which are especially prone to oxidative damage. Unfortunately, free radicals kill brain cells, and the older you get, the more oxidative damage there is to the DNA and fats in your brain.[32]

- **Inflammation** A tight layer of cells called the blood-brain barrier (BBB) separates the brain from normal circulation and prevents harmful substances from entering. However, chronic system inflammation—which can be initiated by cigarette smoking, obesity, disrupted sleep patterns, poor dietary habits, and chronic infection—can compromise the integrity of the BBB. As a result, irritants that would normally be barred from entering the brain have free access. Once inside, they produce inflammatory cytokines, which can hamper the generation of new brain cells.[33,34]

- **Hormonal Imbalance** Throughout the brain are numerous steroid hormone receptors. Having low levels of any of the steroid hormones—including DHEA, estrogen, pregnenolone, and testosterone—can cause memory loss, difficulty concentrating, and confusion.[35] (Just ask any woman going through menopause!) One study found women with high levels of estradiol (a type of estrogen) had better long-term memory and ability to retrieve information than women with low levels.[36]

- **Insulin Resistance and Diabetes** The brain has very high energy demands, and it uses a lot of glucose to function. When you are insulin-resistant or have full-blown diabetes, your body has trouble moving glucose out of your bloodstream and into your brain cells. As a result, even small perturbations in glucose metabolism can noticeably impact your cognitive function. In fact, diabetes has been linked with lower levels of brain-derived neurotrophic factor (which regulates the development of brain cells),[37] decreased brain volume,[38] and a higher incidence of all types of dementia.[39]

- **Overweight and Obesity** Finally, extra weight can affect brain function. Case in point: one study of diabetics found that those with the highest total fat mass had an almost two-fold decline in cognitive performance compared to those with the lowest.[40] Another study found that women with higher body mass indexes had decreased gray matter volume—and did worse on tests of executive functioning—than normal-weight women.[41] Belly fat may be particularly deadly. Even normal-weight women who carried extra fat around the midsection had greater risk of cognitive impairment and probable dementia than those who didn't.[42]

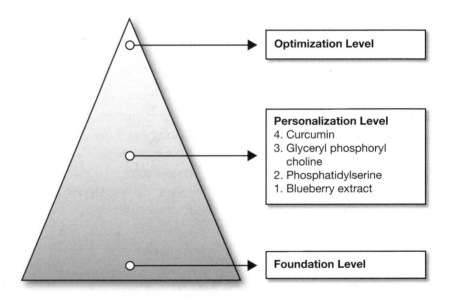

Optimization Level

Personalization Level
4. Curcumin
3. Glyceryl phosphoryl choline
2. Phosphatidylserine
1. Blueberry extract

Foundation Level

Primary Recommended Supplements

1. **Blueberry extract:** Blueberries have been in the limelight lately because they have proven brain-supporting properties. Animal and human studies have shown blueberry consumption improves learning, memory, and overall cognitive performance.[43,44,45] The dark blue fruit appears to work in several ways, including combating oxidative stress,[46] preventing the breakdown of the key memory

neurotransmitter acetylcholine,[47] stimulating the production of new brain cells in the hippocampus,[48] and enhancing insulin sensitivity.[49]

2. **Phosphatidylserine:** Once thought to be merely the outside container of the cell, researchers now realize the cell membrane plays an active role in cell signaling. In the brain, phosphatidylserine (PS) and DHA work together to facilitate communication between brain cells.[50] Two double-blind, placebo-controlled human studies found that supplementing with PS improves cognitive function in older adults with cognitive impairment.[51,52] In another small study, subjects' recall of words was improved by 42 percent after taking PS.[53]

3. **Glyceryl phosphoryl choline:** Glyceryl phosphoryl choline (GPC) is a safe, well-tolerated precursor of acetylcholine.[54] It's naturally present in all the cells of your body, but as you age, you produce less of this vital chemical. Fortunately, you can replenish your supplies with supplemental GPC. A review of thirteen published studies with a total of more than 4,000 subjects found that GPC improved neurological function and relieved symptoms of cerebral deterioration.[55]

4. **Curcumin:** Curcumin is a compound found in turmeric, one of the mainstay spices of curry. Turmeric has long been used in traditional Ayurvedic and Chinese medicines, and population research shows a link between curry consumption and better cognitive function in elderly Asian subjects.[56] This may be because curcumin reduces oxidative stress and inflammation, thus protecting brain cells from damage.[57,58]

Secondary Recommended Supplements

- Acetyl-L-carnitine
- Bacopa
- Resveratrol
- Huperzine A

Alzheimer's Disease

Alzheimer's disease is a heartbreaking neurodegenerative disorder characterized by a progressive decline in cognitive function. As it advances, memory erodes, and so does the ability to carry out simple everyday tasks. It ultimately results in death. So far, there is no cure for Alzheimer's disease, so a diagnosis can feel like a life sentence.

What is happening inside the brain of a person with Alzheimer's disease? It is being suffocated by a buildup of proteins, known as plaques (beta-amyloid proteins in between nerve cells) and tangles (tau proteins inside nerve cells). Scientists believe that these plaques and tangles gum up normal communication between nerve cells.

With an increase in the aging population, the worldwide prevalence of Alzheimer's disease has increased remarkably and is expected to continue to do so. In the United States right now, there are 5.2 million people aged sixty-five and over with the disease.[59] That number is expected to triple to 11 to 16 million by 2050.[60]

The risk factors for Alzheimer's disease remain elusive; however, some include advanced age, family history of the disease, serious head injury, and a history of heart disease. And researchers are still trying to figure out what causes it.

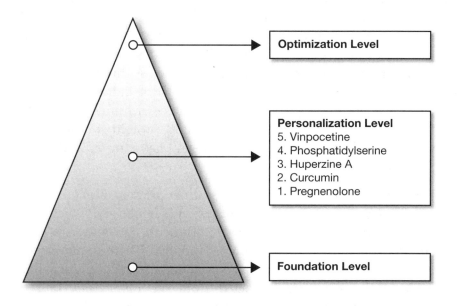

The current thinking is that Alzheimer's disease is the consequence of several convergent factors that should sound familiar to you if you read the last chapter, including oxidative stress, inflammation, and mitochondrial dysfunction. Intriguing emerging research implicates chronic infection with several pathogenic organisms in its development and progression. This makes sense if you think about it, because chronic infection means chronic inflammation, and chronic inflammation destroys healthy tissue.[61] Declining hormone levels associated with age as well as vascular dysfunction (poor blood vessel function resulting in impaired blood flow) may also play a role.[62]

Primary Recommended Supplements

1. **Pregnenolone:** As I mentioned in Chapter 5, this hormone is the "mother hormone" of other steroidal hormones, giving rise to DHEA, progesterone, testosterone, estrogen, and cortisol. As you get older, your levels of pregnenolone steeply decline. Since it has been shown to influence the release of acetylcholine—a neurotransmitter necessary for memory—pregnenolone may be helpful for improving recall in those with Alzheimer's disease.[63,64] It also promotes new nerve growth, which is important, since the disease kills off nerve cells.[65]

2. **Curcumin:** Population studies have shown that long-term use of nonsteroidal anti-inflammatory drugs (NSAIDs) can reduce the risk of developing Alzheimer's disease. Of course, the downside is that they cause gastrointestinal, liver, and kidney toxicity. Curcumin might offer a natural alternative. Animal research has shown that curcumin lowered levels of plaque in the brain by up to 50 percent.[66] It may have the same effect in humans: one study found it reduced levels of beta-amyloid protein (found in brain plaque) in healthy adults.[67] Yet it doesn't have the side effects typical of NSAIDS.

3. **Huperzine A:** There are two kinds of neurotransmitters: excitatory, which increase the firing of neurons, and inhibitory, which do the opposite. If the receptors for excitatory neurotransmitters are overstimulated, neurons can be damaged or killed. There is some speculation that excitotoxicity is involved in the development of Alzheimer's disease. Huperzine A, extracted from the plant *Huperziaserrata*, reduces excitotoxicity.[68] Taking huperzine A has been shown to improve the standardized cognitive test scores of Alzheimer's patients.[69]

4. **Phosphatidylserine:** This constituent of cell membranes has not only been shown to be effective in alleviating age-related cognitive decline. Numerous double-blind human clinical trials have shown that phosphatidylserine is an effective treatment for Alzheimer's disease.[70,71,72]

5. Vinpocetine: An extract of the periwinkle flower, vinpocetine is a promising supplement for dementia. Two reviews of human trials found that vinpocetine improved the cognitive performance of dementia patients, as well as their ability to carry out daily activities.[73,74]Vinpocetine may protect the brain from oxidative stress caused by amyloid beta or block receptors thought to be involved in the genesis of the disease.[75,76] Vinpocetine also relaxes blood vessels and reduces platelet aggregation, which could improve blood circulation in the brain.[77,78,79]

Secondary Recommended Supplements

- Gamma E tocopherol (vitamin E)

- Ginkgo biloba

- Panax ginseng

Parkinson's Disease

Like Alzheimer's disease, Parkinson's disease is also a neurodegenerative disorder. Progression of the disease usually leads to characteristic symptoms such as tremors, muscle rigidity, bradykinesia (slowness and difficulty with movements), poor balance, sleep disturbances, and loss of coordination. Eventually, cognitive decline occurs, and, in the advanced stage of the disease, dementia arises.

All of these symptoms result from the depletion of dopamine-producing cells in a region of the brain called the *substantia nigra*. Dopamine is a fascinating neurotransmitter that shapes our decision-making in two ways: it strengthens brain circuits that induce action ("go" circuits), and it weakens brain circuits that block action ("stop" circuits).[80,81] When the brain has insufficient dopamine, actions—such as movement—become much harder to initiate.

Up to 1 million Americans live with Parkinson's disease, with 60,000 new cases diagnosed each year. Thousands more have the disease but remain undiagnosed. Men are more likely to be affected than women, and the risk increases substantially after age fifty to sixty; however, 4 percent of patients are diagnosed under the age of fifty.[82]

Researchers aren't sure what causes Parkinson's disease, but both genetic and environmental factors—including exposure to certain toxins such as pesticides and herbicides—appear to play a role. Emergent research also implicates oxidative stress, inflammation, and dysfunctional mitochondria (the same suspects behind Alzheimer's disease) as major contributors. Interestingly, caffeine consumption is protective against Parkinson's disease, possibly because it reduces the death of dopamine-producing brain cells.[83]

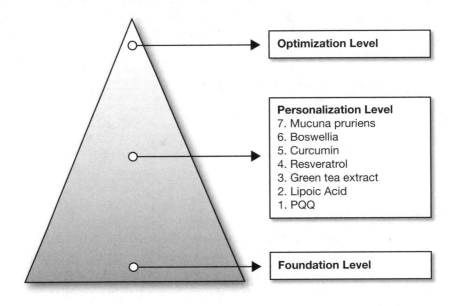

Primary Recommended Supplements

1-2. PQQ and Lipoic Acid: It's now well accepted that mitochondrial dysfunction plays a role in the development of Parkinson's disease. When the mitochondria become damaged, they can contribute to the malfunction and death of brain cells that manufacture dopamine.[84] Cell studies have shown that lipoic acid, an antioxidant, can protect cells from mitochondrial dysfunction.[85] PQQ, a newly discovered antioxidant vitamin, protects existing mitochondria *and* promotes the biogenensis of new mitochondria.[86] No wonder a human study found PQQ improved memory and other higher brain functions in adults with forgetfulness.[87]

3-4. Green tea extract and resveratrol: Where there is inflammation, there is oxidative stress. Both resveratrol and green tea are powerful antioxidants that quench free radicals, putting a stop to the oxidation-inflammation cycle. Animal research has shown that resveratrol reduces mitochondrial damage and loss of dopamine-producing cells in Parkinson's disease.[88] Likewise, pretreating mice with green tea extract or EGCG (the active constituent of green tea) before inducing Parkinson's disease through chemical injection prevented the cellular changes associated with the disease.[89,90,91]

5-6. Curcumin and boswellia: In the brain of Parkinson's disease patients, inflammation contributes to the death of dopamine-producing cells. The key inflammatory mediator involved in this process is called NF-kappaB. Boswellia and curcumin are powerful anti-inflammatory agents that block NF-kappaB.[92,93] Both have both been shown to have neuroprotective effects on dopamine-producing brain cells.[94,95,96]

7. Mucuna pruriens: This herb has been used for thousands of years in Ayurveda and naturally contains L-dopa. As a precursor to dopamine, L-dopa can increase concentrations of this critical neurotransmitter in the brain. Not only does mucuna improve motor control among Parkinson's patients, it works more quickly (within 35 minutes) and is longer-lasting (4.6 hours) than conventional (that is, synthetic) drug preparations of L-dopa, yet doesn't have the same side effects.[97,98,99,100]

Secondary Recommended Supplements

- Melatonin
- Creatine
- N-acetyl cysteine
- Acetyl-L-carnitine

■ CANCER

Cancer is probably the scariest diagnosis for people to receive today. We all know someone who has died because of it. And there's something inherently unnerving about feeling that your own body has turned against you.

As you probably know, cancer is the uncontrolled growth of abnormal cells. These cells develop when their DNA becomes damaged. Normally, a cell with damaged DNA is either repaired or dies. (In fact, certain immune cells, called natural killer cells, are always scanning the body looking for cancer cells to kill.) However sometimes things don't go the way they're supposed to and the cancer cell not only lives, but also starts to make new cells with damaged DNA.

Any number of things can cause injury to the cells' DNA. Smoking, heavy alcohol use, poor diet, inactivity, pathogens, and exposure to UV radiation are some of the more well-known ones. But as we discussed in Chapter 1, carcinogens in our environment abound. In fact, a group of scientists who met at a conference hosted by the United Nations in 2004 stated that "[the use of] industrial chemicals has been incriminated as a major cause of increasing cancer rates and other chronic diseases."[101] And unfortunately, it's very difficult to limit your exposure to this toxic onslaught.

Not surprisingly, cancer is becoming increasingly more common. In fact, cancer is now the nation's number-one killer of people under eighty-five.[102] If you're a woman, your chances of getting cancer in your lifetime are one in three, and your chances of dying from it are one in five.[103] Men, you're even worse off: there's a one in two chance you will get cancer in your lifetime and a one in four chance that it will kill you.[104]

In this chapter, I'll discuss nutritional supplements that can improve your chances of beating cancer and help you stay cancer-free. I've prioritized therapies that are substantiated in published scientific literature or that represent cutting edge treatment strategies. My goal here is to share information with you so that you and your doctor can evaluate which approach may be suited toward your particular case.

In the following pages, you'll see a general cancer Supplement Pyramid, as well as several cancer-specific pyramids. Anyone with cancer will want to take the supplements in the general cancer pyramid because they apply to everybody. Then, you'll want to customize your treatment plan by adding supplements from the pyramid specific to your type of cancer.

General Cancer Supplement Pyramid

Note: The supplements recommended for the general cancer pyramid are equally important; therefore, they are not numbered. If you have cancer, I suggest you take them all.

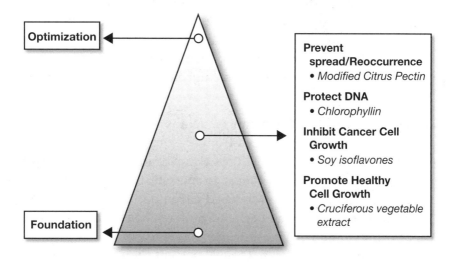

Primary Recommended Supplements

Cruciferous vegetable extract: It's widely known that fruits and vegetables are protective against cancer development. But even more protective than total fruit and vegetable intake is total consumption of cruciferous vegetables, such as broccoli, cabbage, cauliflower, Brussels sprouts, kale, and bok choy. Crucifers, rich in phytonutrients called isothiocynates, protect against cancer by altering estrogen metabolism, protecting against free radicals, aiding the body's detoxification process, slowing tumor growth, and inducing apoptosis (programmed cell death) of cancer cells.[105]

Soy isoflavones: Certain plants, most notably soy, contain constituents called phytoestrogens. These plant estrogens are so similar to human estrogen that they can occupy the same receptor sites, thus blocking the actions of the hormone in the body. This may reduce the risk of hormone-associated cancers such as breast, uterine, and prostate. But in addition to their role in reducing estrogen activity, soy isoflavones also inhibit cancer cell growth by blocking an enzyme that stimulates cell proliferation.[106] *Caution:* Because of soy isoflavones' ability to interfere with hormones, you should not take them if you are currently on hormone therapy for an estrogen-positive cancer.

Chlorophyllin: All cancers start with damage to cellular DNA. Therefore, preventing DNA damage is of critical importance in cancer prevention. Chlorophyllin, derived from the green pigment chlorophyll, may help. Animal research has shown it inhibits carcinogens from binding with DNA and causing mutations.[107] One study in a Chinese population at high risk of liver cancer found chlorphyllin reduced a biomarker of DNA damage.[108]

Modified citrus pectin: Most cancer deaths occur after the original cancer has metastasized, or spread from one organ or tissue to another, distant site.[109] Therefore, it is of prime importance to try to keep the tumor localized. In order for cancer to metastasize, cancer cells must first clump or bind together. Modified citrus pectin, a complex polysaccharide obtained from the peel and pulp of citrus fruits, helps keep cancer cells from binding. MCP has been found to decrease metastasis of melanoma to the lungs by more than 90 percent.[110]

Secondary Recommended Supplements

- Watercress
- Coriolus
- Curcumin
- Reishi

Note: The following sections provide supplement recommendations for specific cancers. These are to be taken in addition to the supplements in the general cancer pyramid.

Breast Cancer Supplement Pyramid

Breast cancer is the most common cancer found in women, accounting for one of every three cancer diagnoses. Every year, 230,000 American women are diagnosed with breast cancer and 39,600 women die of the disease.[111] But it's not just a woman's disease. In 2002, the American Cancer Association estimates that 1,500 men will be diagnosed with breast cancer and 400 will die as a result. I believe we can reduce those numbers. The following scientifically backed supplements can help you or a loved one beat breast cancer and remain.

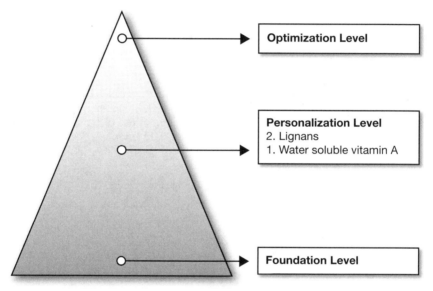

Note: The pyramid graphics for specific cancers only list the primary supplement suggestions. That's because the general cancer pyramid listed previously is the complete one.

Prostate Cancer Supplement Pyramid

Prostate cancer is the most common cancer found in men.[112] Nearly 240,000 men are diagnosed with prostate cancer every year in the United States, and the disease kills 30,000 American men yearly. In fact, if you are a man, your lifetime chance of developing prostate cancer is about one in six. The good news is that the disease is nearly 100 percent survivable if detected early and if appropriate therapy, including supplements, is started early.

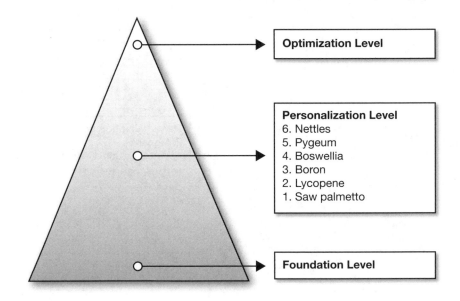

Lung Cancer Supplement Pyramid

Lung cancer is primarily caused by smoking, although it does sometimes develop in nonsmokers, especially if they have worked with asbestos or harmful chemicals.

Not counting skin cancer, lung cancer is the second-most common cancer in both men and women, but by far the leading cause of cancer death. It is estimated that in 2013 nearly 230,000 new cases of lung cancer will be diagnosed in the United States, and there will be an estimated 160,000 lung cancer deaths.[113]

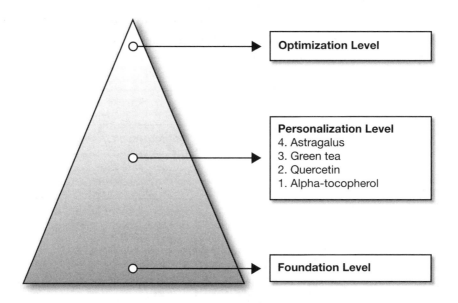

The statistics regarding conventional treatment outcomes for lung cancer remain disappointing. Therefore, if you have lung cancer, you should consider vitamin and mineral supplementation combined with other alternative therapies to help control it, maintain your quality of life, and prolong your survival. Taking vitamin and mineral supplements is associated with longer survival and quality of life in lung cancer patients. In fact, non-small cell lung cancer patients who supplement with vitamins and minerals have a median survival of 4.3 years from time of diagnosis versus just 2 years for those who don't.[114]

Liver Cancer Supplement Pyramid

Liver cancer is not nearly as common as breast or prostate cancer, but it is much more deadly. For all stages combined, the relative five-year survival rate for liver cancer is just 15 percent,[115] whereas for breast cancer it's 85 percent[116] and for prostate cancer it's nearly 100 percent.[117] Yet every decade, more and more Americans are diagnosed with this disease. That may be because obesity and type 2 diabetes are both risk factors for liver cancer, and both have also been increasing for decades. In 2013, about 30,600 new cases of liver cancer will be diagnosed—the majority in men—and about 21,600 people will die of the disease.[118]

In most cases, supplements are supportive only, and how effective they are will depend on what stage the disease is in. The suggestions below are helpful for both primary liver cancer and other cancers that have spread to the liver.

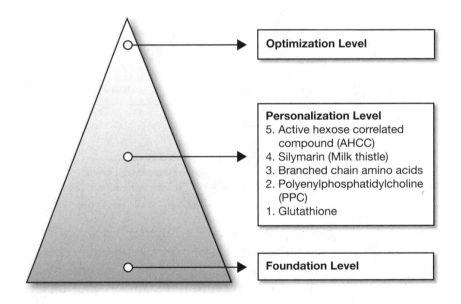

Optimization Level

Personalization Level
5. Active hexose correlated compound (AHCC)
4. Silymarin (Milk thistle)
3. Branched chain amino acids
2. Polyenylphosphatidylcholine (PPC)
1. Glutathione

Foundation Level

Brain Cancer Supplement Pyramid

One of the scariest cancers, brain cancer is more common that you might think. Every year, about 23,100 malignant tumors of the brain or spinal cord are diagnosed in the United States, and about 14,100 people will die of these tumors annually.[119] Many more benign tumors are found each year. Secondary brain tumors—tumors that started somewhere else and metastasized to the brain—are four times as common than primary brain tumors. So add another 100,000 cases a year and you get an idea of the total number of people who will be diagnosed with brain cancer each year.

Survival rates depend greatly on what kind of tumor a person has and how old he or she is. For example, the five-year relative survival rate for a forty-year-old with ependymoma/anaplastic ependymoma is 91 percent, but the five-year relative survival rate for a sixty-year-old with glioblastoma is just 4 percent.[120] Many patients wisely seek complementary therapies, including supplements, hoping to improve their odds.

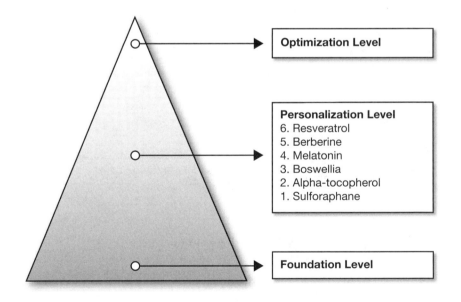

Colon Cancer Supplement Pyramid

Not counting skin cancer, colorectal cancer is the third most common cancer in both men and women is this country, and it's the second-leading cause of cancer-related deaths.[121] There are 102,400 new cases of colon cancer and 40,300 cases of rectal cancer diagnosed each year. The good news is that fewer people are dying from the disease than twenty years ago, due to earlier detection. (That's why you want to get your yearly colonoscopy once you turn fifty!)

The outlook for colon cancer patients diminishes dramatically if the cancer has metastasized to other organs or lymph nodes before detection. But I believe the following supplements, along with conventional treatment, can help you or a loved one beat it and remain cancer-free.

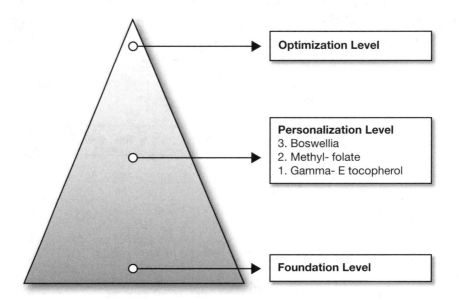

Unfortunately, there are too many types of cancer to cover in this chapter. If you or someone you love has a type of cancer that is not included in this chapter, call a Life Extension health advisor, who will help advise you as to which supplements best suit your individual needs.

■ CHRONIC FATIGUE AND CHRONIC PAIN

Chronic Fatigue Syndrome

For years, chronic fatigue syndrome was dismissed by the medical establishment as an invention of hypochondriacs. Fortunately, this mysterious medical condition is now recognized as a bona fide disease. The main distinguishing feature of chronic fatigue syndrome is debilitating fatigue that is long-lasting and that does not go away with rest. It tends to arise suddenly in otherwise active individuals.

According to the Centers for Disease Control, three criteria must be met in order for a diagnosis of chronic fatigue syndrome to be made.[122] A person must suffer from extreme fatigue lasting six months or more that is not related to ongoing exertion or other medical conditions. The fatigue must be severe enough that it causes a significant reduction in previous activity levels. And four of the following symptoms must also be present:

- Post-exertion malaise lasting more than twenty-four hours

- Unrefreshing sleep

- Significant impairment of short-term memory or concentration

- Muscle pain

- Multi-joint pain without swelling or redness

- Headaches of a new type, pattern, or severity

- Tender lymph nodes

- A sore throat that is frequent or recurring

Typically, there is no evidence of muscle weakness or joint or nerve abnormalities in chronic fatigue syndrome. In addition, it is not considered a psychological disorder, although it may have psychological elements such as depression.

Chronic fatigue syndrome affects approximately 1 to 4 million Americans, only 20 percent of whom have been diagnosed.[123] It primarily strikes women in their forties and fifties, and it tends to run in families, so there may be a genetic component.[124,125,126] The cause of CFS remains unknown, and there is no test that can measure for it. However, in recent years researchers have learned more about the disease. They believe it may have multiple, interlocking causes or triggers, including:

- **Infectious disease.** To date there is no specific correlation between any infectious agent and CFS. Anecdotally, many CFS sufferers believe that their condition began with a flu-like illness.

- **Immune disorders.** Many patients with CFS have impaired immune function, although it is unclear whether these conditions were caused by CFS itself.[127]

- **Dental amalgam toxicity.** Some research shows a possible correlation between dental amalgam, metal toxicity, and CFS symptoms. In one study, eighty-three patients reported long-term health improvement following the removal of dental metal.[128]

- **Oxidative stress.** Studies suggest that oxidative stress may play a role in the development of CFS.

- **Endocrine system disorders.** Stress, both physical and emotional, can lead to imbalances of hormones and neurotransmitters. CFS may be associated with low cortisol levels and increased serotonin function.

- **Low blood pressure.** Low blood pressure is a common finding in CFS. Orthostatic hypotension (low blood pressure that occurs when going from a lying to a standing position) is also a common symptom in chronic fatigue patients.

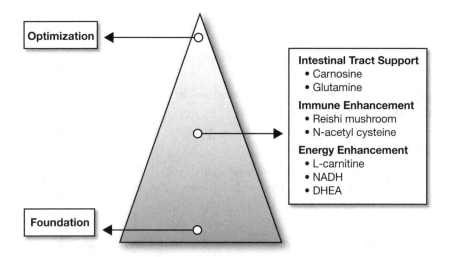

Optimization

Intestinal Tract Support
- Carnosine
- Glutamine

Immune Enhancement
- Reishi mushroom
- N-acetyl cysteine

Energy Enhancement
- L-carnitine
- NADH
- DHEA

Foundation

Primary Recommended Supplements

The supplements recommended for the chronic fatigue syndrome pyramid are equally important; therefore, they are not numbered. If you have chronic fatigue syndrome, I suggest you take at least one supplement from each of the three categories listed.

1. For Energy Enhancement

DHEA: Often called the "youth hormone," DHEA is the most abundant hormone precursor in the body and an intermediate in the production of sex hormones. A pilot, open-label study of patients with chronic fatigue syndrome found that 89 percent of them had suboptimal production of DHEA and that DHEA supplementation significantly improved CFS symptoms.[129]

Caution: Because it is a steroid hormone, you should not supplement with DHEA if you have any type of hormone-related cancer.

NADH: Like CoQ_{10}, NADH is a coenzyme that is essential for the production of cellular energy through ATP generation. A small, double-blind, placebo-controlled study in CFS patients found that NADH supplementation caused improvements in 31 percent of patients, compared to just 8 percent for placebo.[130]

L-carnitine: L-carnitine is an amino acid that helps shuttle fatty acids into the mitochondria where they can be burned for energy. A head-to-head study comparing L-carnitine to the drug amantadine in CFS patients found L-carnitine improved twelve of the eighteen studied parameters of the disease, while amantadine did not improve any.[131]

2. For Immune Enhancement

N-acetyl cysteine: As mentioned previously, oxidative stress may play a role in the development of CFS. N-acetyl cysteine is powerful antioxidant that acts as a precursor to glutathione, the body's "master antioxidant." Glutathione levels decline with age, and glutathione may be depleted in CFS patients.[132]

Reishi mushroom: Many patients with CFS have impaired immune function. Reishi is a medicinal mushroom with impressive immune-boosting power. It has been shown in laboratory research to increase the number and function of virtually all types of immune cells, including dendritic cells, natural killer cells, B cells, and T cells.[133,134]

3. For Intestinal Tract Support

Glutamine: This conditionally essential amino acid is the preferred energy source for enterocytes, the cells that line the gastrointestinal tract. A study in athletes found that those suffering from chronic fatigue had a persistent decrease in the amount of amino acids in their blood—mainly glutamine.[135]

Zinc-carnosine: There is some evidence that leaky gut syndrome may play a role in CFS. Patients with CFS have been found to have increased levels of antibodies that are produced in response to harmful gut flora in their blood, indicating these bacteria are entering the bloodstream through a damaged intestinal wall.[136] Zinc-carnosine bolsters the ability of the gastric lining to repair itself, so it may help resolve leaky gut syndrome.[137]

Secondary Recommended Supplements

- Rhodiola
- R-lipoic acid
- N-acetyl cysteine (NAC)
- Gamma linolenic acid (GLA)

Chronic Pain

Just like inflammation, pain can be either acute or chronic. Acute pain is short lived. It's your body's way of making you aware of an injury so that you don't cause further damage to the affected area. Once the injury heals, the pain goes away. Chronic pain, on the other hand, can last for months or years. In most cases, it is not protecting you from further injury. Instead, it makes your nerve cells hyperresponsive to stimuli, signaling pain when there is no threat of damage.

Chronic pain is more widespread than you might imagine. According to the Institute of Medicine, 100 million adults in the United States suffer from the condition.[138] Sometimes it starts with an injury, surgery, or infection. But for some people, it has no known origin.

In addition to the physical discomfort of chronic pain, there are also emotional consequences. It's not uncommon for chronic pain sufferers to experience anxiety, stress, depression, and anger. The pain frequently disrupts their daily activities and negatively impacts their personal relationships. Adding to the frustration, chronic pain is often resistant to conventional medical treatments. Moreover, taking prescription drugs for chronic pain has grave side effects.

The good news is that there are supplements that can offer you hope for managing chronic pain and making you less dependent on over-the-counter and prescription medications. These natural remedies can offer relief by targeting some of the fundamental mechanisms behind pain—without debilitating side effects.

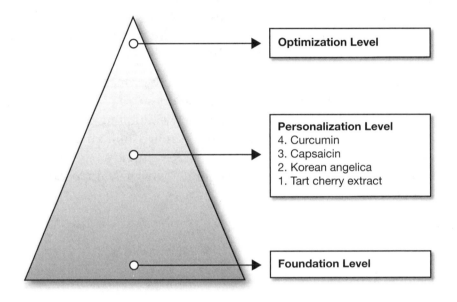

Primary Recommended Supplements

1. **Tart cherry extract:** When nerve cells become hypersensitized to stimuli, they release inflammatory chemicals that heighten the pain response. Tart cherries are a natural source of numerous anti-inflammatory phytonutrients. A placebo-controlled, crossover human clinical study found that tart cherry juice significantly reduced the pain of exercise-induced muscle damage versus placebo.[139]

2. **Korean angelica:** This herb has been widely used in traditional Asian medicine to relieve pain associated with menstruation, migraines, and other injuries.[140] Modern research has identified that it contains a medicinal compound called decursinol, which has been shown through animal research to have pain-relieving properties. Decursinol is thought to work in several ways, including tamping down inflammation[141,142] and inhibiting the sensation of pain.[143,144]

3. **Capsaicin:** In addition to taking supplements to manage chronic pain, you can also use a topical cream containing capsaicin, the compound that gives cayenne and chili peppers their hot taste. When capsaicin is regularly applied to a part of the body, it depletes a chemical called substance P. This chemical is released when tissues are damaged and creates the sensation of pain. By depleting substance P, capsaicin provides some, though not usually total, relief from pain. It has been shown to be an effective analgesic for low-back pain, neuropathic pain, arthritis, and fibromyalgia.[145,146,147,148,149]

4. **Curcumin:** The active constituent of the herb turmeric, curcumin is a powerful natural anti-inflammatory that doesn't have the side effects of typical NSAIDs. It acts as an analgesic by inhibiting pain hypersensitivity.[150] A double-blind, placebo-controlled human study found curcumin improves pain and fatigue after surgery.[151] And several studies have shown it improves joint tenderness in people with rheumatoid arthritis.[152,153]

Secondary Recommended Supplements

- DL-phenylalanine
- Gamma linolenic acid (GLA)
- Ginger extract
- Saffron extract

■ DIABETES

Diabetes is a disease in which the body cannot properly process glucose (blood sugar). It is characterized by either an inability to produce or use insulin—a hormone that transports glucose from the blood into the cells.

After you eat, your blood sugar levels rise. In a perfect world, your pancreas secretes insulin, which helps your body make use of this new fuel. Some of it goes to your cells to power activity right now. Some of it is stored in your liver and muscles as glycogen, which provides cellular fuel between meals when your blood sugar levels are low. And some of it is stored as fat for long-term energy reserves. Insulin orchestrates all of this.

In type 1 diabetes, which accounts for 5 to 10 percent of all cases, the body attacks and destroys the cells in the pancreas that make insulin.[154,155] Since people with type 1 diabetes can't make insulin, insulin replacement therapy is essential. In type 2 diabetes, the body produces plenty of insulin, but gradually becomes resistant to it and is no longer able to use it efficiently. Risk factors for type 2 diabetes include aging, obesity, family history, physical inactivity, ethnicity, and insulin resistance.

Type 2 diabetes is a slowly progressing disease that goes through identifiable stages. In the early stages of the disease, both insulin and glucose levels are elevated. In the later stages, insulin levels are reduced while glucose levels are extremely elevated. Few people are aware of this crucial distinction, yet therapy for type 2 diabetes should be tailored to disease stage.

America is in the midst of a diabetes epidemic. Currently, nearly 26 million people in the United States, or 8 percent of the population, have diabetes—7 million of whom are undiagnosed.[156] Over the past twenty years, the number of adults diagnosed with diabetes has more than doubled. And type 2 diabetes, once confined to adults, is being increasingly discovered in children. Because it increases the risk of heart disease, stroke, and kidney disease, diabetes is the seventh leading cause of death in this country.[157] It can also cause blindness and painful peripheral nerve damage, sometimes requiring amputation.

Glycation and oxidative stress are central to the damage caused by diabetes. Unfortunately, neither of these factors is taken into consideration by conventional diabetes treatment, which is generally concerned only with blood sugar control.

As you may remember from Chapter 6, glycation is a process whereby sugars bond to proteins without the benefit of an enzyme to control the reaction. Proteins that have been glycated are known as advanced glycation end products (or AGEs). They have been linked with the development of a number of age-related diseases.

One well-known AGE among diabetics is glycated hemoglobin, or HbA1c. Hemoglobin is an oxygen-carrying protein in red blood cells. If your HbA1C level is elevated, it indicates that your blood sugar levels have been high enough for long enough to create alarming numbers of these mutant proteins.

Lowering your levels of HbA1C can have a dramatic impact on your health. In a large human trial, each 1 percent reduction in HbA1c correlated with a 21 percent reduction in risk for any complication of diabetes, a 21 percent reduction in deaths related to diabetes, a 14 percent reduction in heart attack, and a 37 percent reduction in microvascular complications.[158]

As if glycation weren't bad enough, it also produces free radicals that create oxidative stress in the system. Unfortunately, high levels of oxidative stress can damage your nerves, blood vessels, and heart muscle. So it goes without saying that a significant portion of the diabetes Supplement Pyramid is focused on preventing glycation and reversing oxidative stress.

The five main actions of the supplements in the diabetes pyramid are:

1. Improving dietary sugar metabolism

2. Improving insulin sensitivity

3. Preventing glycation reactions

4. Reversing oxidative stress

5. Preventing post-meal sugar spikes

While you don't have to take every single supplement recommended, I suggest choosing at least one supplement from each group for the best protection.

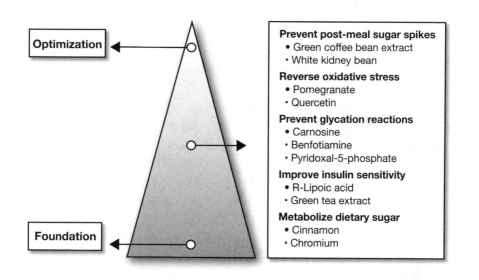

Primary Recommended Supplements

The supplements recommended for the diabetes pyramid are equally important; therefore, they are not numbered. If you have diabetes, I suggest you take at least one supplement from each of the three categories listed.

1. To Metabolize Dietary Sugar

Cinnamon: Cinnamon is one of the world's most popular spices, but it also has a long tradition of medicinal use across various cultures. Double-blind, placebo-controlled human studies have shown it helps reduce both fasting blood sugar and post-meal blood sugar in diabetic subjects.[159,160] In one study, fasting blood sugar dropped by 10.3 percent after four months.[161] Cinnamon extract is a safer form of the herb than cinnamon powder.

Chromium: An essential trace mineral, chromium plays a significant role in sugar metabolism, and diabetics are more likely to be deficient in it.[162] A review of fifteen studies of chromium supplementation in people with impaired glucose tolerance found chromium helped improve insulin efficiency and/or blood lipid profiles.[163] Multiple placebo-controlled studies have found chromium helps improve both fasting blood sugar and levels of HbA1 (a measure of average blood sugar over time).[164,165]

2. To Improve Insulin Sensitivity

R-lipoic Acid: Lipoic acid is an antioxidant naturally found in the body. Human clinical research has shown it increases the body's sensitivity to insulin.[166] In fact, one study found it enhanced insulin's ability to clear glucose out of the system by an astonishing 50 percent compared to controls.[167] The most effective form of lipoic acid is R-Lipoic acid, which is twice as potent as alpha-lipoic acid.

Green Tea Extract: Green tea contains many antioxidant compounds, including EGCG. If you're diabetic, green tea can help you in multiple ways. In a well-designed trial of sixty borderline diabetics, subjects who took green tea extract had better blood sugar management than control subjects.[168] It's also been shown to protect pancreatic cells, increase the release of insulin, and improve insulin resistance in animal and human studies.[169,170]

3. To Prevent Glycation Reactions

Carnosine: Carnosine is a substance found in brain and muscle tissue that helps inhibit glycation and the formation of dangerous AGEs.[171] Diabetics have been shown to have lower-than-average levels of carnosine.[172,173] That can have serious health implications, because carnosine has been shown to offer protection against multiple conditions that are aggravated by high blood sugar, such as atherosclerosis, cataracts, blindness, and loss of sensory nerve function (neuropathy).[174–178]

Befotiamine: Benfotiamine is a fat-soluble form of thiamine (vitamin B_1). Since cell membranes are made out of fat, it can enter the cells more easily.[179] Thiamine is well known to help prevent glycation reactions and the accumulation of AGEs, but research shows bentotiamine is even more effective at blocking these dangerous substances.[180] Multiple human studies have found that benfotiamine reduces symptoms of neuropathy in diabetic subjects and improves blood vessel function.[181,182,183]

Pyridoxal-5-phosphate: The active, body-ready form of vitamin B_6, pyriodoxal-5-phosphate has been shown to possess impressive anti-glycation powers in several preliminary test-tube studies.[184,185] One study comparing various forms of B_6 found that pyridoxal-5-phosphate was the best at inhibiting lipid glycation and also outperformed the drug aminoguanidine.[186] Human research is still needed, but pyridoxal-5-phosphate appears to be a promising treatment for complications of diabetes.

4. To Reverse Oxidative Stress

Pomegranate Extract: Since diabetics suffer from higher levels of oxidative stress, it's no surprise that the antioxidant superstar pomegranate extract can help. One study found that after three months of taking pomegranate juice, diabetic subjects' oxygen radicals had decreased by 71 percent while their cellular antioxidants were up by 141 percent.[187] Pomegranate also lowers post-meal blood sugar levels, reduces cardiac risk factors, and helps prevent glycation reactions.[188,189,190]

Quercetin: Another antioxidant that's great for diabetics is quercetin, a flavonol found in apples, berries, broccoli, kale, yellow onions, and tea. A study in rats induced to develop diabetes found that quercetin had several positive effects. First, it reduced their blood glucose levels. Second, it lowered the amount of damaging free radicals in their systems. And third, it brought their levels of several antioxidants up to normal levels.[191]

5. To Prevent Post-Meal Sugar Spikes

Green Coffee Bean Extract: What's the difference between roasted and green coffee beans? Chlorogenic acid (or CGA)! This unique substance, destroyed when coffee beans are roasted, appears to prevent post-meal spikes in blood sugar by blocking two enzymes: amylase, which breaks down carbohydrates (thus minimizing glucose absorption), and glucose-6-phosphate, which is involved in glucose generation by the liver.[192,193] The results are dramatic. One human study found that taking green coffee bean extract (standardized to contain 50 percent CGA) prior to a glucose challenge reduced blood sugar levels by 32 percent after two hours.[194]

White Kidney Bean Extract: *Phaseolus vulgaris,* or white kidney bean (sold under the brand name Phase 2), also blocks the enzyme amylase, so it too prevents blood sugar spikes.[195] A study on diabetic rats found that not only did the animals' blood sugar levels remain more stable when they were fed white kidney bean extract, but they also ate less food.[196] Human studies are also impressive, showing decreases of up to 67 percent in post-meal blood glucose levels.[197,198,199]

Secondary Recommended Supplements

- Blueberry
- L-carnitine
- NAC
- Soluble fibers

■ CHRONIC OBSTRUCTIVE PULMONARY DISEASE

Primarily affecting smokers, chronic obstructive pulmonary disease (COPD) is a respiratory condition in which airflow is obstructed, making it difficult to breathe. It is a progressive disease, meaning it gets worse with time. COPD is the third leading cause of death in this country, topped only by heart disease and cancer.[200] It's also tremendously under-diagnosed—the majority of people with COPD don't know they have it.[201]

There are two main types of COPD: emphysema and chronic bronchitis. In emphysema, the walls of the alveoli (tiny air sacs at the ends of the bronchioles responsible for the exchange of oxygen and carbon dioxide in the lungs) become damaged. This results in fewer and larger air sacs—and less gas exchange. In chronic bronchitis, the airways are continually inflamed. As a result, the lining of the airways thickens and mucous is produced in abundance, leading to the classic smoker's cough. Most people with COPD have both emphysema and chronic bronchitis.

COPD develops slowly over time. At first, you may not have any symptoms. But then you may notice a cough that doesn't go away or that produces a lot of mucous. Or perhaps you notice you're short of breath, especially when you exercise. Or you find that you're getting sick more often than you used to. Wheezing and chest tightness are also common symptoms.

The very most important thing you can do prevent COPD or keep it from getting worse is to stop smoking. However, you don't have to be a smoker to develop COPD. The disease is the body's response to continual exposure to lung irritants. The most common lung irritant contributing to COPD in the United States is cigarette smoke, but COPD can also be caused by breathing in air pollution, chemical fumes, and workplace dust.

Once COPD develops, you can't fully reverse it. Therefore, the goal of treatment is to slow or prevent its progression, improve exercise tolerance, improve health status, and reduce mortality. That's where the COPD Supplement Pyramid can help.

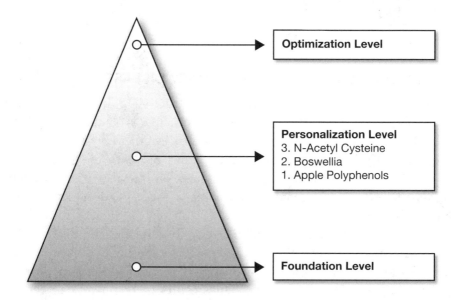

Optimization Level

Personalization Level
3. N-Acetyl Cysteine
2. Boswellia
1. Apple Polyphenols

Foundation Level

Primary Recommended Supplements

1. **Apple Polyphenols:** An apple a day may keep COPD away. That's the result of a recent study, which found that smokers who emphasized fruits and vegetables—especially apples—in their diet cut their risk of developing COPD almost in half.[202] Researchers believe the protective effect comes from the antioxidants, called polyphenols, that apples contain. That notion was recently confirmed in a study specifically on apple polyphenols, which found that mice pretreated with apple polyphenols before being exposed to cigarette smoke had lower levels of oxidative stress in their lungs than control mice.[203]

2. **Boswellia:** COPD is a disease characterized by inflammation. The East Indian herb boswellia contains a compound known as 3-O-acetyl-11-keto-ß-boswellic acid (AKBA), which blocks the activity of two inflammatory enzymes: 5-lipoxygenase (5-LOX) and cathespin.[204,205] 5-LOX causes the bronchial tubes to constrict, which may explain why boswellia increases lung function in people with asthma.[206] Cathespin is involved in the pathological process that leads to COPD, and inhibiting it reduces smoke-induced inflammation of the airways.[207]

3. **N-Acetyl Cysteine (NAC):** Smoking creates a lot of tissue-damaging free radicals. Fortunately, N-acetyl cysteine acts as a precursor to glutathione, the body's "master antioxidant," so it counteracts oxidative stress among people with COPD.[208] Even more interesting, NAC also has the unique ability to dissolve mucus.[209] Not surprisingly, it's been shown in multiple studies to improve symptoms and lung function in people with COPD.[210,211,212]

Secondary Recommended Supplements

- Resveratrol

- Sulforaphane

- Panax Ginseng

■ HEART DISEASE

Heart disease is an umbrella term. It refers to a number of different conditions that can affect either the health of your blood vessels or your actual heart muscle. The leading cause of mortality in the United States among both men and women, heart disease accounts for one out of every four deaths.[213] I've put together some sample pyramids for the most common risk factors and conditions that fall under the scope of heart disease.

Risk Factor: Cholesterol

You've probably heard that one of the main risk factors for heart disease is having high levels of "bad" cholesterol and low levels of "good" cholesterol. This is a very simplified, and not quite accurate, version of the truth.

As you may remember from Chapter 5, there is, in fact, only one kind of cholesterol. What makes it "good" or "bad" is not the cholesterol itself, but the carrier (or lipoprotein) that is transporting it throughout the body. LDL, which stands for low-density lipoprotein, is considered bad because it deposits cholesterol in the tissues, thus contributing to hardening of the arteries. HDL, which stands for high-density lipoprotein, is thought of as good because it scoops up excess cholesterol from the tissues, preserving arterial flexibility.

Even more important than the kind of lipoproteins that are present in your body, though, is their particle size. Recall that when LDL particles are small and dense, they are more *"atherogenic"*—meaning they're more likely to harden your arteries—than larger, fluffier ones. On the other hand, when HDL particles are small and dense, they are actually more *protective* because they appear to be better at removing cholesterol from the endothelium (the lining of the blood vessels).[214,215]

High LDL-cholesterol

Primary Recommended Supplements

1. **Red Yeast Rice:** An extremely well-researched supplement, red yeast rice is a traditional preparation of rice combined with the yeast *Monascus purpureus*. When the yeast ferments the rice, it produces metabolites called monacolins, including monacolin K, which is chemically identical to the prescription drug Lovastatin. A comprehensive review of ninety-three well-controlled studies including

nearly 10,000 patients found RYR lowers LDL cholesterol to the same degree as statin drugs.[216]

Caution: Because monacolin K is chemically identical to Lovastatin, it has the potential to deplete coenzyme Q_{10} (CoQ_{10}), just like statin drugs do. Therefore, if you take a red yeast rice supplement, you'll want to make sure you're taking your foundational CoQ_{10} supplement too.

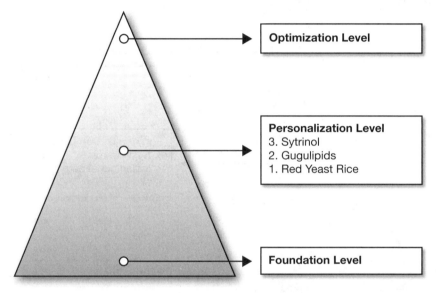

Optimization Level

Personalization Level
3. Sytrinol
2. Gugulipids
1. Red Yeast Rice

Foundation Level

2. **Guggulipids:** Certain plants contain compounds called phytosterols. These compounds are so structurally similar to cholesterol, they compete with it for the same absorption sites in the intestines, and thus lowering LDL levels. Guggulipid is a fatty extract of the gum of the Commiphora mukul tree that contains the phytosterols gugguler-stones E and Z. Most, but not all, studies on guggulipid have found it significantly lowers LDL cholesterol.[217]

3. **Sytrinol:** Sytrinol is the branded name for a proprietary formula derived from citrus and palm fruit extracts. Three human clinical trials have been carried out on Sytrinol so far—all with impressive results. The most recent study, which involved 120 men and women with moderately elevated cholesterol levels, found Sytrinol reduced LDL cholesterol by 27 percent compared to placebo after twelve weeks.[218]

Secondary Recommended Supplements

- Policosinol

- Black tea theaflavin

- Artichoke leaf

Low HDL-cholesterol

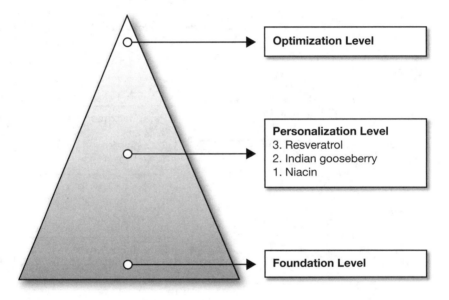

Primary Recommended Supplements

1. **Niacin:** In small does, the B vitamin niacin helps metabolize carbohydrates, but in large doses, it can significantly raise HDL levels—in some cases by 30 to 35 percent.[219,220] A recent meta-analysis, which pooled the results of seven previous studies, found patients taking niacin suffered fewer heart attacks.[221] You'll want to talk to your doctor before starting on high-dose niacin, though, because it can cause side effects.

2. **Indian gooseberry:** Also known as amla, Indian gooseberry is famous for its high content of vitamin C. Since vitamin C is a powerful antioxidant, it's not surprising that Indian gooseberry protects LDL from oxidation.[222,223] (That's critical, because it's not LDL, but *oxidized* LDL, that contributes to atherosclerosis.) Human research has

shown Indian gooseberry also boosts levels of protective HDL in both normal and diabetic subjects.[224]

3. Resveratrol: Found in grape skins and red wine, resveratrol is a phytonutrient that has anti-atherogenic properties, meaning it prevents hardening of the arteries.[225] Animal research has found resveratrol works in several ways, including increasing HDL levels and reducing triglycerides.[226]

Secondary Recommended Supplements

- Green tea
- Dark chocolate

Risk Factor: Homocysteine

In 1968, a Harvard researcher noticed an interesting thing. Children with a genetic defect causing them to have sharply elevated levels of an amino acid called homocysteine had arteries so clogged, they looked like those of middle-aged people with arterial disease. This was the first indication that homocysteine might be bad for the heart.

Now it's official: homocysteine is an independent risk factor for heart disease. This harmful amino acid is synthesized from another amino acid known as methionine. In an ideal world, about half of the homocysteine your body produces would be converted back into methionine through a process called remethylation, and the other half would be turned into the beneficial amino acid cysteine through a process called transsulfuration.

The catch is that both of these processes depend on B vitamins: remethylation can't happen without folate and vitamin B_{12}, and transsulfuration can't happen without vitamin B_6. If any of these B vitamins are in short supply, then dangerous levels of homocysteine can build up in the body. Plus, numerous factors increase homocysteine levels, including smoking, certain medications, coffee consumption, excessive alcohol intake, lack of exercise, obesity, stress, and various disease states.

A healthy level of homocysteine is about 6 μmol/L. That's the amount you can expect to find in preteen girls and boys. After puberty, levels rise—and they keep rising as we age.[227] That's not good, because homocysteine damages the delicate lining of the arteries and high levels are linked to congestive heart failure.

Clinical testing laboratories consider a homocysteine value between 5 and 15 µmol/L as healthy, but I think that upper limit is too high. A good target for people over age fifty is to keep homocysteine levels around 7–8 µmol/L.

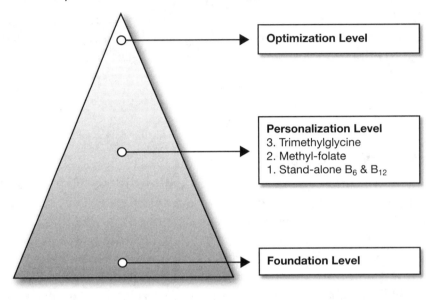

Primary Recommended Supplements

1–2. Vitamins B_6, B_{12}, and Methyl-folate: Because of their role in metabolizing homocysteine, this trio of B vitamins is critical for lowering it in the body. If you have elevated homocysteine, you'll want to take additional amounts of these vitamins in addition to what's found in your foundational multivitamin. You may have heard that B vitamins effectively lower homocysteine levels, but have no effect on cardiovascular disease risk.[228,229,230] However, these studies failed to use high enough doses of B vitamins to reduce study participants' homocysteine levels to the optimal target range of 7–8 µmol/L. That's crucial, because even having a homocysteine value above 6.3 µmol/L puts you at increased risk of atherosclerosis, heart attack, and stroke.[231,232]

3. Trimethylglycine: In addition to B vitamins, trimethylglycine is also important in converting homocysteine back to methionine. Research is still in the initial stages, but data from the Framingham Offspring Study found that people who ingested the most TMG had the lowest levels of circulating homocysteine and vice versa. And TMG supplementation has been shown to reduce homocysteine values in healthy people by about 9 percent.[233]

Secondary Recommended Supplements

- SAMe
- N-acetyl cysteine

Risk Factor: Fibrinogen

If you're over age fifty, one of the greatest threats to your health is the formation of abnormal blood clots in your arteries. Some blood clotting is normal and necessary. After all, if your blood didn't clot at all you could bleed to death from a simple cut. However, if you have a lot of plaque buildup in your arteries, pieces can break free and cause abnormal clots.

The most common type of heart attack occurs when a blood clot (also called a thrombus) blocks a coronary artery that feeds the heart muscle. The most frequent form of stroke happens when a blood clot obstructs an artery that nourishes the brain. If either one of these organs is deprived of oxygen for even a very short time, permanent damage or death can occur.

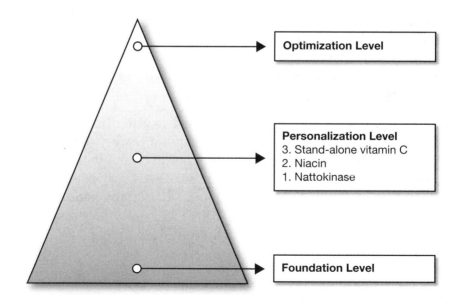

Optimization Level

Personalization Level
3. Stand-alone vitamin C
2. Niacin
1. Nattokinase

Foundation Level

All too often, heart attacks and strokes appear to happen out of the blue, with no warning signs. So how do you tell if you're at increased risk? An excellent indicator of excessive blood clotting is a substance called fibrinogen. Produced by the liver, this protein helps blood clots to form. It's been established that people with elevated levels of fibrinogen are at increased risk for heart attack and stroke.[234] In fact, if your fibrinogen is high, you're more than twice as likely to die of a heart attack than someone whose fibrinogen is low.[235]

Clinical testing laboratories generally agree that normal values for fibrinogen range from 150–400 mg/dL.[236] I would suggest getting yours between 295–369 mg/dL. The supplements in the fibrinogen pyramid can help you do just that.

Primary Recommended Supplements

1. **Nattokinase:** Derived from the traditional Japanese soy food natto, nattokinase is an anti-clotting enzyme. It works by reducing the production of coagulation factors such as fibrinogen in the body. In fact, one human study found that supplementing with nattokinase daily for two months caused a decrease of 7 to 10 percent in fibrinogen levels.[237] Bonus: it also reduces the viscosity of the blood and lowers blood pressure in people with early-stage hypertension.[238,239]

2. **Niacin:** When it comes to heart health, niacin is most well known for its positive effects on cholesterol. But several human clinical studies show this B vitamin also helps lower fibrinogen levels.[240,241,242] Just remember, high-dose niacin can cause side effects, so don't start on niacin therapy without talking to your doctor first.

3. **Vitamin C:** One of the most effective ways to lower fibrinogen levels may be the simple vitamin C. It only works at levels you can achieve with supplementation beyond a daily multivitamin though. In fact, even a dosage of 1,000 mg—more than sixteen times the daily value—doesn't affect fibrinogen levels. But at 2,000 mg daily, patients with a history of heart attack witnessed a 45 to 63 percent increase in fibrinolysis (fibrinogen breakdown) activity.[243]

Secondary Recommended Supplements

- Capsaicin
- Ginger

Risk Factor: Triglycerides

If you asked the average person what the biggest risk factor for cardiovascular disease is, they'd probably tell you high cholesterol. But the truth is, elevated triglycerides are even more of a threat. In fact, decades ago researchers discovered that among heart disease patients, elevated triglycerides were far more common than high cholesterol.[244] It's only recently, though, that this fact has been given any mainstream attention.

Triglycerides are a form of fat created in response to eating carbohydrates, particularly simple carbs such as white flour products and sugary foods. They accumulate in various organs, where they exert numerous harmful effects, most prominently in heart tissue.[245] Triglycerides contribute to atherosclerosis, increasing your risk of heart disease and stroke. Frequently, high triglycerides point to other problems in the body, such as insulin resistance, inflammation, high blood pressure, and abdominal obesity.

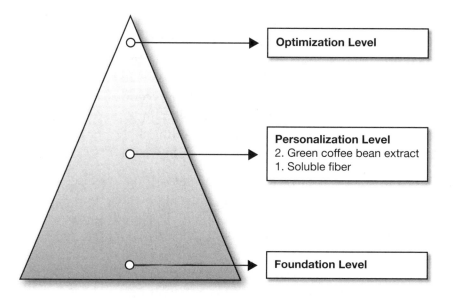

However, since the popular theory a few decades ago (which still persists to this day) was that fat was responsible for clogged arteries—not carbohydrates—most researchers and health authorities did not focus on reducing triglycerides but instead on saturated fat. Ironically, the low-fat, high-carbohydrate diets that were recommended during the

1980s and 1990s to reduce the incidence of heart disease actually raised triglycerides, and with them, heart disease risk.[246]

Normal triglyceride values are generally deemed to be anything below 150 mg/dL, while levels over 200 mg/dL are designated as high. The American Heart Association has higher standards, recommending that people achieve an optimal level of 100 mg/dL or lower. I'm with the AHA on this one: shoot for 80 mg/dL.

Primary Recommended Supplements

One of the best natural ways to treat elevated triglycerides is through supplementation with omega-3 fatty acids. In fact, a recent meta-analysis of forty-seven placebo-controlled studies concluded that fish oil effectively lowers triglyceride levels.[247] Other research has found that the average decline is significant, resulting in reductions of 25 to 30 percent![248] So remember, the following supplements are recommended in addition to your daily omega-3 supplement, which is part of the Foundation Level of your Supplement Pyramid.

1. **Soluble fiber:** As you probably know, there are two types of fiber: insoluble and soluble. Insoluble fiber, the kind that is not digestible, is good for constipation, because it adds bulk to the intestines. Soluble fiber, which turns into a gel when exposed to water, acts as a sponge that binds lipids such as cholesterol and triglycerides, increasing their elimination from the body. One double-blind, placebo-controlled human study found that 14 grams of soluble fiber per day reduced triglycerides by 21.6 percent after just eight weeks.[249]

2. **Green coffee bean extract:** In the diabetes section, we discussed how green coffee bean extract appears to prevent post-meal spikes in blood sugar by blocking two enzymes: amylase and glucose-6-phosphate.[250,251] Since excess blood sugar is converted into triglycerides, it follows that GCA would also reduce these harmful fats. That's exactly what animal research has found so far: mice administered green coffee bean extract experienced a reduction in liver triglycerides.[252]

Risk Factor: Hypertension

Your blood pressure measures how much force is being exerted on your blood vessel walls as blood travels through them. It's determined by two things: how much blood your heart pumps and how wide your arteries are. (Atherosclerosis not only hardens your arteries but also makes them narrow.) You can think of it like water flowing through a hose. If the hose is wide and the water is turned on low, there won't be much pressure. But if the hose is narrow and the water is on full blast, the walls of the hose are going to have a lot of stress put on them.

No doubt you've heard that high blood pressure, or hypertension, is an independent risk factor for heart disease—more important than elevated LDL cholesterol, C-reactive protein, triglycerides, and obesity.[253,254] But like many cardiovascular risk factors, it can go silently undetected for years. That's why regular checkups are so important.

Just don't buy into the reference range for healthy blood pressure commonly promoted by mainstream medicine. According to this standard, blood pressure is considered high when it surpasses 139/80 mmHg. However, in 2006, researchers found that blood pressure levels ranging from 120–129/80–84 mmHg were associated with an 81 percent higher risk of cardiovascular disease compared to levels less than 120/80 mmHg, and those between 130–139/85–89 mmHg with a 133 percent greater risk![255] I suggest keeping your blood pressure at or below 115/75 mmHg, which studies estimate can slash your risk of death due to stroke by 30 to 40 percent and your risk of death due to heart disease or other vascular causes by 30 percent.[256]

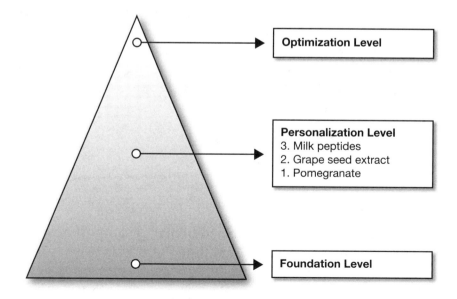

Factors that may contribute to high blood pressure include high sodium intake, low potassium intake, obesity and insulin resistance, stress, a sedentary lifestyle, smoking, and excess alcohol consumption. Low levels of vitamins D and K may also play a role in its development.

The good news is that it's very easy to monitor your blood pressure, and with appropriate lifestyle changes and supplementation, you can control it without medication. (However, if you are currently taking blood pressure drugs, you'll want to consult with your doctor before making any changes to your regimen.)

Primary Recommended Supplements

1– 2. **Pomegranate juice and grape seed extract:** If you have hypertension, your blood vessels are constricted. Both pomegranate and grape seed extract are natural vasodilators, meaning they help your vessels relax. One human study lasting four weeks found that grape seed extract initiated an average drop in blood pressure of -12/-7 mmHg.[257] And drinking pomegranate juice has been shown to decrease systolic blood pressure (the top number) by 8 mmHg after two weeks and 21 mmHg after one year.[258,259]

3. **Milk peptides:** Perhaps one of the reasons a warm glass of milk is so soothing is that it contains peptides that help relax the blood vessels. Two tripeptides in particular—isoleucine-prolyl-proline (IPP) and valyl-propyl-proline (VPP)—have been shown in several human studies to lower blood pressure.[260] They work in much the same way as prescription hypertension medications (although much less powerfully), by inhibiting ACE, an enzyme that causes the blood vessels to constrict.[261,262,263]

Secondary Recommended Supplements

- Olive leaf extract
- L-arginine

Condition: Atherosclerosis

Arteries—blood vessels that carry blood from the heart to the rest of the body—are supposed to be flexible and clear of debris. In atherosclerosis, however, the arteries become rigid and coated in plaque. As a result blood flow, carrying life-giving oxygen, is impeded. Nearly all heart attacks, strokes, and peripheral vascular disease can be attributed to atherosclerosis.

That's the simple explanation. But if you really want to understand atherosclerosis, you need to learn a little bit more about the anatomy of the arteries.

Your arteries are lined by a thin layer of cells known as the endothelium. Endothelial cells are delicate; they can be damaged easily. Once there is a tear in the endothelium, small, dense LDL particles can slip through and get stuck. There, they are more prone to oxidation by free radicals.

Your immune system doesn't like oxidized cholesterol (rightly so). So it sends immune cells to the scene to absorb them. Unfortunately, immune cells bloated with oxidized cholesterol (called foam cells) aren't any better for you than oxidized cholesterol. In fact, they just create a big sticky mess called arterial plaque.

In a desperate attempt to contain the plaque, smooth muscle cells within the arterial wall multiply and form a hard cover over the affected area. Now, things have gone from bad to worse, because this extra layer of tissue narrows the arteries even more, further reducing blood flow and oxygen. If the plaque ruptures, it can create a blood clot that completely blocks blood flow to the heart, resulting in a heart attack, or the brain, resulting in a stroke.

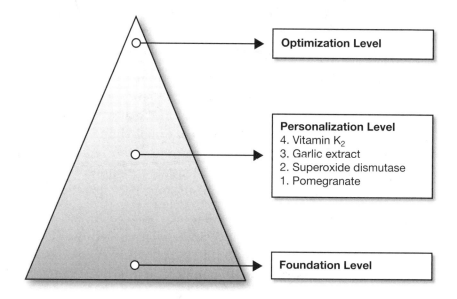

Optimization Level

Personalization Level
4. Vitamin K_2
3. Garlic extract
2. Superoxide dismutase
1. Pomegranate

Foundation Level

As many as 35 percent of Americans currently have atherosclerosis.[264] While it used to be thought of a disease that affected aging adults, research indicates that two out of three Americans have some plaque buildup by the time they turn thirty-five.[265] Therefore, it's essential to take steps now—no matter what your age—to slow this pathological process.

Primary Recommended Supplements

1. **Pomegranate extract:** The simple pomegranate can have a dramatic effect on atherosclerosis. Specifically, pomegranate juice caused a 35 percent reduction in arterial thickening in a three-year study (while controls saw a 9 percent *rise*).[266] As we just discussed, pomegranate acts as a vasodilator, relaxing the blood vessels. But it also has the unique ability to elevate levels of an enzyme called PON-1, which protects LDL cholesterol from oxidation.[267] And finally, it prevents oxidized LDL cholesterol from being taken up by immune cells, thus halting the process of plaque development.[268,269]

2. **Superoxide dismutase:** The body's most important antioxidant defense enzyme, superoxide dismutase (SOD) helps the body fend off dangerous oxygen free radicals that can constrict blood vessels and compromise the function of endothelial cells.[270,271] Researchers have found that heart patients have lower than average SOD levels, along with higher levels of oxidative stress.[272] One impressive study found that a form of SOD derived from cantaloupe was able to not just slow or halt the progress of atherosclerosis, but actually *reverse* it.[273]

3. **Garlic extract:** Garlic may not ward off vampires, but it does protect against atherosclerosis. Animal and human studies alike show that garlic extract can reduce plaque buildup in the arteries and prevent arterial calcification.[274,275,276] A four-year double-blind, placebo-controlled trial in patients with atherosclerotic plaque buildup found high-dose garlic powder not only attenuated plaque deposits, but actually caused a regression of plaque in some participants.[277]

4. **Vitamin K_2:** Once known only for its role in bone health, vitamin K is essential for preserving arterial flexibility. That's because it directs calcium *away* from arteries, and *to* the bone, where it belongs.[278,279] Animal studies have shown that vitamin K_2 (but not K_1) can impede the progress of atherosclerosis.[280,281]And population studies have

shown a definite correlation between high intake of vitamin K_2 (but not K_1) and reduced coronary calcification and heart disease.[282,283]

Secondary Recommended Supplements

- Carnitine and/or arginine
- Ginkgo
- Resveratrol

Condition: Congestive Heart Failure

Your heart is a pump that's divided into two sections. The left side of your heart collects fresh blood and pumps it through the aorta to the rest of your body, delivering the oxygen your cells need. The right side of your heart collects the "used" blood once it's circulated through your body and pumps it to the lungs where it can get reoxygenated.

If your heart's pumping action is weak, as is the case in congestive heart failure, your blood moves at a slower than normal rate, and your heart can't work fast enough to meet the oxygen and nutrient needs of your body. As a result, you may get short of breath and have trouble exercising, feel dizzy and weak, and your arms, legs, ankles, feet, lungs, and other organs may become congested with fluid.

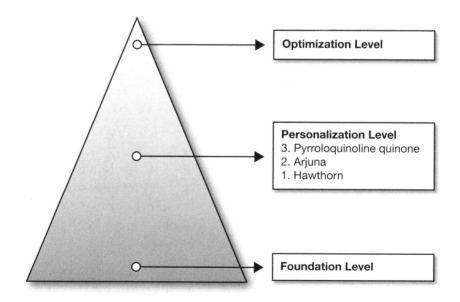

Optimization Level

Personalization Level
3. Pyrroloquinoline quinone
2. Arjuna
1. Hawthorn

Foundation Level

Congestive heart failure is a serious condition that affects 5.7 million Americans and causes more than 55,000 deaths each year.[284] In fact, only 50 percent of people diagnosed with congestive heart failure are still alive five years later.[285] Over the last few decades, we've done well as a country in battling heart disease. Unfortunately, heart failure is a glaring exception, as it is on the rise and has even been called an epidemic by some researchers.[286]

Congestive heart failure can be caused by any number of conditions that damage the heart muscle, including coronary artery disease, heart attack, diabetes, cardiomyopathy, and any condition that causes the heart to work too hard, such as high blood pressure. In treating heart failure, we want to focus on strategies that help the heart muscle contract with more power.

Primary Recommended Supplements

The hearts of people with congestive heart failure have lower levels of coenzyme Q_{10} than those of healthy people, and research has shown CoQ_{10} supplementation is an excellent treatment for the disease.[287,288] So remember, the following supplements are recommended *in addition* to your daily CoQ_{10} supplement, which is part of the Foundation Level of your Supplement Pyramid.

1. **Hawthorn:** Hawthorn offers proof that herbal remedies can be powerfully effective in treating serious disease states. It's been shown to strengthen the heart muscle, decrease cardiac symptoms (such as shortness of breath and fatigue), and increase exercise tolerance in people with congestive heart failure.[289,290,291] In a large-scale, double-blind study of heart failure patients, hawthorn reduced sudden deaths by 39.7 percent compared to placebo![292]

2. **Arjuna:** The bark of the arjuna shrub has traditionally been used in Ayurvedic medicine to support heart health. Two controlled clinical trials of arjuna in congestive heart failure patients found it dramatically improved their symptoms and quality of life. In one study, 100 percent of the patients reduced their symptoms from severe to moderate with arjuna.[293] In another, 100 percent of those with moderate symptoms had no symptoms at all by the study's end![294]

3. **Pyrroloquinoline quinone:** New vitamins aren't discovered every day, but scientists recently identified one. It's called pyrroloquinoline

quinone, or PQQ for short. PQQ protects your mitochondria from damage and promotes the formation of new mitochondria.[295] How does this impact heart health? Mitochondria supply energy to every cell of your body, and your heart is an energy-demanding organ. Researchers think PQQ could lead to improvements in cardiac strength. Indeed, a study found that compared to normal heart tissue, that of patients with end-stage heart failure had 40 percent less mitochondrial DNA.[296]

Secondary Recommended Supplements

- D-ribose
- Taurine

■ INSOMNIA

Insomnia is the most common sleep disorder. According to the Centers for Disease Control, it affects 50 to 70 million Americans.[297] Insomniacs generally fall into one of two categories: people who have trouble falling asleep and people who have trouble staying asleep.

Insomnia can be acute or chronic. Acute insomnia, which lasts from one night to a few weeks, is usually attributable to some change in life circumstances or environment, whether that's life stress, illness, emotional or physical discomfort, environmental factors—such as noise, light, or temperature—medications, or changes in sleep schedule. Chronic insomnia is diagnosed when a person has insomnia at least three nights a week for a month or longer. Depression, anxiety, chronic stress, and pain or discomfort at night can all cause chronic insomnia, but sometimes it just strikes people for no apparent reason.

It's obvious that insomnia can decrease your quality of life. After all, it's hard to seize the day when you're feeling groggy. However, it can have much more serious repercussions on your health. Did you know, for example, that not getting enough sleep increases your risk of the following?

- Being obese[298]
- Getting a cold or flu[300,301]
- Breast cancer[304]
- Becoming resistant to insulin[299]
- Arterial calcification[302,303]
- Mortality[305]

This is serious stuff. According to one study, people who slept six or fewer hours a night increased their mortality risk by 70 percent compared to those who got seven or eight hours of shut-eye nightly![306]

Despite the dramatic toll insomnia takes on us as a nation, conventional treatment options remain far from ideal. That's where nutritional supplementation can play a helpful role.

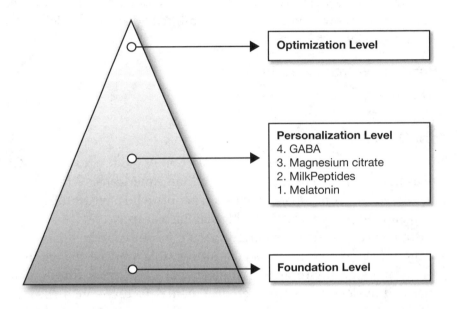

Primary Recommended Supplements

1. **Melatonin:** Healthy sleep is regulated by hormones. When it gets dark, the pineal gland of your brain releases melatonin, a hormone that induces sleep. When the sun comes up, your production of melatonin shuts off. Research has shown that melatonin works as well as conventional drugs for inducing sleep—without the side effects—by helping reset the sleep-wake cycle.[307,308] It can both reduce the time it takes to fall sleep and the number of times people awake during the night.[309,310]

2. **Milk peptides:** Your mother may have been right that drinking a warm glass of milk can help you fall asleep. Peptides, made by breaking down milk protein with enzymes, relieve stress-related symptoms, so they may help with stress-induced insomnia.[311] Indeed, one study found that milk peptides improved sleep quality, decreased

the time it took to fall asleep, and helped subjects function better during the day.[312]

3. **Magnesium citrate:** Magnesium depletion is associated with decreased melatonin production and may play a role in insomnia.[313] The more sleep is restricted, the more intracellular concentrations of magnesium go down.[314] A combination of magnesium, melatonin, and zinc has been shown to improve several parameters of sleep— including ease of getting to sleep, quality of sleep, and total time spent sleeping—in the elderly compared to placebo.[315] It's also help-ful for relieving insomnia related to periodic leg movements and rest-less leg syndrome.[316]

4. **GABA:** There are four kinds of brain waves: beta waves (indicative of a stressed and awake state), alpha waves (associated with being relaxed and awake), theta waves (characteristic of a meditative or day-dreamy state), and delta waves (produced only during sleep). GABA, short for gamma-aminobutryric acid, is an amino acid that has been shown to decrease beta wave activity by 50 percent, while increasing alpha wave activity by 50 percent, thus supporting a tran-sition from stressed to relaxed.[317] Best of all, it works within one hour.

Secondary Recommended Supplements

- Tryptophan
- Lemon balm
- Passionflower

■ MOOD DISORDERS

Depression

Everyone feels sad at times or grieves over a loss. People commonly comment that they are feeling depressed, but true depression is not a temporary state of mind. It is a medical illness that requires treatment.

Depression is characterized by a feeling of sadness that does not go away and a loss of interest in life. It can be mild, moderate, or severe. In severe cases, depression can cause such overwhelming despair that it interferes with day-to-day activities and makes life seem not worth liv-ing. It is often accompanied by fatigue, difficulty concentrating, physical pain, reduced sex drive, insomnia or excessive sleeping, increased or decreased appetite, and feelings of irritability or agitation.

More common that you might think, depression is estimated to affect one in ten adults in the United States.[318] It strikes women more than men and people of color more than Caucasians.[319] However, nearly half the population can expect to experience an episode of depression in their lifetime.[320]

As with many diseases, it's not certain what causes depression. Brain-imaging studies have unveiled that depressed patients tend to have abnormalities in the regions that regulate emotions, motivation, and long-term memory.[321,322] It's unclear whether these changes are the cause or the result of depression though. Depression may result from a disruption in the body's production or reaction to certain neurotransmitters, brain chemicals that powerfully influence mood.[323] There are also certain genes that make a person more vulnerable to depression.[324]

But not all cases of depression are physiological in nature. Stressful life events—such as the death of a loved one, divorce, and even job loss—can trigger depressive episodes. In addition, if you experienced profound loss or emotional trauma during childhood, you may be more vulnerable to developing depression later in life.

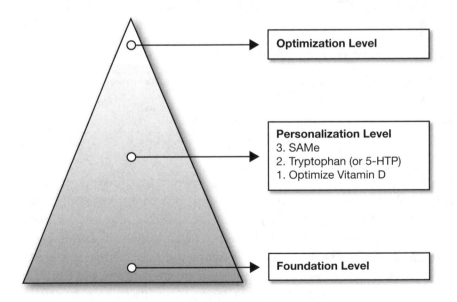

Primary Recommended Supplements

1. Vitamin D: Vitamin D is not technically a vitamin but a hormone.

And knowing how much hormones can impact how we feel, it's not surprising that low levels of vitamin D have been linked to an increased risk of depression in both younger and older adults.[325,326] In fact, you have an 85 percent higher chance of being depressed if you are deficient in vitamin D![327] Therefore, before you decide you have a mental illness, make sure you don't have a simple nutrient deficiency! Get your vitamin D level tested and, if necessary, optimize it with a vitamin D supplement.

2. **L-tryptophan and 5-HTP:** While researchers don't believe that depression is caused by a deficiency in the neurotransmitter serotonin, it does appear that some type of serotonin imbalance plays a role. L-tryptophan and 5-HTP (5-hydroxytryptophan) are both precursors to serotonin, increasing its production. Acute tryptophan depletion can cause depression,[328,329] and several human clinical studies have found that 5-HTP is as effective for depression as standard antidepressant drugs.[330,331]

3. **SAMe:** A compound of methionine and ATP that naturally occurs in the body, SAMe (short for S-adenosylmethionine) influences the metabolism of neurotransmitters such as serotonin and dopamine.[332] Several well-controlled human studies have shown that SAMe alleviates symptoms of depression, yielding results better than placebo or comparable to standard antidepressant drugs.[333,334,335,336]

Secondary Recommended Supplements

- St. John's wort
- Inositol
- Saffron

Anxiety

Anxiety serves a useful purpose in nature. Characterized by the fear that something bad will happen, it occurs in response to situations that threaten our sense of security. We may feel anxious about losing a job or home, or worry that a spouse is cheating, or fear that a medical test may come back positive. Occasional anxiety is a signal. It tells us that it's time to take action to either prevent the feared situation from happening or to prepare ourselves in case it does.

However, when anxiety occurs inappropriately in response to normal, everyday events, it can become a debilitating condition known as generalized anxiety disorder (GAD). People who have GAD are constantly "primed"—their fear response is continually heightened in anticipation of an impending threat to their physical or psychological well-being. Unlike occasional anxiety, GAD is a serious mental illness that can interfere with a person's ability to lead a normal life.

According to the Anxiety and Depression Association of America, anxiety disorders are the most common mental illness in the United States. Approximately 40 million adults—or a shocking 18 percent of the population—are affected.[337] Of those, 6.8 million have GAD.[338] (Other anxiety disorders include obsessive-compulsive disorder, panic disorder, post-traumatic stress disorder, social anxiety disorder, and phobias.)

The main symptoms of GAD are crippling fear and worry about everyday life events. It's as if the anxiety is always there as a backdrop, looking for things to project itself upon, whether that's work, family, health, school, relationships, or money. People with GAD may also have restlessness, irritability, tense muscles, headaches, sweating, difficulty concentrating, nausea, tiredness, and problems sleeping.

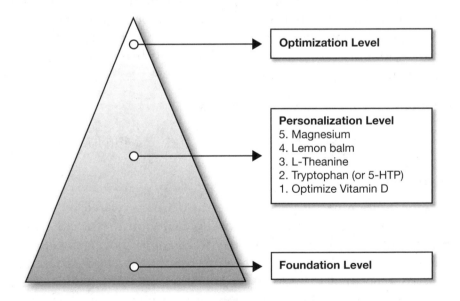

A number of factors are suspected to contribute to GAD. Genes may play a role, as it appears that having a family member with GAD increases your chances of suffering from the disease. Brain chemistry may also be involved. People with GAD have abnormal levels of certain neurotransmitters that regulate mood. And finally, just like depression, stressful life events can trigger GAD.

Primary Recommended Supplements

1. **Vitamin D:** In addition to being linked to an increased risk of depression, vitamin D deficiency is also associated with a higher chance of suffering from anxiety.[339] It's not clear whether low vitamin D levels somehow alter brain chemistry to trigger feelings of anxiety, or whether having anxiety depletes vitamin D stores, but either way, if you have GAD, you should get your vitamin D level tested and, if necessary, optimize it with a vitamin D supplement.

2. **5-Hydroxytryptophan or 5-HTP:** Just as in depression, serotonin imbalance is thought to be involved in the development of anxiety disorders. As mentioned previously, L-tryptophan and 5-HTP are precursors to serotonin. Human research has demonstrated that tryptophan depletion increases feelings of anxiety, so it's reasonable to assume that replenishing the body's stores would alleviate symptoms of GAD.[340,341] Indeed, one human clinical trial found that 5-HTP induced a moderate reduction in symptoms of anxiety disorders.[342]

3. **L-Theanine:** How anxious you feel is directly related to how quickly your brain waves are oscillating. Alpha brain waves are indicative of a relaxed state of wakefulness, as opposed to beta waves, which are generated when you are alert, problem-solving, or stressed. An amino acid found in green tea, L-theanine induces the production of alpha brain waves.[343] This may explain why students with high anxiety who took a single dose of L-theanine showed improved attention and reaction times—yet slower heart rates—compared to similarly stressed students who took a placebo.[344,345]

4. **Lemon Balm:** As you may remember from the section on insomnia, GABA is a calming amino acid. Test-tube research has shown that lemon balm, a member of the mint family, contains compounds that strongly suppress the breakdown of GABA, which may prolong its antianxiety effects.[346] In a double-blind, placebo-controlled human study, a single dose of lemon balm alleviated the anxiety of a twenty-minute stress-inducing test.[347]

5. **Magnesium:** If you suffer from any type of anxiety disorder, you could be deficient in magnesium. In fact, when researchers want to study anxiety, they use mice that have been bred to be magnesium-deficient.[348] Adrenaline, produced when you are under stress, decreases stores of this essential mineral. And, in a vicious cycle, low magnesium levels magnify stress.[349] Several human studies have shown that magnesium, in combination with a variety of different ingredients, decreases symptoms of anxiety.[350,351,352]

Secondary Recommended Supplements

- GABA
- Saffron
- SAMe
- Valerian
- Ashwagandha

■ OSTEOARTHRITIS

There are three types of joints in your body: fibrous joints, which are joined by fibrous tissue; cartilaginous joints, which are joined by cartilage; and synovial joints, which aren't directly joined at all. Unlike the other two types of joints, the bones in a synovial joint are separated by a cavity that is filled with synovial fluid and encased by the synovial membrane. Examples of synovial joints include the elbows, wrists, fingers, shoulders, hips, and knees.

The less joined a joint is, the more it moves. Since synovial joints are the least joined, they have the most movement—and the most potential for injury.

Osteoarthritis is a very common degenerative joint disease characterized by inflammation, structural damage, and functional impairment within the synovial joints. The most common symptoms are joint pain and stiffness, as well as decreased range of motion. The leading cause of disability in the United States, arthritis affects one out of every five American adults.[353] People who are obese are more likely to suffer from arthritis because of the stress excess weight puts on the joints.[354]

In a healthy joint, a slick layer of cartilage covers the ends of both bones, so they slide against one another seamlessly. Both rheumatoid arthritis, which is an autoimmune disease, and osteoarthritis, which is not, are due to the degradation of joint cartilage. The pain you feel when you have arthritis is the result of bone grinding against bone.

While the prevailing theory regarding the development of osteoarthritis is that cartilage is simply "worn down" over time, I have a different explanation: inflammation. Inflammation is caustic. It's like acid. It destroys healthy tissue. If inflammatory chemicals are chronically coursing through your system, they will eat away at your cartilage, causing osteoarthritis.

I believe there are three keys to successfully managing osteoarthritis. First, you need to stop the inflammation that lies at the heart of this disease. Second, you need to provide support for the structure of your joints. And while it seems counterintuitive, you have to keep moving. So many older adults stop exercising because their joints hurt. But I like to teach that your joints hurt because you *don't* exercise! In fact, every time you flex your joints, you move waste products out of the joints and let oxygen and nutrients in.

The osteoarthritis Supplement Pyramid can help you ease inflammation and provide joint structure support. You're going to have to handle the exercise part on your own!

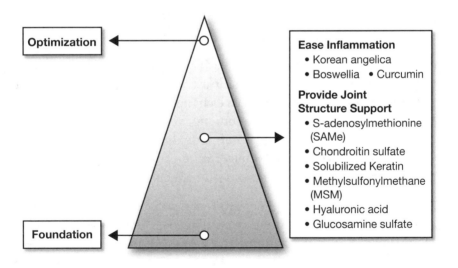

Primary Recommended Supplements

The supplements recommended for the osteoarthritis pyramid are equally important; therefore, they are not numbered. If you have osteoarthritis, I suggest you take at least two supplements listed under joint structure support and at least one supplement listed under easing inflammation.

1. To Provide Joint Structure Support

Glucosamine Sulfate: The most well-known ingredient for relieving arthritis symptoms, glucosamine sulfate is a constituent of joint cartilage. While anti-inflammatory agents stop the destructive process that degrades cartilage, glucosamine may actually repair cartilage by stimulating the synthesis of chondrocytes (cartilage cells).[355] (This is why it may take up to eight weeks to have an effect.) The majority of published studies on glucosamine show it's effective in relieving osteoarthritis, particularly of the knee.[356] The current thinking is that the sulfate form is more effective than the HCl form.

Hyaluronic Acid: Cartilage cells secrete hyaluronic acid (HA) and use it to build more cartilage. Researchers believe it helps arthritis patients because it interferes with pain mediators and decreases the production of enzymes that destroy healthy cartilage.[357] Originally, HA was only available by injection. Luckily, it can now be taken orally, in which case it's made more effective by mixing it with phospholipids.[358] Human and animal research has shown oral HA can reduce joint pain and swelling.[359,360]

Methylsulfonylmethane (MSM): MSM is rich in sulfur. That's relevant, because scientists believe sulfur compounds may ease pain and put the brakes on the degenerative changes of osteoarthritis by stabilizing cell membranes and scavenging free radicals. A double-blind, placebo-controlled clinical trial of patients with osteoarthritis of the knee found MSM reduced their pain and improved their physical function.[361] Even better, it has no side effects.[362]

Solublized Keratin: Another sulfur-rich substance, keratin is a naturally occurring protein found in cartilage.[363,364] A placebo-controlled clinical trial found that solubilized keratin reduced pain in subjects with arthritis compared to placebo.[365] Animal research has shown it activates two important antioxidant defense enzymes—glutathione peroxidase and superoxide dismutase—thus protecting joint tissue.[366]

Chondroitin sulfate: If you've heard of glucosamine, chances are you've heard of chondroitin, because the two are frequently used together, with good results. Chondroitin sulfate is a glycosaminoglycan, which is a fancy way of saying a building block of connective tissue, such as joint cartilage. Therefore, it provides your body with what it needs to make new joint cartilage. Several studies have shown that chondroitin sulfate relieves the pain of osteoarthritis and helps slow its progression.[367,368,369]

SAMe: SAMe is a compound of methionine and ATP that naturally occurs in the body. Human studies have shown it can reduce pain and stiffness and increase functioning among arthritis patients.[370,371,372] What's more, research indicates SAMe may be as effective—and safer—than nonsteroidal anti-inflammatory drugs (such as aspirin and ibuprofen).[373] Scientists haven't pinpointed how SAMe works, but they believe it may stimulate the production of cartilage, reduce inflammatory mediators, and/or increase the production of antioxidants liklutathione.[374]

2. To Ease Inflammation

Curcumin: The active constituent of turmeric, curcumin is a powerful anti-inflammatory agent. A special preparation of curcumin known as Meriva, in which curcumin is complexed with phospholipids for enhanced bioavailability, has been clinically shown effective for the management and treatment of osteoarthritis.[375,376] How does it work? By dialing down the activity of two inflammatory mediators: NFkappaB and cyclooxygenase.[377]

Boswellia: An herb with a long history of use in the East Indian tradition of Ayurveda, boswellia is also profoundly anti-inflammatory. In addition to blocking NF-kappaB,[378]boswellia constituents also inhibit 5-lipoxygenase, a pro-inflammatory enzyme.[379] Several human studies have found boswellia extract, standardized to the key constituent AKBA, reduces symptoms of osteoarthritis, such as pain and dysfunction.[380,381,382]

Korean Angelica: Widely used in traditional Asian medicine to treat the pain of arthritis, *Angelica gigas Nakai* contains a special constituent called decursinol.[383,384]This medicinal compound is thought to act within the central nervous system to relieve pain.[385,386] Like curcumin, Korean Angelica's analgesic powers may come from its ability to dial down both NF-kappaB and cyclooxygenase.[387,388]

■ OSTEOPOROSIS

It's natural for bones to lose some of their density over time. In fact, you achieve your peak bone mass at around age thirty. However, when bones lose enough density to become porous, thin, and prone to fracture, a diagnosis of osteoporosis is made.

Don't underestimate the seriousness of this bone-ravaging disease. Losing just 10 percent of the bone mass in your hip more than doubles your risk of hip fracture.[389] A fracture may not sound like that big a deal, but one in five people who sustain a hip fracture die within a year.[390] In fact, a fifty-year-old woman is as likely to die from a hip fracture as she is from breast cancer.[391]

And men, you're not off the hook. Osteoporosis used to be thought of as an aging woman's disease that was due to a postmenopausal decline in estrogen (which is known to be bone protective). It was traditionally treated with hormone replacement therapy in the hopes of mitigating this estrogen loss. Unfortunately, the truth behind the disease is much more complicated. Like many age-related conditions, osteoporosis doesn't have a singular cause or affect just one specific population. It's a complex disease caused by a web of interrelated factors—and it can strike both women and men.

Women are more likely to develop osteoporosis than men, but by no means is it a "woman's disease." Fully one-third of those affected by osteoporosis—about 2.8 million—are men.[392] According to the International Osteoporosis Foundation, one in three women over age fifty will experience an osteoporotic fracture in her remaining lifetime, as will one in five men.[393] In fact, if you're a guy, your chance of sustaining a fracture due to osteoporosis is about the same as your chances of getting prostate cancer.[394] And here's more bad news: men who get fractures are much more likely to die of them than women.[395]

We now know that osteoporosis stems from more than just hormonal imbalance. Multiple factors appear to contribute to its development, including a sedentary lifestyle,[396] nutrient deficiencies,[397,398] insulin resistance,[399,400] glycation,[401,402] oxidative stress,[403,404] and inflammation.[405] If you want to successfully prevent and treat osteoporosis, you need to address all of these factors, regardless of your gender. That's the goal of the osteoporosis Supplement Pyramid.

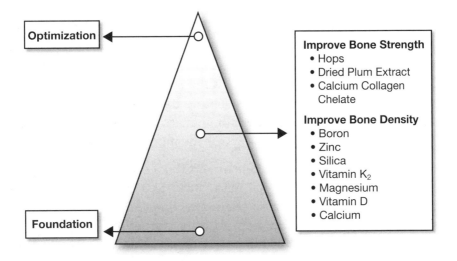

Improve Bone Strength
- Hops
- Dried Plum Extract
- Calcium Collagen Chelate

Improve Bone Density
- Boron
- Zinc
- Silica
- Vitamin K_2
- Magnesium
- Vitamin D
- Calcium

Primary Recommended Supplements

1. To Improve Bone Density

Note: You can find many of the ingredients below in a comprehensive bone health formula.

Calcium: If you're only familiar with one nutrient for bone health, it's probably calcium—with good reason. Calcium is the predominant mineral in bone; it's what makes bone hard. Calcium supplementation has been shown to promote bone growth in children,[406] improve bone mineral density in people of all ages,[407,408,409] and reduce bone resorption (or breakdown) in men and women.[410,411,412] However, calcium does not work alone. In fact, taking calcium *without* its co-nutrients (particularly vitamin K) may do more harm than good!

Vitamin D: Have you ever wondered why vitamin D is added to milk? The reason is because vitamin D enhances the body's absorption of calcium from the intestines.[413] As a result, the combination of calcium and vitamin D is especially effective at preventing bone loss.[414,415] A shocking 77 percent Americans do not have sufficient blood levels of vitamin D.[416] This may explain why, compared to other nations, America's calcium intake is high, yet so is our rate of osteoporosis.[417] Get your vitamin D level tested and, if necessary, optimize it with a vitamin D supplement.

Magnesium and Vitamin K: Magnesium and vitamin K act as escorts for calcium, guiding it to the bones where it's needed. Magnesium regulates calcium transport and reduces bone turnover.[418] A two-year study of postmenopausal women showed it improved bone density and reduced fractures.[419] Vitamin K directs calcium toward the bones and away from the arteries, preventing dangerous arterial calcification.[420] Plus, it helps build the protein matrix calcium needs to attach to bone once it gets there.[421,422] K_2 is the more bioavailable form.[423]

Silica and Zinc: Bones are made up mostly of calcium and collagen, a protein that's needed for calcium to "stick" to the skeletal framework. Because both silica and zinc stimulate collagen synthesis, this duo of nutrients helps calcium complete its journey by making sure it attaches to your bones.[424] Human and animal studies show silica promotes bone density and prevents bone loss.[425,426,427] Adequate zinc intake has been associated with better bone mineral density in young women,[428] and low zinc intake has been associated with greatly increased fracture risk in middle-aged to elderly men.[429]

Boron: On the bone health team, boron is the cleanup hitter—the one who bats fourth in the lineup to clean up the bases. Why? Because it supports the actions of calcium, magnesium, and vitamin D. Boron helps the body preserve its stores of calcium and magnesium[430] and amplifies the actions of vitamin D. A study of rats deficient in vitamin D found that when given boron, they were better able to utilize what little vitamin they had.[431]

2. To Enhance Bone Strength

Calcium Collagen Chelate: In the same way that earthquake-resistant buildings need to be bendable enough to withstand seismic shifts and resist collapse, bone needs to be flexible enough to absorb compression forces and resist stress fractures. That's the job of collagen. Calcium collagen chelate binds calcium to collagen, providing the two major elements of bone in one compound. Animal research has shown that calcium collagen chelate improves bone strength and flexibility better than either calcium or collagen given alone or together.[432]

Dried Plum Extract: Dried plums, or prunes, are famous for keeping you regular, but they're also good for your bones. Polyphenols in this fruit have been shown to suppress bone breakdown, enhance bone-building activity, and increase collagen cross-linking (the more collagen in your bones is cross-linked, the stronger your bones will be).[433,434,435] Dried plum extract has been shown to promote bone formation and increase bone mineral density, in one study it even restored bone loss previously thought to be irreversible! [436,437,438]

Hops: When you think hops, you probably think beer, but this herb is also a promising supplement for osteoporosis. The active constituents in hops act as selective estrogen receptor modulators. That means they boost the helpful actions of estrogen (such as preventing bone loss)—but not the worrisome ones (such as increasing breast cancer risk). Animal and laboratory studies suggest hops may enhance bone mineral density by increasing the gene expression and differentiation of bone-forming cells.[439,440,441]

■ OVERWEIGHT AND OBESITY

No doubt you've heard the startling statistics: 33.1 percent of American adults are overweight (with a body mass index of 25 to 29.9) and an additional 35.7 percent are obese (with a body mass index of 30 or above).[442] Together, that's more than two-thirds of the population! It's not just an American problem though. Around the world, the prevalence of obesity nearly doubled from 1980 to 2008.[443]

Being overweight or obese doesn't just negatively impact your self-esteem. It interferes with restful sleep, contributes to digestive disorders, and can lower your overall quality of life. Even more troubling, it raises your risk of multiple chronic diseases, including diabetes, cardiovascular disease, arthritis, and certain kinds of cancer.[444] This helps explain why excess body weight increases your risk of early death.[445]

Now, that's not to say that just because you are overweight you are doomed to have health issues. There is a fair amount of research that indicates it is possible to be both fat and fit. In fact, fitness is a better indicator of mortality than fatness. The results of a large eight-year study by the Cooper Institute in Dallas, Texas, for example, show that men who were overweight but fit (as measured by treadmill tests) were two times less likely to die over the study period than men who were thin but out of shape.[446]

However, statistically, your best bet is to get in good cardiovascular shape *and* maintain a healthy weight. But here's what I want to make clear: Regardless of the diet plan you decide to follow or the surgery you may intend to have, there are some weight-gain mechanisms you'll need to reverse in order to experience lasting results. Recent scientific investigation has shed light on why we get fat, and it's much more complex than the overly simplistic "We eat too much and exercise too little" message promoted by the government, the media, and just about everyone you talk to. That's what the overweight and obesity Supplement Pyramid is all about.

Let's take a look at some age-related weight-gain mechanisms.

1. High rate of carbohydrate absorption

While it was once thought that "a calorie is a calorie"—meaning that a calorie of protein counts the same as a calorie of carbohydrates—a substantial body of research now refutes this concept. The reason has to do with insulin, which is secreted in response to high-carbohydrate meals.

You may know that insulin helps transport glucose out of the blood and into the cells. But did you realize that when insulin levels are elevated, your body holds on to fat? As a result, the more carbs you eat—particularly simple carbs like white flour and sugar—the less fat you'll burn. The same is not true of fat or protein.

2. Insulin resistance

Sometimes people become insulin-resistant, meaning their bodies no longer respond to the hormone the way they should. As a result, their blood glucose levels remain high and their cells don't get the fuel they need. Insulin resistance is a key characteristic of diabetes.

Numerous factors can cause insulin resistance, including excess weight, physical inactivity, normal aging, sleep problems, and certain diseases and medications.[447] When the cells do not respond to normal levels of insulin, the pancreas is forced to pump out even more, resulting in a state known as hyperinsulinemia. Because insulin signals the body to store fat instead of burn it, hyperinsulinemia leads to additional weight gain.

3. Low resting metabolic rate

A missing link for successful long-term weight loss is boosting your resting metabolic rate (RMR), which determines how many calories you burn when resting.

There is quite a bit of natural variation in RMR, which explains why some people can eat whatever they want without gaining weight, while others seem predisposed toward weight gain. Unfortunately, as you age, your RMR decreases, so you have an even harder time burning off the same amount of calories you once did.

4. Improper fat cell signaling

There are many reasons why people gain weight, but if you are putting on pounds despite eating less (particularly fewer carbs), exercising, and following other practices that should in theory lead to weight loss, then your problem could be age-related.

Weight gain occurs when adipocytes, or fat cells, become bloated with triglycerides.

Unfortunately, the aging process adversely affects the fat cell command signal network, which regulates the size and number of adiopcytes. If you're doing everything right but still not losing weight, three critical command signals we need to restore to normal include:

- Leptin, a hormone that signals to the brain that you're full

- Adiponectin, a protein that regulates how much fat is stored in your adiopcytes

- Glycerol-3-phosphate dehydrogenase, an enzyme that converts sugar into fat

5. Low brain serotonin

You probably associate serotonin with mood, but this neurotransmitter also affects appetite. When your brain is flooded with serotonin, you feel full faster.

Just like it's possible to be deficient in a vitamin or mineral, you can also be deficient in serotonin. And you know what happens when you don't have enough of this feel-full brain chemical? You binge on carbohydrates—the very type of food that leads to weight gain.[448]

This reaction is probably stress-related. When you are chronically stressed, your level of cortisol increases and your level of serotonin decreases. Your body tries to prepare you to fight or flee the stressful circumstance by encouraging you to eat food that will turn into energy quickly: carbohydrates! Therefore, the best way to counteract this instinctual response is to raise your serotonin level.

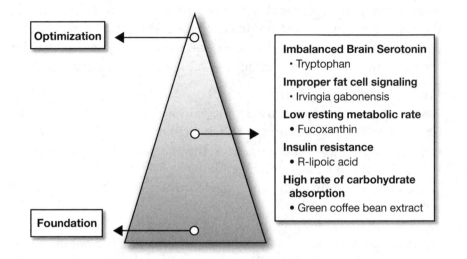

Primary Recommended Supplements

If you are unsure which of the supplements below to take for weight loss, call Life Extension advisors. They will help you identify which weight gain mechanisms you are likely facing and then help you decide which supplements are best for you. They are not numbered because they are equally important.

1. To Slow Carbohydrate Absorption

Green Coffee Bean Extract: As we discussed in the diabetes section, green coffee bean extract helps manage blood glucose levels. It also has serious weight loss benefits. A recent double-blind study of obese adults found that over a six-week period, green coffee bean extract caused an average weight loss of 17.6 pounds and an average decrease in body fat of 4.44 percent compareo placebo![449]

2. To Increase Insulin Sensitivity

R-Lipoic Acid: If you are resistant to insulin, then lipoic acid is a critical supplement for you. Lipoic acid is a naturally occurring anti-oxidant in the body that increases the body's sensitivity to insulin and dramatically increases its ability to clear glucose out of the blood.[450,451] I recommend R-lipoic acid—the form that is produced by the body—over alpha-lipoic acid, which is not nearly as available.

3. To Increase Resting Metabolic Rate

Fucoxanthin: In animal models, fucoxanthin, a carotenoid from brown seaweed, increases energy expenditure. How? By activating a factor called UCP1 that induces thermogenesis (the process of heat production, which burns calories).[452] As a result, it jump-starts weight loss. In fact, a sixteen-week trial of obese women found taking a combination of fucoxanthin plus pomegranate seed oil, in combination with a reduced calorie diet, caused an average weight loss of thirteen to fifteen pounds compared to placebo.[453]

4. To Improve Fat Cell Signaling

Irvingia gabonensis: A mango-like fruit from West Africa, *Irvingia gabonensis* is believed to inhibit adipogenesis, or the development of fat cells.[454] Three published human studies have found it significantly decreases body fat stores, weight, and waist circumference.[455,456,457] Overweight and/or obese study subjects who took *Irvingia gabonensis* before meals for ten weeks experienced a 6.3 percent decrease in body fat percentage compared to just 1.9 percent for those who took a placebo.[458]

5. To Increase Brain Serotonin Levels

Tryptophan: As we discussed previously, serotonin regulates appetite, and tryptophan is a precursor (or building block) of serotonin. Unfortunately, when you restrict calories, you also reduce your circulating tryptophan level by 14 to 23 percent.[459] This may in turn lower your serotonin level, causing you to feel hungry and eat more. Several studies have shown that when people take tryptophan before a meal, they eat fewer calories.[460,461]

Secondary Recommended Supplements

- Saffron extract
- Mangosteen extract
- *Sphaeranthus indicus*
- 7-keto DHEA
- Green tea extract

CHAPTER 8

Personalized Supplement Pyramid Case Studies

I've presented a lot of information in this book, and I don't want to overwhelm you. So let's take a look at some examples of different individuals and see how building a personalized Supplement Pyramid works in real life.

Case Study 1: John

John is a forty-nine-year-old business executive. He is married with three kids and works seventy hours per week. He admits he is out of shape and stressed out. John's diet is poor. He frequently eats on the run, and rarely is the food fresh. Currently, he's taking a low-dose, generic multivitamin and, when he remembers, generic fish oil soft gels.

Step 1: John decides to start out slowly. He researches the recommended supplement companies using Appendix A and chooses a higher-quality multivitamin and fish oil product, which he vows to take daily. He's going to hold off on taking CoQ_{10} and a probiotic for now.

Step 2: After two weeks, John admits he feels better on the new multivitamin and regular fish oil regimen. This inspires him to start building the Personalization Level of his Supplement Pyramid. He takes the family medical inventory and comes up with the following results:

Body System	Result	Recommended Supplements
Heart	Father died of heart attack	Pomegranate extract; Stand-alone vitamin D₃; Aged garlic extract
Lungs	No family history	
Blood pressure & blood vessels	He is prehypretensive; Mother is hypertensive	Pomegranate extract; Grape seed extract; Olive leaf extract
Cancer & precancerous lesions	No family history	
Diabetes & metabolic disorders	No family history	
Brain & nerves	No family history	
Bones & joints	No family history	
Immune problems	No family history	
Kidneys	No family history	
Eyes, ears, nose & throat	No family history	

Step 3: John then takes the personal medical inventory and writes down the following:

Body System	Result	Recommended Supplements
Inflammatory & pain syndromes	No personal history	
Low energy & fatigue	He is tired from overwork	Rhodiola; Glutathione; Magnesium citrate
Overweight & obesity	He is slightly overweight	Irvingia extract; Fucoxanthin; Green coffee bean extract
Muscles & skin	No personal history	
Gastrointestinal system	No personal history	
Low thyroid	No personal history	
Urinary tract & bladder infections	No personal history	
Depression	No personal history	

Body System	Result	Recommended Supplements
Anxiety	He occasionally feels work-related anxiety	GABA; Lemon balm; Valerian

Step 4: John isn't ready to take a lot of supplements just yet, so he makes some choices. He decides to take pomegranate extract for his heart and grape seed extract for his blood pressure. He rereads Chapter 4 and learns that CoQ_{10}, one of the foundation supplements he skipped, is good for the heart and for energy, so he decides he should probably take it after all. But he's not particularly worried about his weight and his anxiety is infrequent, so he decides to take GABA only as needed for sleep. He figures if he sleeps better, he may not need to take anything for energy.

Here is John's initial pyramid:

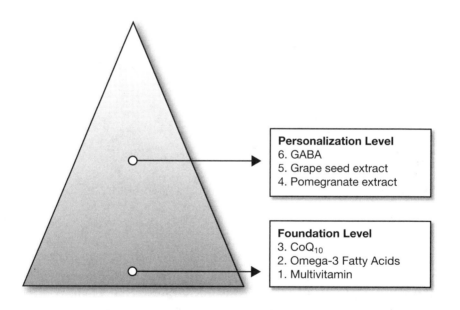

Personalization Level
6. GABA
5. Grape seed extract
4. Pomegranate extract

Foundation Level
3. CoQ_{10}
2. Omega-3 Fatty Acids
1. Multivitamin

He decides to stick with this regimen for three months and then reevaluate.

Step 5: After three months, John has a doctor's appointment. He reports that his energy is better. While his blood pressure is down slightly, it's still too high. This encourages him to dive into the medical quizzes. He comes up with the following results:

Body System	Quiz Score	Recommended Supplements
Heart & circulation	4 points	Pomegranate extract; Stand-alone vitamin D$_3$; Aged garlic extract
Cancer	0 points	
Diabetes & metabolic disorders	4 points	Chromium and/or cinnamon extract; Green coffee bean extract
Brain & nerves	0 points	
Memory	1 point (excellent)	
Blood pressure & blood vessels	4 points	Pomegranate extract; Grape seed extract
Hormone imbalances	1 "yes"	Get hormone levels tested
Inflammatory conditions	1 "yes"	Curcumin
Bones	1 point	
Respiratory	0 points	
Eyes	0 points	
Joints	0 points	
Kidneys & urinary tract	0 points	
Chronic infections	0 "yeses"	
Chronic fatigue	3 points	Rhodiola; Glutathione
Fibromyalgia & pain syndromes	0 points	

Step 6: John is already taking pomegranate and grape seed extracts, and he feels like he's got his heart and blood pressure needs covered with those two supplements. (He also got his vitamin D level checked at the doctor and he's within normal range.) But he is prediabetic, so he decides it's a good idea for him to take cinnamon extract. He also decides it's time to add the final product to his Foundation Level: probiotics. He scored fairly low on the inflammation quiz, so he doesn't feel like he needs to take curcumin. And his energy has been better, so at this point, he's going to skip the rhodiola and glutathione. Now, his Supplement Pyramid looks like this:

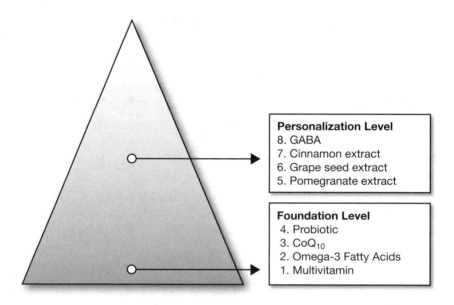

Personalization Level
8. GABA
7. Cinnamon extract
6. Grape seed extract
5. Pomegranate extract

Foundation Level
4. Probiotic
3. CoQ$_{10}$
2. Omega-3 Fatty Acids
1. Multivitamin

In six months to a year, John plans on testing his levels of hormones and inflammatory markers. He really likes his regimen and can't wait to see how it influences his blood pressure and blood sugar at his next doctor's appointment. Seeing how happy he is, his wife Amy decides to build her Supplement Pyramid too.

Case Study 2: Amy

Amy is forty-two and in great physical shape. She eats a mostly plant-based diet. Despite taking care of three kids, she has an easygoing attitude, which she attributes to her exercise program and healthy diet. Like John, she takes a generic multivitamin. But she takes fish oil and CoQ$_{10}$ (as ubiquinone) regularly.

Step 1: After reading Chapter 4, Amy decides to complete the Foundation Level of her pyramid by adding a probiotic supplement. She also upgrades her multivitamin to one with ideal doses and more bioavailable forms, chooses a higher-quality fish oil product, and switches the form of CoQ$_{10}$ she takes from ubiquinone to ubiquinol (which is more bioavailable).

Step 2: Amy doesn't need any convincing to build the Personalization Level of her Supplement Pyramid, so she digs right in. She takes the family medical inventory and gets the following results:

BODY SYSTEM	RESULT	RECOMMENDED SUPPLEMENTS
Heart	No family history	
Lungs	No family history	
Blood pressure & blood vessels	No family history	
Cancer & precancerous lesions	Mother and aunt died of colon cancer	Cruciferous vegetable extract; Stand-alone vitamin D_3; Reishi mushroom or curcumin extract
Diabetes & metabolic disorders	No family history	
Brain & nerves	No family history	
Bones & joints	No family history	
Immune problems	No family history	
Kidneys	No family history	
Eyes, ears, nose & throat	No family history	

Step 3: Amy then takes the personal medical inventory and writes down the following:

BODY SYSTEM	RESULT	RECOMMENDED SUPPLEMENTS
Inflammatory & pain syndromes	No personal history	
Low energy & fatigue	No personal history	
Overweight & obesity	No personal history	
Muscles & skin	No personal history	
Gastrointestinal system	No personal history	

Body System	Result	Recommended Supplements
Low thyroid	No personal history	
Urinary tract & bladder infections	No personal history	
Depression	No personal history	
Anxiety	No personal history	

Step 4: Based on this information, Amy decides to add cruciferous vegetable extract to her supplement regimen to protect against colon cancer. (However, her risk is relatively low because of her healthy diet.)

Here is Amy's initial pyramid:

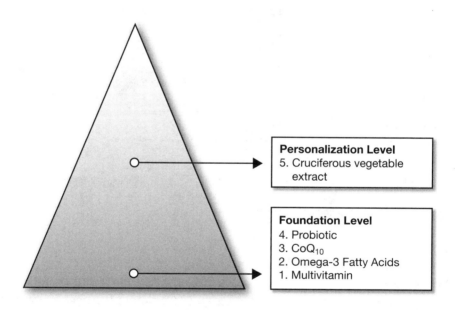

Personalization Level
5. Cruciferous vegetable extract

Foundation Level
4. Probiotic
3. CoQ$_{10}$
2. Omega-3 Fatty Acids
1. Multivitamin

Step 5: Amy feels pretty healthy, but she completes the medical quizzes just to double-check. They reveal the following:

Body System	Quiz Score	Recommended Supplements
Heart & circulation	0 points	
Cancer	2 points	Cruciferous vegetable extract; Stand-alone vitamin D$_3$

Body System	Quiz Score	Recommended Supplements
Diabetes & metabolic disorders	0 points	
Brain & nerves	0 points	
Memory	7 points (needs work)	Blueberry extract; Magnesium threonate
Blood pressure & blood vessels	2 points; "yes" to varicose veins and spider veins	Pomegranate extract; Diosmin
Hormone imbalances	no "yeses"	
Inflammatory conditions	no "yeses"	
Bones	2 points	Stand-alone vitamin D$_3$
Respiratory	1 point	
Eyes	0 points	
Joints	0 points	
Kidneys & urinary tract	1 point	
Chronic infections	0 "yeses"	
Chronic fatigue	2 points	Rhodiola; Glutathione
Fibromyalgia & pain syndromes	1 point	

Step 6: Amy is already taking cruciferous vegetable extract. Since she had two separate quizzes recommend stand-alone vitamin D$_3$, she decides to get her blood level tested and supplement if necessary. She knows she is somewhat forgetful, so she decides to add blueberry extract to her pyramid. She'd also like to do something about those spider veins on her legs, so she chooses to try diosmin. And even though she scored a "2" on the chronic fatigue quiz (1 point for being female and 1 point for being between the ages of forty and fifty), she doesn't feel fatigued, so she's going to skip the rhodiola and glutathione. Now, her Supplement Pyramid looks like this:

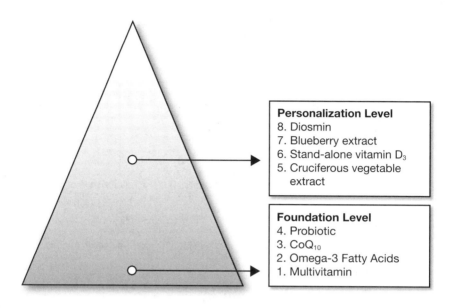

Personalization Level
8. Diosmin
7. Blueberry extract
6. Stand-alone vitamin D_3
5. Cruciferous vegetable extract

Foundation Level
4. Probiotic
3. CoQ_{10}
2. Omega-3 Fatty Acids
1. Multivitamin

Case Study 3: Diego

Diego, age sixty-three, is a bit of a health nut. He eats a healthy organic diet, plays tennis three to four times a week, and engages in regular weight lifting. He meditates daily so his stress level is low. But he's noticed over the years that his energy and sex drive have dropped considerably, and he sometimes suffers from mild depression. Diego reads several health magazines, and every time he reads about the latest, greatest nutritional supplement, he adds it to his regimen. So now he is taking seventeen different products, but he can't remember why he's taking them all, or if they are doing him any good! After reading this book, he decides to start over from scratch.

Step 1: Diego is already taking the four foundational products recommended in Chapter 4, and now he remembers why he's taking them. He feels good about the brands he originally chose so he sticks with them.

Step 2: Diego takes the family medical inventory and comes up with the following results:

BODY SYSTEM	RESULT	RECOMMENDED SUPPLEMENTS
Heart	No family history	
Lungs	No family history	
Blood pressure & blood vessels	No family history	
Cancer & precancerous lesions	No family history	
Diabetes & metabolic disorders	No family history	
Brain & nerves	Father has Alzheimer's disease	Fat-soluble vitamin B_1 and B_{12}; Blueberry extract; Magnesium L-threonate
Bones & joints	Mother has osteoporosis	Stand-alone vitamin D_3
Dedicated bone formula		
Immune problems	No family history	
Kidneys	No family history	
Eyes, ears, nose & throat	No family history	

Step 3: Diego then takes the personal medical inventory and writes down the following:

BODY SYSTEM	RESULT	RECOMMENDED SUPPLEMENTS
Inflammatory & pain syndromes	No personal history	
Low energy & fatigue	He is low on energy	Rhodiola; Glutathione; Magnesium citrate
Overweight & obesity	No personal history	
Muscles & skin	No personal history	
Gastrointestinal system	No personal history	
Low thyroid	No personal history	
Urinary tract & bladder infections	No personal history	
Depression	He suffers from mild depression	Tryptophan or 5-HTP; SAMe; Saffron extract
Anxiety	No personal history	

Step 4: Diego is already taking a high-potency multivitamin, so he decides he probably doesn't need extra vitamin B_1 and B_{12}. However, he thinks it would be a good idea to add extra magnesium to his regimen because of his family history of Alzheimer's disease and because his multivitamin only provides 100 mg per day (a quarter of the daily value). He is not particularly worried about osteoporosis, which his mother has, because he eats a calcium-rich diet and regularly engages in weight-bearing exercise, so he skips those supplement recommendations. But after reading Appendix B, he decides rhodiola may raise his energy levels and 5-HTP could lighten his mood.

Here is his initial pyramid:

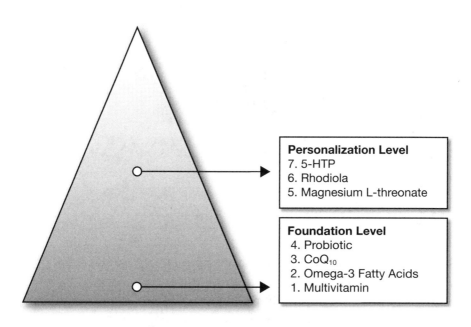

Personalization Level
7. 5-HTP
6. Rhodiola
5. Magnesium L-threonate

Foundation Level
4. Probiotic
3. CoQ_{10}
2. Omega-3 Fatty Acids
1. Multivitamin

Step 5: Diego is excited to complete the medical quizzes because he wants to design a supplement program this is custom-tailored to his specific needs. The results reveal the following:

BODY SYSTEM	QUIZ SCORE	RECOMMENDED SUPPLEMENTS
Heart & circulation	1.5 points	
Cancer	0 points	

Body System	Quiz Score	Recommended Supplements
Diabetes & metabolic disorders	1 point	
Brain & nerves	1 point	
Memory	5 points (good)	Consider blueberry extract
Blood pressure & blood vessels	0 points	
Hormone imbalances	5 "yeses"	Get a complete thyroid panel; Get a complete hormone panel
Inflammatory conditions	no "yeses"	
Bones	1.5 points	
Respiratory	1 point	
Eyes	1 point	
Joints	1 point	
Kidneys & urinary tract	0 points	
Chronic infections	0 "yeses"	
Chronic fatigue	1 point	
Fibromyalgia & pain syndromes	0 points	

Step 6: Diego is not too worried about his memory. But after taking the quiz on hormonal imbalances, he starts to suspect that maybe his low energy is due to insufficient thyroid or testosterone levels. He decides to get a complete thyroid panel and a complete male hormone panel.

While he's at it, Diego gets some other blood tests as well, including a comprehensive metabolic panel (to cover all the basics), isoprostane testing (to check his levels of oxidative stress), and a specialized micronutrient profile (to detect any nutritional deficiencies). He also completes a Food Safe Allergy test to determine if he has any food sensitivities.

Several weeks later, Diego learns some interesting things from his blood tests. His testosterone levels are very low, so instead of taking rhodiola for his low energy, he adds DHEA and pregnenolone supplements to his pyramid. His thyroid hormone levels are normal. All of his metabolic markers are within the ideal range, but his level of oxidative stress is on the high side. He calls Life Extension advisors, and they recommend that he take pomegranate extract to bring it down. His vitamin B_{12} status is inadequate, so he decides to take those B vitamins after all. And it turns out that he has food sensitivities to wheat and eggs, so he vows to cut those foods out of his diet.

The 5-HTP seems to be helping with his depression, so he wants to keep taking it.

Now, his Supplement Pyramid looks like this:

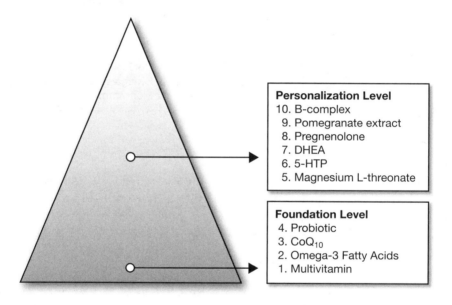

Personalization Level
10. B-complex
9. Pomegranate extract
8. Pregnenolone
7. DHEA
6. 5-HTP
5. Magnesium L-threonate

Foundation Level
4. Probiotic
3. CoQ_{10}
2. Omega-3 Fatty Acids
1. Multivitamin

Step 7: After three months on his new regimen, Diego is feeling great. He gets his testosterone and isoprostane levels retested, and everything is headed in the right direction. He's ready to complete the Optimization Level of his pyramid, so he rereads Chapter 6 and is pleased to find out that he has already taken the most important anti-aging actions: optimizing his hormones and reducing his oxidative stress. The next two anti-aging recommendations are to ease inflammation and prevent glycation reactions, so he adds boswellia extract and benfotiamine (fat-soluble B_1) to his Optimization Level.

Diego's final completed pyramid looks like this:

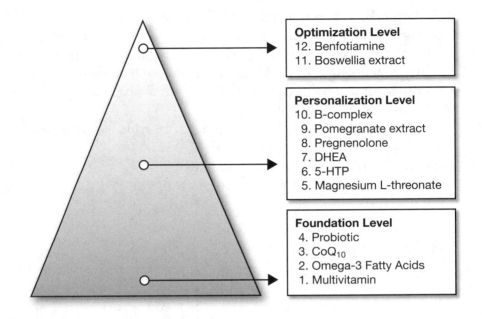

Optimization Level
12. Benfotiamine
11. Boswellia extract

Personalization Level
10. B-complex
 9. Pomegranate extract
 8. Pregnenolone
 7. DHEA
 6. 5-HTP
 5. Magnesium L-threonate

Foundation Level
 4. Probiotic
 3. CoQ_{10}
 2. Omega-3 Fatty Acids
 1. Multivitamin

Case Study 4: Carla

Carla has never taken a nutritional supplement in her life. She never felt like she had to. But now that she's fifty-four, her poor diet and lack of exercise are catching up with her. Carla never used to have to worry about her weight, but she's put on about twenty pounds in the last decade. Plus, her joints are starting to bother her, and she gets indigestion frequently.

Carla has a friend who is very health conscious and recommended that supplements could help her feel better without making drastic changes to her lifestyle. She's open, but she's also not about to start taking twelve products a day like Diego. She just wants to start on some basics, lose weight, and ease her knee pain and indigestion.

Step 1: Carla can see the wisdom in taking a multivitamin, especially since her diet is not the best. She's also heard a lot about fish oils—including that they're anti-inflammatory, which could help with her joint pain—so she decides to give them a try. She's going to skip the CoQ_{10}. But she suspects the probiotics could help her digestive issues, so she adds those to her Foundation Level.

Step 2: Carla doesn't have the patience to complete all the medical quizzes or undergo any blood testing. She'd rather just fill out the medical inventories and be able to quickly scan what might benefit her. Here are the results of her family medical inventory:

Body System	Result	Recommended Supplements
Heart	Mother died of stroke	Pomegranate extract; Stand-alone vitamin D_3; Aged garlic extract
Lungs	No family history	
Blood pressure & blood vessels	No family history	
Cancer & precancerous lesions	No family history	
Diabetes & metabolic disorders	Father has diabetes	Chromium; Green coffee bean extract; R-Lipoic acid
Brain & nerves	No family history	
Bones & joints	She has joint pain	Methylsulfonylmethane (MSM); Glucosamine
Immune problems	No family history	
Kidneys	No family history	
Eyes, ears, nose & throat	No family history	

Step 3: Carla then takes the personal medical inventory and comes up with the following results:

Body System	Result	Recommended Supplements
Inflammatory & pain syndromes	No personal history	
Low energy & fatigue	No personal history	
Overweight & obesity	She is twenty pounds overweight	Irvingia extract; Fucoxanthin; Green coffee bean extract
Muscles & skin	No personal history	
Gastrointestinal system	She has frequent indigestion	Zinc-carnosine; Artichoke leaf extract; Picrorhiza kurroa extract
Low thyroid	No personal history	
Urinary tract & bladder infections	No personal history	

Body System	Result	Recommended Supplements
Depression	No personal history	
Anxiety	No personal history	

Step 4: Carla is really only concerned with the health issues she is facing directly, so she decides to ignore the suggestions from her family medical inventory. She really wants to drop some weight, so she adds irvingia extract to her Personalization Level. She's excited to find out about supplements that can take away her joint pain, so she also decides to start on MSM. If that's not working after two months, she'll add glucosamine. Reading Appendix B, artichoke leaf looks interesting for indigestion, but she wants to wait and see if the probiotics do anything before she adds it to her pyramid.

Here is Carla's pyramid:

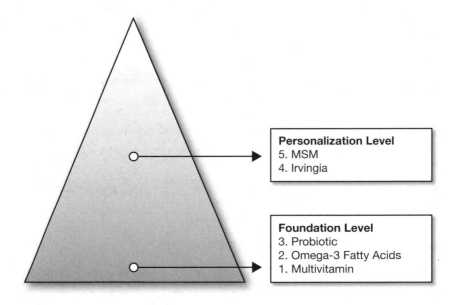

Personalization Level
5. MSM
4. Irvingia

Foundation Level
3. Probiotic
2. Omega-3 Fatty Acids
1. Multivitamin

Five supplements seems like a lot to Carla, since she's not used to taking any. But she feels that if they actually make a difference in how she looks and feels, it will be worth it.

Hopefully these case studies have helped you understand how to create your own Supplement Pyramid. Next case study . . . you!

CHAPTER 9

Your Own Personalized Supplement Pyramid

Hopefully, the case studies in Chapter 8 have been helpful to you. As you can see, the Supplement Pyramid is both highly individualized—and totally dynamic. You can decide to start slowly, with only the Foundation Level supplements, or you can choose to do everything at once: the Foundation Level, the Personalization Level, and the Optimization Level. You can build your pyramid based solely on recommendations from the family and personal medical inventories, or you can complete all the medical quizzes and get extensive blood testing for more targeted suggestions. You can choose to take every supplement recommended for a particular body system, or you can opt to take just one or none at all. It's totally up to you and what you feel comfortable with. The beauty of this system is that you can always change it up to suit your needs.

As a physician specializing in nutritional supplements, I have witnessed firsthand the difference that the right vitamins, minerals, omega-3 fats, probiotics, antioxidants, and herbs can make to our health and well-being. I hope this book has inspired you to take your health to the next level, and that I've made it simple for you to put together your own personalized Supplement Pyramid. You may find it's the best thing you ever did for yourself!

MY SUPPLEMENT PYRAMID

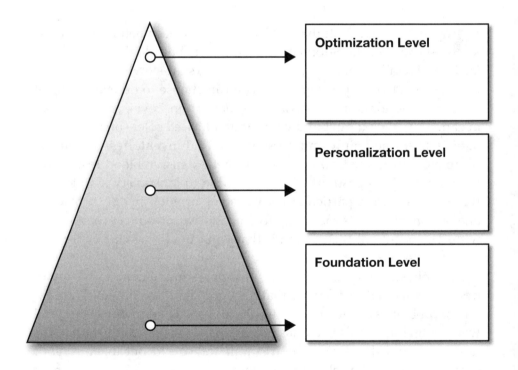

Conclusion

Hopefully you're now well on your way to creating a personalized supplement pyramid—one that is uniquely tailored to your specific health needs and goals. First and foremost, build upon the foundational supplements, starting with a high-quality, ideally dosed multivitamin. Working up, add omega-3 fish oils, ubiquinol CoQ_{10}, and probiotics. These four supplements are foundational to your health as they help every cell and tissue throughout your body.

Once the foundation is in place, continue to work up the pyramid by completing the inventories and then the quizzes. As you see fit, add the suggested products into your pyramid in order of importance, moving from the bottom up. Lastly, consider the suggested products at the optimization level for counteracting the leading theories of aging.

Remember, your pyramid is dynamic and will change as you change. I suggest retaking the quizzes a couple times a year and make the appropriate changes to your pyramid as your quiz scores change.

BUILD YOUR SUPPLEMENT PYRAMID ONLINE

Build your personalized supplement pyramid online at www.mysupplement pyramid.com. You can complete your inventories and take all of the quizzes by creating a FREE online account. All of your supplement suggestions, quizzes, and inventories are stored digitally in place for easy access.

Recommended Nutritional Supplement Companies

After completing your personalized supplement pyramid, it's time to purchase products. Chapter 3 covers how to choose high-quality products. To help you find the best products, I've put together some information on my favorite supplement companies. These are companies I buy from and have come to trust.

Source Naturals

Source Naturals has introduced numerous award-winning formulas, recognized for their excellence in independent surveys and nutritional analyses. In addition to Wellness, these award-winners include Life Force Multiple, Mega-Kid Multiple, Inflama-Rest, the Skin Eternal line, Higher Mind, Essential Enzymes, Male Response, and more. Source Naturals' comprehensive Bio-Aligned Formulas help bring the power of alignment to your body. When formulating, they evaluate the underlying causes of system imbalances, and then provide targeted nutrition to interdependent body systems. Their line of more than 600 products also includes well-researched, single-entity nutrients in their highest quality and most bioavailable forms. Their nutritional supplements are at the leading edge of today's Wellness Revolution. This transformation in health consciousness also includes new perspectives in diet, lifestyle, emotional and spiritual development, and complementary health care. Source Naturals Strategy for Wellness provides education that empowers individuals to take responsibility for their health, rather than relying solely on outside medical authority. The result is people who are more productive and fulfilled, and a world that is stronger and healthier. For more information, visit www.sourcenaturals.com.

Country Life

Country Life is a leader and authority in natural health, and in 2011, they celebrated their fortieth anniversary. Their internationally popular, top-selling products include a broad and deep offering of natural supplements and beauty care including full lines of Certified Gluten Free vitamins, mineral supplements, fish oils, specialty products, and more. The Company operates NSF GMP compliant manufacturing and distribution facilities for their brands, which include Country Life Vitamins, Desert Essence, Biochem Sports, and Iron-Tek. A commitment to strict and current Quality Control protocols ensures fresh product and reliable label claims. For more information, visit www.country-life.com.

NOW Foods

In 1948, with the natural food and supplement industry in its infancy, entrepreneur Paul Richard paid $900 for the purchase of Fearn Soya Foods—a Chicago-based manufacturer of grain and legume-based products. This began a six-decade legacy of providing health-seeking consumers with high-quality, affordable nutrition products. Still a family-owned company today, NOW manufactures and distributes more than 1,400 dietary supplements, natural foods, sports nutrition, and personal-care products. For more information, visit www.NowFoods.com.

Rainbow Light Nutritional Systems

Rainbow Light began in 1981 by offering consumers a nutritious spirulina supplement and went on to become the first-ever food-based supplement brand. During nutritional content testing procedures in those early days, their researchers discovered that spirulina, when exposed to a light spectrophotometer, refracted all the colors of the rainbow. In addition to their simple beauty, these rainbow colors revealed the full spectrum of nutritional constituents present in spirulina. Inspired by the power of nature revealed in this nourishing food base, their brand name was born. Since then, Rainbow Light has become a natural products leader and today, certified organic spirulina is still their primary food base. For thirty years, their targeted, food-based supplements have been delivering measurable health benefits and positive improvements in daily energy and vitality you can feel. For more information, visit www.rainbowlight.com.

Carlson Laboratories

Founded by John and Susan Carlson in 1965, J. R. Carlson Laboratories, Inc. has been a family owned and operated business for over forty-five years. Carlson Laboratories is a good company, dedicated to providing only the highest quality nutritional supplements.

Carlson Laboratories began with one vitamin E formula. Since then, the line has grown to become the most complete line of natural vitamin E products in the world. Carlson Laboratories' product range has expanded through the years to meet the nutritional needs of their customers. Their product lines now include award-winning Norwegian fish oils, a full line of vitamins, minerals, amino acids, special formulations, and nutritional supplements.

Carlson Laboratories' professional sales force offers individual and personalized services including staff training, brochures, posters, sample packets, and in-store promotions to increase sales. Carlson Laboratories also sponsors radio shows, free lectures, and more. For more information, visit www.carlsonlabs.com.

Gaia Herbs

Gaia Herbs is one of the top herbal and plant extract manufacturers in the world. They back up their claims of purity and potency with an industry-first, herb traceability program. This is essentially proof of their product's label claims. For more information, visit www.gaia herbs.com.

Garden of Life

A solid company that believes raw, whole food nutrition, from organically grown sources, is more beneficial for health than isolated nutrients. When coupled with exercise, a diet that includes the consumption of raw, live foods, particularly those containing probiotics, enzymes, and products of their fermentation, is the foundation for a healthy lifestyle. Garden of Life's commitment to health goes beyond offering some of the most effective nutritional products in the world. They are interested in building relationships with people to help them transform their lives to attain extraordinary health. By combining the best of nature and science, the Garden of Life brand offers a path to healthy living with premium products that are supported by education and innovation. For more information, visit www.gardenoflife.com.

Jarrow Formulas

Jarrow Formulas, which is based in Los Angeles, California, is a formulator and supplier of superior nutritional supplements. The company was founded in 1977 and incorporated in 1988. Today it markets its products in the United States, Mexico, Canada, and throughout the world. Jarrow Formulas' mission is reflected in its motto "Superior Nutrition and Formulation."

Jarrow Formulas' complete line of nutritional products includes vitamins, minerals, probiotics, standardized herbal concentrates, amino acids, enzymes, and enteral nutrition products. Both retailers and consumers are assured of purity, value, and potency when choosing these products.

The company is active in monitoring governmental regulatory affairs, which affect the nutritional industry. It also vigorously promotes the rights of Americans to free access to dietary supplements. Jarrow Formulas funds research studies on important nutritional products such as CoQ_{10}, to ensure that customers receive the full biological value of these products. For more information, visit www.jarrow.com/index.

Life Extension

Life Extension is an organization whose long-range goal is the extension of the healthy human life span. In seeking to control aging, their objective is to develop methods to enable us to live in vigor, health, and wellness for an unlimited period of time. Life Extension is offering you a free, six-month Life Extension Foundation membership. Simply call toll-free 1–866–491–4989, or visit www.lef.org/freemem to activate your free membership today.

Life Extension was established in the early 1980s, but its founders have been involved in the anti-aging field since the 1960s. Life Extension publishes the very latest information on anti-aging and wellness in its monthly publication, *Life Extension* Magazine, the *Disease Prevention and Treatment* book of integrative health protocols, the *Life Extension Update* e-mail newsletter, and the *Daily Health Bulletin* at their website. All to support more informed health choices.

In addition to a wealth of information, Life Extension offers 350+ premium-quality vitamins, minerals, hormones, diet, and nutritional supplements, and even skin-care products, which are often the fruits of research reported on or funded by the Life Extension Foundation.

Based on current scientific research, Life Extension is continually formulating and upgrading its science-based multivitamin, vitamin, and nutritional supplement formulas to include the latest novel ingredients that are years ahead of mainstream offerings.

Life Extension's stringent approach to quality assurance and 100 percent Satisfaction Guarantee makes its supplements the "gold standard" of the industry.

As a Life Extension member, you'll receive:

- The full-color monthly *Life Extension* Magazine that reports on the latest health and wellness research.

- Toll-free phone access to an integrative staff of health advisors (naturopaths, nutritionists, nurses, personal trainers, and other health professionals) available every day to answer your health questions and concerns, and to assist you in formulating your personal regimen of diet, exercise, and supplements. They can be reached at 1-866-491-4989.

- 25 to 50 percent discounts on premium-quality Life Extension products, plus 2,000 other health-related products.

- A 24/7/365 call center for ease of ordering (or the convenience of shopping online).

- A mail-order blood testing service that costs a fraction of what commercial blood labs charge, with blood draws performed in a convenient local LabCorp facility near you (some restrictions apply).

- Access to the independent, full-service Life Extension Pharmacy, including compounded prescriptions, offering a unique knowledge of pharmaceuticals and nutraceuticals, as well as remarkable prescription savings.

Learn how you can access all of the above services, as well as receive discounts on dietary supplements and blood testing, by joining the Life Extension Foundation—free for six months. Simply call toll-free 1–866–491–4989 or visit www.lef.org/freemem to activate your free membership today.

New Chapter

New Chapter supplements are whole food. They call their vitamin, mineral, and herbal supplements "whole-food complex"—something your body easily recognizes and absorbs. Sourced from nature's bounty of organic fruits, vegetables, herbs, and superfoods, and cultured in probiotics to deliver the full spectrum of nature's benefits. For more information, visit http://www.newchapter.com/.

Twinlab

Twinlab Corporation manufactures and distributes several hundred different vitamin, mineral, and herbal supplements and nutritional products, thus making it an industry leader. While about 63 percent of its products are sold in health food stores, the firm is increasing sales through mass retailers and supermarket chains as well, including Wal-Mart and Albertson's.

In addition to nutritional products, the company publishes *Muscular Development* magazine and a variety of books on nutrition and fitness. Although 94 percent of Twinlab sales are in the United States, its products are sold in seventy nations. Twinlab operates two production and distribution plants: its historic facility in Ronkonkoma, New York, and one in American Fork, Utah, built in the 1990s. For more information, visit www.twinlab.com.

Recommended Nutrients

Below is a brief description of all of the nutrients suggested in the book, including what it is and how it can benefit you. For more information on each nutrient, you can use the following resources:

Life Extension: www.lef.org

Healthnotes and PCC Natural Markets:
www.pccnaturalmarkets.com/health/2402003

Memorial Sloan-Kettering Cancer Center:
www.mskcc.org/mskcc/html/11570.cfm

University of Maryland Medical Institute:
www.umm.edu/altmed/index.htm

5-HTP (5-Hydroxytryptophan)
Intermediate metabolite between the amino acid tryptophan and serotonin. It improves sleep, enhances mood, and modulates stress.
Average dose: 50–100 mg/day.

7-Keto DHEA
A natural metabolite of the hormone DHEA that has been shown to safely increase thermogenesis, improve fat loss, and help maintain healthy body weight when combined with a diet and exercise program.
Average dose: 100 mg/day.

Acai Extract

Potent antioxidant. Acai palm trees grow along the rich waters of the South American Amazon River. The berries are full of antioxidants and have been used for thousands of years to increase energy, stamina, and vitality. Acaí provides vitamins B_1, B_2, B_3, E, C, potassium, calcium, omega fatty acids, and valuable trace minerals. Supports a healthy immune system.
Average dose: 500–1,000 mg/day.

Acetyl-L-Carnitine (ALC)

Amino acid intermediate. Supports brain function by crossing the blood-brain barrier to combat oxidative stress and promote energy production in brain and central nervous system tissues. It also supports the release and synthesis of acetylcholine, enhances the release of dopamine from neurons and helps it bind to dopamine receptors.
Average dose: 500 mg/day.

Active Hexose Correlated Compound

An alpha-glucan-rich nutritional supplement produced from the mycelia of shiitake mushrooms. It supports a healthy immune system and liver function.
Average dose: 750 mg/day.

Aged Garlic Extract

Potent antioxidant. Supports many parts of the cardiovascular system, including blood pressure control and healthy lipid and cholesterol levels. Supports a healthy immune system.
Average dose: 1,000–4,000 mg/day.

Alpha Linoleic Acid

An important omega-3 fat that eases inflammation and promotes healthy heart and brain function. It converts into the longer chained omega-3 fats, EPA and DHA. It is often sourced from Perilla oil.
Average dose: 1,000–2,000 mg/day.

Andrographis Paniculata

An herbal extract that supports the immune system and may help fight against bacterial and viral infections.
Average dose: Daily dose is 50–100 mg/day. During an infection, the dose can increase to 300 mg/day.

Apple Polyphenols

Antioxidants found in white fleshy fruits like apples may help reduce the risk of stroke and other cardiovascular diseases. New research shows they may be helpful in gastroesophageal reflux disease, asthma, and for improving lung function.
Average dose: 600 mg/day.

Arginine

An amino acid essential to a healthy cardiovascular system, wound healing, helping the kidneys remove waste products from the body, and maintaining immune and hormone function.
Average dose: 500–700 mg/day.

Aronia Extract

Potent antioxidant. Supports healthy cells and tissues, including the heart, brain, and immune system.
Average dose: 450 mg/day.

Artichoke (Leaf) Extract

Plant extract that helps to support healthy blood sugar levels and healthy liver and gallbladder function.
Average dose: 500–1,500 mg/day.

Ashwagandha

An Indian herb that counters some of the oxidative damage generated by nervous tension. Ashwagandha has been the subject of animal studies and is believed to confer improvements in well-being and a healthy outlook in humans.
Average dose: 250 mg/day.

Astaxanthin

Natural pigmented antioxidant. Protects against free radical–induced DNA damage, repairs UVA-irradiated cells, and inhibits inflammatory cell infiltration. It also helps support vascular health within the eye and improves visual acuity. Astaxanthin may play a preventative role in eye fatigue.
Average dose: 2–6 mg/day.

Astragalus

Herbal extract. Support healthy immune system and may protect against bacterial and viral infections.
Average dose: 400 mg/day.

B-Complex, Stand-alone Supplement

B vitamins are essential for healthy cell growth and repair and cell energy production from fats, carbohydrates, and protein. They support healthy nerve function, a healthy cardiovascular system, and can protect the body from the damaging effects of excess sugar.
Average dose: Usually dosed as B-50, B-75, or B-100.

Bacopa

An Ayurvedic herb that enhances clear thinking and supports memory function.
Average dose: 250–500 mg/day.

Berberine

A natural compound found in goldenseal, giving the herb its yellow color. It helps maintain healthy cell growth and may have anticancer properties. Also supports the heart and immune system.
Average dose: 550 mg/day from goldenseal.

Beta-Carotene

Potent antioxidant and a precursor to vitamin A. It is essential for growth and reproduction, maintaining healthy vision, and supporting protein synthesis and cell differentiation.
Average dose: 5,000–25,000 IU based on individual need and doctor's suggestion.

Bilberry

Potent antioxidant. Supports healthy eye function and may be neuroprotective.
Average dose: 100 mg/day.

Bitter Melon Extract

Bitter melon is a fruit used for supporting digestion. It is also used for maintaining healthy blood sugar, kidneys, and liver function. May be supportive for people with HIV/AIDS.
Average dose: 500 mg/day.

Black Cohosh
Herbal extract. Helps reduce the severity of hot flashes, and promotes hormonal balance in women. Encourages a positive mood.
Average dose: 100–500 mg/day.

Black Cumin Seed Oil
Plant-based oil that provides immune support and promotes healthy inflammatory response.
Average dose: 500 mg/day.

Black Tea Extract with Theaflavins
Eases inflammation and protects against LDL oxidation and favorably affects endothelial function, thus helping to maintain healthy circulation.
Average dose: 350 mg/day extract of which 25 percent is theaflavins.

Blueberry Extract
Potent antioxidant. Helps support healthy brain function and reduce the risk of metabolic syndrome.
Average dose: 400–1,200 mg/day.

Boron
A mineral with several functions, including optimizing calcium metabolism for healthy bones and joints, supports steroid hormone levels, and supports a healthy prostate.
Average dose: 1–3 mg/day.

Boswellia Extract
Plant extract. Eases chronic inflammation and supports a healthy immune system.
Average dose: 100 mg/day of which 20% is AKBA.

Branched Chain Amino Acids (BCAAs)
Special class of amino acids. Provide energy and may serve as fuel sources for skeletal muscles during periods of metabolic stress. BCAAs have been used with success to support liver function. A study in 2008 also showed BCAA supplementation improved insulin resistance and glucose tolerance in certain people. A current mouse study showed restoring brain BCAA concentrations to normal had the effect of reinstating normal brain function by helping brain cells connect to each other and function efficiently.
Average dose: 2 grams/day.

Broccoli Extract
Favorably affects estrogen metabolism and cell division.
Average dose: 400 mg/day.

Butterbur
Herbal extract. Helps to maintain nasal comfort and head cavity comfort.
Average dose: 100–200 mg/day.

Calcium Collagen Chelate Complex
A chelated compound of calcium and hydrolyzed collagen peptides (type I collagen) designed to enhance bone collagen support while supporting optimal bone mineral density and strength.
Average dose: 1–3 grams/day.

Capsaicin
Potent antioxidant. It's used to treat minor aches and pains of the muscles and joints. It may also be used to treat nerve pain. Capsaicin works by decreasing a certain natural substance in your body (substance P) that helps pass pain signals to the brain. It may also help to reduce the risk of blood clots by decreasing fibrinogen levels.
Average dose: 600 mg/day or 40,000 heat-units.

Carnitine
Amino acid intermediate. Helps maintain cellular metabolic activity by assisting in the intracellular transport of fatty acids from the cell fluid into mitochondria, inhibits excess accumulation of cellular debris, supports a healthy concentration of nitric oxide for optimal arterial (endothelial cells) function, helps the body maintain healthy body fat composition, supports insulin sensitivity and healthy blood sugar levels, and supports brain cells' natural defenses against age-related memory and cognitive decline.
Average dose: 1,000–2,000 mg/day.

Carnosine
Small protein (dipeptide). Potent antioxidant and antiglycation agent. It acts as a pH buffer, it can keep on protecting muscle cell membranes from oxidation under the acidic conditions of muscular exertion. It enables the heart muscle to contract more efficiently. It also helps to support a healthy gastrointestinal lining.
Average dose: 500–2,000 mg/day.

Chromium, Stand-alone Supplement

A mineral. It plays an important role in maintaining healthy blood sugar levels. Chromium is recognized by the FDA as a treatment for type 2 diabetes.

Average dose: 250–500 mcg/day.

Chrysin

A plant-based antioxidant (bioflavonoid) found in passionflower (Passi-flora coerula), that promotes healthy testosterone levels and lean muscle mass by inhibiting aromatase, the enzyme that converts testosterone to estrogen.

Average dose: 500 mg/day.

Cinnamon Water-based Extract

It contains polyphenols (plant-based antioxidants) that activate glucose detection systems, enabling them to support healthy blood glucose, induces satiety (the feeling of being full), which inhibits overconsumption and optimizes after-meal blood sugar spikes.

Average dose: 175 mg/day.

Coriolus Mushroom Extract

It's a mushroom with anticancer and immune boosting properties.

Average dose: 600–1,800 mg/day.

Cranberry Extract

Potent antioxidant. Cranberries support a healthy urinary tract. Clinical research demonstrates that cranberries' natural antioxidants (proanthocyanidins) are powerful antioxidants that can reduce oxidative stress.

Average dose: 500 mg/day.

Creatine

A small protein that elicits improvements in exercise performance and may be responsible for the improvements of muscle function and energy metabolism seen under certain conditions. It optimizes energy metabolism and inhibits tissue damage by stabilizing cellular membranes.

Average dose: 1,000–2,000 mg/day.

Cruciferous Vegetable Extract

Usually contains extracts from broccoli, cauliflower, cabbage, and Brussels sprouts. When combined, they help protect cellular DNA and have anticancer and hormone-supporting properties.

Average dose: 500 mg/day.

Curcumin Extract

An extract from turmeric spice, curcumin eases chronic inflammation and may have anticancer properties. Evidence shows it may support healthy bowels and joint function. It may also help maintain normal healthy platelet function and has immune supporting effects. Other studies show curcumin's potential in supporting healthy brain function and offering neuro-protection.

Average dose: 400 mg/day (if it is Curcumin BCM-95).

D-Glucarate

The salt form of a weak acid, it is found in grapefruit, apples, oranges, broccoli, and Brussels sprouts.[486,487] D-glucarate supports the body's cleansing system—a detoxification mechanism called glucuronidation. The human body uses glucuronidation to make a large variety of substances more water-soluble, and, in this way, allow for their subsequent elimination from the body through urine or feces (via bile from the liver). May also help maintain hormonal balance.

Average dose: 200 mg/day.

Dark Chocolate Extract

Potent antioxidant. Maintains healthy lipids, cholesterol, and blood pressure.

Average dose: 120 mg/day.

DHEA

Considered by many doctors to be the anti-aging hormone. It has been shown that DHEA often declines by 75 to 80 percent from peak levels by age seventy, leading to hormonal imbalances that can affect one's quality of life. The marked decline in serum DHEA with age is believed to play a role in health problems associated with aging. Optimal, youthful levels can help support your immune system, metabolism, and muscle mass.

Average dose: varies based on blood serum testing.

DIM (di-indolyl-methane)

Found in cruciferous vegetables, DIM favorably modulates estrogen metabolism and induces liver detoxification enzymes to help neutralize potentially harmful estrogen metabolites and xenoestrogens (estrogen-like environmental chemicals).
Average dose: 100–200 mg/day.

Diosmin

A potent antioxidant. Maintains tone and elasticity of your veins, healthy blood flow through your capillaries, eases the inflammatory effects of free floating biochemical compounds, and safeguards collagen and elastin against oxidative damage.
Average dose: 600 mg/day.

Dried Plum Extract

See Plum Extract.

EDTA (Ethylene Diamine Tetra-acetic Acid)

An amino acid–like compound that supports detoxification through excretion of toxins heavy from the body. It works by chelating (binding or capturing) certain trace minerals, metals, and oxidative compounds for transporting out of the body. It may help support a healthy gastrointestinal tract and cardiovascular system.
Average daily oral dose: 250–500 mg/day.

Elderberry Extract

Potent antioxidant. Supports a healthy immune system and may protect against bacterial and viral infections.
Average dose: 800–2,400 mg/day.

Fat-soluble Vitamin B_1 (Benfotiamine)

Supports healthy blood sugar metabolism and helps protect the body's tissues against advanced glycation end products and oxidative stress.
Average dose: 250–1,000 mg/day.

Fat-soluble Vitamin B_{12} (Methylcobalamin)

Essential for cell growth and repair and proper nerve cell functioning, and promotes healthy homocysteine levels.
Average dose: 1–5 mg/day.

Fucoxanthin

A compound from brown seaweed kelp. It activates the uncoupling protein-1 in white fat, which results in increased fat burning. It supports healthy body fat composition and weight.

Average dose: 600 mg/day in three divided doses.

GABA (Gamma Amino Butyric Acid)

A neurotransmitter that crosses the blood-brain barrier and increases alpha brain waves and decreases beta waves, which results in relaxation and improved sleep.

Average dose: 200 mg/day.

Gamma E Tocopherol

The term "vitamin E" refers to a family of eight related, lipid-soluble, antioxidant compounds widely present in plants. The tocopherol and tocotrienol subfamilies are each composed of alpha, beta, gamma, and delta fractions having unique biological effects. Prestigious scientific journals have highlighted gamma E tocopherol as one of the most critically important forms of vitamin E for those seeking optimal health benefits, including improved colon health, brain function, and protection against heart disease and Alzheimer's disease.

Average dose: 200 IU/day (total of 400 IU/day of all tocopherols).

Gamma Linolenic Acid (GLA)

It's a healthy omega-6 fatty acid that helps ease inflammation and may play a role in increasing energy and well-being for people with chronic fatigue syndrome.

Average dose: 500 mg–1 gram/day.

Ginger Extract

Ginger has been shown to do the following: support stomach, liver, and intestinal health; support healthy fibrinogen and blood platelet levels; promote healthy inflammation response and ease pain; contains herbal anti-aging constituents that inactivate free radicals; and treat motion sickness.

Average dose: 150–300 mg/day.

Ginkgo Biloba

One of the oldest trees known and has been used to support health for nearly 2,800 years. Ginkgo has been found to do the following: support

healthy circulation; help maintain the normal function and tone of blood vessels; support healthy oxygen and glucose metabolism in the brain; stabilize capillaries and make them less fragile; support normal coagulation of blood; support healthy aging in the brain
Average dose: 120 mg/day.

Ginseng
See Panax Ginseng.

Glucosamine
An amino sugar for joint function and repair.
Average dose: 2,000 mg/day.

Glutathione
Potent antioxidant. It is a small protein that supports liver function and the immune system.
Average dose: 100–500 mg/day.

Goldenseal
See Berberine.

Grape Seed Extract
Potent antioxidant. Supports healthy blood pressure control, supports a healthy immune system and helps maintain healthy testosterone levels by blocking its conversion into estrogen.
Average dose: 100 mg/day.

Green Coffee Bean Extract
Green coffee beans contain the antioxidant chlorogenic acid. This extract has been shown to improve post-meal sugar spikes and may aid in weight loss.
Average dose: 200– 400 mg/day, of which 50 percent is chlorogenic acid.

Green Tea Extract
This extract has been shown to provide many benefits including the following: reduces oxidative stress; has fluid-stabilizing properties; possibly promotes healthy weight; boosts liver detoxification; helps maintain healthy cell proliferation; helps maintain healthy blood cholesterol, LDL, and triglyceride levels; enhances immune function.
Average dose: 725 mg/day.

Hawthorn Extract
Plant extract that contains specific bioflavonoid complexes targeted to help promote normal circulation and efficient heart muscle function. Studies indicate that the constituents in hawthorn support: strong contractile force of human heart muscle; protection for heart muscle cells from oxidant damage; normal gene expression to promote cardiovascular health; improved cardiovascular performance.
Average dose: 500 mg/day or 30 mg of oligomeric proanthocyanidins.

Hibiscus Extract
Potent antioxidant. It's been shown to provide support for urinary system health.
Average dose: 100–200 mg/day.

Holy Basil
An herb that promotes a healthy inflammatory response. It demonstrates cell-protective properties with respect to cells of the breast, oral cavity, colon, prostate, skin, and liver. They have also been studied worldwide for their effect on normal cell growth. May help reduce symptoms of irritable bowel syndrome.
Average dose: 500–1,000 mg/day.

Hops
A plant extract that contains a phytoestrogen (8-prenylnaringenin) that offers natural female support during menopause.
Average dose: 120 mg/day.

Horsetail Extract
Herbal extract. Silicon is an element that helps to strengthen bones, improves bone density, and contributes to overall bone health. Because horsetail contains high amounts of silicon, the herb may help to harden brittle nails and help support healthy bone density. The silicon content may also help to strengthen connective tissues.
Average dose: 400 mg/day.

Huperzine A
This standardized extract from the Chinese club moss is an all-natural herbal supplement that has been shown to maintain healthy levels of acetylcholine and to promote optimal memory function.
Average dose: 200–400 mcg/day.

Hyaluronic Acid
A natural compound in humans that supports joint lubrication, skin hydration, and skin repair.
Average dose: 100 mg/day.

Indian Gooseberry
A plant extract that helps maintain healthy levels of all three key blood lipids—LDL, HDL, and triglycerides. It also eases chronic inflammation by reducing inflammatory markers like C-reactive protein.
Average dose: 500 mg/day.

Inositol
A primary component of cellular membrane phospholipids and is involved in a number of biological processes. Inositol has been found to be essential for calcium and insulin signal transduction, and serotonin-activity modulation. Research indicates inositol is beneficial for stabilizing moods.
Average dose: 1,000 mg/day.

Iodine
A health-promoting trace element essential for life. Its primary biological role lies in the production of the thyroid hormones. It's a natural antibiotic and helps promote healthy breast tissue.
Average dose: 1 mg/day.

Irvingia gabonensis
Plant extract. Helps to maintain healthy weight by decreasing hunger and minimizing sugar's impact on body fat accumulation.
Average dose: 300 mg/day in two divided doses.

Japanese Honeysuckle
Supports healthy immune function and may protect against bacterial and viral infections.
Average dose: Not well established. Speak with your doctor.

Korean Angelica (Decursinol)
Helps ease pain and improves fluid regulation by inhibiting activation of a DNA transcription factor associated with inflammation.
Average dose: 200 mg/day.

Lactoferrin
A protein that helps to support healthy gut bacteria and a healthy immune response.
Average dose: 300 mg/day.

Lemon Balm
An herb that enhances mood and relieves everyday stress and sleep problems. It may also offer smokers relief from the mental stress of quitting, aid in leveling mood swings, and help reduce the emotional hunger associated with dieting.
Average dose: 300 mg/day.

Lignans
A plant-based antioxidant that helps to reduce excess estrogen and dihydrotesterone effects (DHT). It helps guard against dangerous lipid peroxidation and helps ease chronic inflammation.
Average dose: 50–100 mg/day.

Lipoic Acid
Potent antioxidant. It helps support healthy blood sugar levels and healthy insulin function. It helps support normal nerve function and a healthy cardiovascular system. For the best results, supplement with the active "R" form.
Average dose: 150–300 mg/day.

Lutein
A carotenoid that reduces photo-damage to the macula, a dense region of rods and cones in the retina, and supports healthy eye function. May have anticancer and heart protective properties.
Average dose: 5–10 mg/day.

Lycopene
Potent antioxidant. Supports healthy cholesterol and lipid levels and healthy prostate function.
Average dose: 10–40 mg/day.

Magnesium, Stand-alone Supplement
Magnesium is used in 350 metabolic reactions and influences many body systems, including healthy bone mineralization, muscle contractions, heart rhythm, and nerve function.
Average dose: 250–500 mg/day.

Magnesium Citrate
The form of magnesium most absorbed into your body. Magnesium is used in 350 metabolic reactions and influences many body systems including healthy bone mineralization, muscle contractions, heart rhythm, and nerve function.
Average dose: 250–500 mg/day.

Magnesium-L-Threonate
Unlike other forms of the mineral, magnesium threonate readily crosses the blood-brain barrier and helps support brain cell connections—connections essential to memory and thought processes.
Average dose: 144 mg/day.

Mangosteen
Mangosteen antioxidants may help to maintain healthy weight and body fat composition.
Average dose: 100–200 mg/day.

Mannose (D-Mannose)
A natural sugar that has been studied for its potential ability to support a normal, healthy urinary tract.
Average dose: 1,000 mg/day.

Melatonin
Mostly known as the sleep hormone, melatonin has several functions throughout the body. Research shows it plays an important role in immunity, gastrointestinal health, and central nervous system function.
Average dose: varies from 1–12 mg/day.

Methylfolate
Methylfolate is involved in neurotransmitter synthesis and critical enzymatic reactions throughout the body. By depleting excess homocysteine, methylfolate benefits cardiovascular health and nervous system function. Optimal levels are necessary for healthy cell division and protein synthesis and are especially important for the maintenance of a healthy gastrointestinal tract.
Average dose: 500 mcg–1 mg/day.

Methylsulfonylmethane (MSM)
A sulfur-containing molecule found in various plants and some body tis-

sues. MSM is a vital building block of joints, cartilage, skin, hair, and nails. It is a natural and efficient source of the sulfur that is used by many of the body's structural molecules. Some peer-reviewed clinical research in the United States has shown MSM is safe and effective in increasing joint comfort and supporting a normal range of motion. MSM may also protect against radiation exposure during radiologic procedures.
Average dose: 1,000–3,000 mg/day.

Milk Thistle
See Silymarin.

Mucuna pruriens
A bean-like plant that contains levodopa (L-dopa), which is used to treat Parkinson's disease. L-dopa is changed to the chemical dopamine in the brain. Symptoms of Parkinson's disease occur in patients due to low levels of dopamine in the brain.
Average dose: 500–1,000 mg/day.

N-acetylcarnosine
A small protein (dipeptide) that helps prevent glycation reactions and may protect vision.
Average dose: 1 percent in eyedrops solution.

N-acetyl-cysteine (NAC)
Potent antioxidant that increases glutathione levels. It is the acetylated form of L-cysteine that has been used to maintain healthy secretions within the upper respiratory track and supports the immune and central nervous system.
Average dose: 600–1,800 mg/day.

NADH
A natural coenzyme derived from vitamin B_3 (niacin) is essential for basic metabolism, respiration, the breakdown of sugars and fats, and the production of ATP, the primary energy molecule in our cells.
Average dose: 5–20 mg/day.

Nattokinase
An enzyme that helps to maintain healthy fibrinolytic (clot removing) activity and clotting function and promotes healthy circulation and blood flow.
Average dose: 100 mg/day (from soy natto).

Natural Vitamin E (Stand-alone Supplement)
Maintains cell membrane integrity and reduces cellular aging, acts as a free radical scavenger, maintains healthy platelet aggregation, promotes a healthy nervous system and retina of the eye, maintains healthy cognitive function, and enhances immune function.
Average dose: 200–400 IU/day.

Nettles Root
Testosterone converts to estrogen at higher rates as men age. Prostate cells are sensitive to estrogen's growth stimulatory effects. It helps support prostate cells against the excess estrogen levels.
Average dose: 120–240 mg/day.

Niacin (Vitamin B$_3$)
It helps support healthy blood lipids and cholesterol. It's also critical for energy transfer reactions, particularly the metabolism of glucose, fat, and alcohol.
Average dose: 250–2,000 mg/day.

Olive Leaf Extract
Potent antioxidant. Helps to support healthy blood pressure.
Average dose: 500 mg/day.

Oregano Oil
It helps support a healthy microbial environment in the intestines and initiates a healthy immune response.
Average dose: 460 mg/day.

Panax Ginseng (Korean Ginseng)
An adaptogenic herb that helps people to respond better to stress. May have immune-boosting and cognitive-enhancing properties.
Average dose: 250 mg/day.

Passionflower
An herbaceous vine with tri-lobed leaves that's been used by Native Americans for hundreds of years for helping with insomnia.
Average dose: 250 mg/day.

Phosphatidylserine

A fat-soluble form of serine that's required for normal cellular structure and function. Brain tissues are especially rich in phosphatidylserine (PS), but aging causes a decline in the PS content of cells throughout the body. Research has shown that in addition to improving neural function, PS enhances energy metabolism in all cells, memory, concentration, learning, and word choice.

Average dose: 100 mg/day.

Picrorhiza Extract

A traditional herb grown in the Himalayan Mountains has been shown to help support a healthy liver and stomach. It has potent antioxidative and immune-supporting properties, and plays a role in gastric protection and healthy liver function.

Average dose: 50–100 mg/day.

Pine Bark Extract (Pycnogenol)

It promotes the integrity and normal characteristics of cell membranes, helps support normal DNA function through antioxidant activity, eases inflammation, reduces oxidative stress, and supports cellular metabolism of sugar.

Average dose: 100–200 mg/day.

Plum Extract

Plum antioxidants support osteoblast (bone building cells) activity and function by up-regulating cell-signaling compounds and enhancing expression of an enzyme that is involved in collagen cross-linking—an important step in building bone strength.

Average dose: 100 mg/day.

Policosanol (Alcohol Compounds from Sugar Cane Wax)

Potent antioxidant. It promotes healthy platelet function and helps to maintain cholesterol levels.

Average dose: 10–20 mg/day.

Pomegranate Extract

Potent antioxidant. Supports many parts of the cardiovascular system, including the inner lining of blood vessels called the endothelial cells, nitric oxide production, and blood pressure control.

Average dose: 500 mg/day.

PPC (Poly-enylphosphatidylcholine)
Potent antioxidant. It supports healthy liver function and incorporates into liver cell membranes to help restore its structure and the functioning of corresponding enzymes. This results in an increase in membrane fluidity and transport activity across the membrane. May also support healthy lipid and cholesterol levels and cognitive function.
Average dose: 900–1,800 mg/day.

PQQ (Pyrroloquinoline quinone)
A natural compound that supports healthy cell energy production and maintains healthy mitochondria number. May help support your heart, brain, and muscles.
Average dose: 10–20 mg/day.

Pregnenolone
Precursor to various hormones, such as progesterone, mineralocorticoids, glucocorticoids, androgens, and estrogens. So it can help the body maintain normal hormone levels, which in turn helps numerous body functions.
Average dose: varies based on blood serum testing.

Progesterone
A hormone. Restoring the body's supply of natural progesterone confers multiple health benefits, including balancing blood sugar levels, promoting normal sleep, reducing anxiety, and stimulating new bone growth.
Average dose: varies based on blood serum testing.

Propionyl-L-Carnitine
It enhances fatty acid metabolism, antioxidant activity and increased nitric oxide production. In addition, it promotes optimal blood flow and combats muscle fatigue by increasing energy and sparing glycogen stores.
Average dose: 500 mg/day.

Pygeum
An herbal extract that helps suppress prostaglandin E2, keeping the prostate gland placid and promoting prostate comfort.
Average dose: 100 mg/day.

Pyridoxal-5-Phosphate (P5P)

It's the metabolically active form of vitamin B_6 that has been shown to protect fats and proteins against glycation reactions—a dangerous reaction involving excess blood sugar. Also supports kidney function in diabetics.

Average dose: 100 mg/day.

Quercetin

Potent antioxidant. Helps maintain healthy sinuses during allergy season. Also supports cellular health and function. It's been shown to block inflammation-causing substances. It also helps promote a healthy cardiovascular system by preserving endothelial integrity and supporting healthy blood glucose levels.

Average dose: 500–1,000 mg/day.

Raft Forming Alginate

A suspension containing sodium alginate (polysaccharide in the cell walls of brown algae), sodium bicarbonate, and calcium carbonate used to treat upset stomach and heartburn.

Average dose: Comes prepared in solution that is diluted with water. Follow instructions on the label for proper use.

Red Yeast Rice

Red yeast rice is manufactured by the fermentation of a strain of yeast, *Monascus purpureas*, on rice. It may help maintain normal cholesterol levels, aid in digestion, circulation, and spleen and stomach health.

Average dose: 600–1,800 mg/day.

Reishi Mushroom Extract

This extracts broad-spectrum benefits have been demonstrated in thousands of studies. Reishi has been traditionally used to boost immune system vitality. It enhances the protective activity of the body's hematopoietic stem cells, T-cells, and other crucial immune factors. It also supports the body's production of endogenous antioxidant enzymes—such as superoxide dismutase (SOD), catalase, and glutathione.

Average dose: 980 mg/day.

Resveratrol Extract

Potent antioxidant. Supports a healthy cardiovascular system, including healthy blood pressure control and healthy lipid and cholesterol levels. May have weight loss properties and help improve cognition. Improves longevity in mice models.

Average dose: 250 mg/day of the trans-form.

Rhodiola Extract

An adaptogenic herb that supports a healthy stress response and several measures of mental performance, including associative thinking, short-term memory, concentration, calculation, and speed of audiovisual perception.

Average dose: 250 mg/day.

Ribose (D-ribose)

Can help speed energy recovery, increase energy reserves, and maintain healthy energy levels in heart and muscle tissue.

Average dose: 5–20 grams/day.

Rosmarinic Acid

A natural compound that helps support the immune system by sustaining normal white-blood cell function, including basophil, cytokine, and eosinophil functions. It also helps support healthy liver function, including phase I and II detoxification enzymes.

Average dose: 100–200 mg/day.

Saccharomyces boulardii

A beneficial yeast species that aids in the digestive process. Beneficial bacteria and yeast species are thought to have several presumably beneficial effects on immune function by increasing the number of IgA-producing plasma cells and helping to maintain healthy immune cell function. Saccharomyces may help reduce the symptoms with irritable bowel syndrome and inflammatory bowel disease.

Average dose: 250 mg/day.

Saffron Extract

A spice that helps support a healthy weight by decreasing sugar cravings and between-meal snacking. It also improves mood by increasing the effective time of serotonin within the central nervous system.

Average dose: 176.5 mg/day in two divided doses.

SAMe (S- adenosylmethionine)

An amino acid derivative that supports healthy cell growth, healthy gene expression, and healthy neuronal regeneration. It also helps to maintain stable mood and joint and liver function.

Average dose: 200–1,200 mg/day.

Saw Palmetto

A plant extract rich in bioactive, high-molecular weight compounds, including beta-sitosterol. It has been shown to interfere with DHT activity in the prostate, inhibit alpha-adrenergic receptor activity (to support normal urinary flow), and help *control* inflammatory actions in the prostate gland.

Average dose: 320 mg/day.

Schisandra chinensis

An adaptogenic vine native to Asia with a half-century of research and nearly 400 published studies that validate its system-wide benefits. Researchers have discovered that its fruit specifically supports healthy levels of liver *glutathione*—the cell's own antioxidant defense system.

Average dose: 250 mg/day.

Selenium (Stand-alone Supplement)

A mineral involved in hundreds of biological reactions. Selenium supports a healthy immune system, cardiovascular system, thyroid function, and healthy cell growth.

Average dose: 200–600 mcg/day.

Sesame Lignans

A plant-based antioxidant that helps to reduce excess estrogen and dihydrotesterone effects (DHT). It helps guard against dangerous lipid peroxidation and helps ease chronic inflammation.

Average dose: 100 mg/day.

Silymarin

Extracted from milk thistle and is known to support liver function and detoxification reactions.

Average dose: 600 mg/day.

Sphaeranthus indicus
An adaptogenic herb that may help to maintain healthy weight and body-fat composition.
Average dose: Best in combination with Mangosteen totaling 400 mg/day.

St. John's Wort
An herb that has been shown to inhibit the reuptake of several neuro-transmitters, such as serotonin, dopamine, noradrenaline, and GABA in the brain, and to reduce expression of interleukin-6. Each of these actions can contribute to alleviating low mood status by slowing the recycling of neurotransmitters needed for maintaining emotional balance.
Average dose: 300–600 mg/day.

Strontium
Is a trace mineral whose metabolism is closely linked to that of calcium; it resembles calcium at the molecular level. It supports healthy bone density.
Average dose: 750 mg/day.

Soluble Fibers
Soluble fibers create a unique "sponge-like" matrix then acts to impede excess calories from entering your bloodstream by absorbing water and quickly expanding in the stomach to make you feel full faster. They impede the breakdown of dietary fats by "soaking up" bile acids in the small intestine and shuttling them safely out of the body. Placebo-controlled studies confirm their ability to induce moderate weight loss by reducing the rate of carbohydrate absorption and consistently lowering after-meal elevations in blood glucose, triglyceride, and LDL cholesterol levels.
Average dose: varies based on individual needs.

Sulforaphane
A compound found in broccoli, as well as in other cruciferous vegetables, such as Brussels sprouts, cabbage, and cauliflower. According to the American Institute of Cancer Research, animal studies to date have shown that sulforaphane can dramatically reduce the number of malignant tumors, reproduction, growth rate and size, as well as delay cancer onset. It may also help reduce symptoms of COPD.
Average dose: 1–2 mg/day.

Superoxide Dismutase

Potent antioxidant. Maintains a healthy cardiovascular system by supporting the endothelium and minimizing the thickness of the arterial wall. *Average dose:* 500 mg/day.

Sytrinol (Citrus and Palm Antioxidants)

Helps maintain blood lipid and low-density lipoprotein (LDL) levels. *Average dose:* 300 mg/day.

Tart Cherry Extract

Eases chronic inflammation, maintains muscle function, promotes rapid muscle recovery after exercise, and brings faster relief from the minor aches, discomfort, and stiffness that can follow everyday muscle exertion. *Average dose:* 600–1,200 mg/day.

Taurine

An amino acid found abundantly in the body, particularly throughout the excitable tissues of the central nervous system, where it is thought to have a regulating influence. It promotes optimal blood flow to nervous tissue. It also appears to play an important role in many physiological processes, such as osmoregulation, immunomodulation, and bile salt formation. Recent studies suggested that it might have neuro- and cardio-protective properties and provide protection against oxidative stress. *Average dose:* 1 gram/day.

Thymus Extract

A natural immune organ that supports immune function. *Average dose:* 2–4 mcg/day.

Trimethylglycine (TMG)

A natural compound that promotes healthy levels of homocysteine, a cardiovascular disease risk factor. *Average dose:* 500–1,000 mg/day.

Tryptophan

An amino acid precursor to serotonin, the "feel good" neurotransmitter. It improves sleep, enhances mood, and modulates stress. *Average dose:* 1,000 mg/day.

Type II Collagen
Helps to support healthy joint function and cartilage formation.
Average dose: 10–40 mg/day.

Tyrosine
An amino acid that can be converted into thyroid hormones and in the brain and in the adrenal glands to dopamine, norepinephrine, and epinephrine (adrenaline) hormones that are depleted by stress, overwork, and certain drugs. By replenishing norepinephrine in the brain, mental energy levels may be improved.
Average dose: 500–1,000 mg/day.

Valerian
An herbal extract that traditionally used to help maintain relaxation and promote sleep.
Average dose: 500 mg/day.

Vinpocetine
Derived from vincamine, the major indole alkaloid of the periwinkle plant. When taken orally, vinpocetine is easily absorbed and it can: improve blood supply to the brain; increase oxygen and glucose use by the brain; maintain optimal energy of healthy brains; maintain normal coagulation of blood; maintain healthy levels of some neurotransmitters; promote healthy attention, memory, and concentration.
Average dose: 10–20 mg/day.

Vitamin D (Stand-alone Supplement)
Research has shown that almost every cell in the human body uses vitamin D. It's involved in hundreds if not thousands of biological reactions including bone mineralization, cardiovascular support, immune modulation, and cell growth and repair.
Average dose: varies based on serum blood level.

Watercress
A cousin to cruciferous vegetables, watercress has potential in the realm of cancer prevention and management. The anticancer benefits of watercress may arise from its ability to increase the level of antioxidants in the blood and to protect DNA against damage. In fact, growing evidence suggests that watercress may lower the risk of prostate, colon, and breast cancers, and may counteract certain processes by which cancers proliferate and spread.
Average dose: 50–100 mg/day.

Wormwood

An herb used for various digestion problems such as loss of appetite, upset stomach, gallbladder disease, and intestinal spasms. Wormwood is also used to treat fever, liver disease, and worm infections; to increase sexual desire; as a tonic; and to stimulate sweating.

Average dose: 500–1,000 mg/day.

Zeaxanthin

Natural pigmented antioxidant. Reduces photo-damage to the macula, a dense region of rods and cones in the retina, and supports healthy eye function. May have anticancer and heart protective properties.

Average dose: 2–4 mg/day.

Endnotes

Chapter 1

1 Casagrande S, et al. Have Americans increased their fruit and vegetable intake? The trends between 1988 and 2002. *Am J Prev Med* 2007 Apr;32(4):257–63.

2 Davis, Donald R. Declining fruit and vegetable nutrient composition: What is the evidence? *HortScience* Feb. 2009;44(1). http://depthome.brooklyn.cuny.edu/anthro/faculty/mitrovic/davis_2009_food_nutrient.pdf

3 Philpott, Tom. New research: Synthetic nitrogen destroys soil carbon, undermines soil health. Grist.org. Feb. 24, 2010. http://grist.org/article/2010–02–23-new-research-synthetic-nitrogen-destroys-soil-carbon-undermines/

4 Passwater, Richard A. Why foods alone are failing us: Significant declines found in the nutritional values of vegetables and fruits. *Whole Foods Magazine* July, 2006. www.drpasswater.com/nutrition_library/davis_2.html

5 David, Donald R, 2009.

6 Davis DR, Epp MD, Riordan HD. Changes in USDA food composition data for 43 garden crops, 1950 to 1999. *J Am Coll Nutr* 2004 Dec;23(6):669–82.

7 Winter, Dayna. Are these foods really healthy? *Prevention* Nov. 2011. www.prevention.com/weight-loss/weight-loss-tips/trans-fats-harmful-effects-unhealthy-fats-and-sugars

8 Bowman GL, et al. Nutrient biomarker patterns, cognitive function, and MRI measures of brain aging. *Neurology* 2012 Jan 24;78(4):241–9.

9 Singh-Manoux A, et al. Low HDL cholesterol is a risk factor for deficit and decline in memory in midlife: the Whitehall II study. *Arterioscler Thromb Vasc Biol.* 2008 Aug;28(8):1556–62.

10 Letter report on dietary reference intakes for trans fatty acids. Food and Nutrition Board, Institute of Medicine at the National Academy of Sciences. July 2002. www.uic.edu/depts/mcam/nutrition/pdf/IOMTransFatsummary.pdf

11 Jakszyn P, Gonzalez CA. Nitrosamine and related food intake and gastric and oesophogal cancer risk: a systematic review of the epidemiological evidence. *Word J Gastroenterol* 2006; 12(27):4296–303.

12 Park, Alice. Top 10 common household toxins: Butylated hydroxyanisole. *Time* April 1, 2010. www.time.com/time/specials/packages/article/0,28804,1976909_1976895_1976901,00. html

13 Carcinogenesis bioassay of propyl gallate (CAS No. 121–79–9) in F344 rats and B6C3F1 mice (feed study). National Toxicology Program, Technical Report Series No. 240. U.S. Department of Health and Human Services, Public Health Services, National Institutes of Health. 1982 Dec. http://ntp.niehs.nih.gov/ntp/htdocs/LT_rpts/tr240.pdf

14 Flinders University. Additives to avoid. http://ehlt.flinders.edu.au/education/DLiT/ 2006/food%20additives/theyare/avoid.htm

15 Fu, Rongjie. Selectivity comparison of Agilent Poroshell 120 phases in the separation of butter antioxidants. Agilent Technologies. www.chem.agilent.com/Library/applications/5991–1897EN.pdf

16 National Toxicology Program. Carcinogenesis Bioassay of propyl gallate (CAS NO. 121–79–9) in F344 rats and B6C3f1 mice (feed study). U.S. Department of Health and Human Services. http://ntp.niehs.nih.gov/ntp/htdocs/LT_rpts/tr240.pdf

17 Schardt, David. Sweet nothings: Not all sweeteners are Equal. *Nutrition Action Healthletter, Center for Science in the Public Interest* May 2004. www.cspinet.org/nah/05_04/ sweet_nothings.pdf

18 Center for Science in the Public Interest. *CSPI Reports* Oct. 24, 1997. www.cspinet.org/reports/saccomnt.htm

19 National Cancer Institute. Artificial Sweeteners and Cancer. Reviewed Aug. 5, 2009. www.cancer.gov/cancertopics/factsheet/Risk/artificial-sweeteners

20 Soffritti M, et al. Aspartame induces lymphomas and leukaemias in rats. *European Journal of Oncology* 2005; 10(2):107–116.

21 Lim U, et al. Consumption of aspartame-containing beverages and incidence of hematopoietic and brain malignancies. *Cancer Epidemiol Biomarkers Prev* 2006 Sep;15(9):1654–9.

22 Scherhammer E, et al. Consumption of artificial sweetener- and sugar-containing soda ad risk of lymphoma and leukemia in men and women. *Am J Clin Nutr* 2012 Dec. [Epub ahead of print] http://ajcn.nutrition.org/content/early/2012/10/23/ajcn.111.030833.abstract

23 Schardt, David, 2004.

24 Humphries P, Pretorius E, Naude H. Direct and indirect cellular effects of aspartame on the brain. *Eur J Clin Nutr* 2008;62:451–462.

25 Teff KL, et al. Endocrine and metabolic effects of consuming fructose- and glucose-sweetened beverages with meals in obese men and women: influence of insulin resistance on plasma triglyceride responses. *J Clin Endocrinol Metab* 2009 May;94(5):1562–9.

26 Ouyang X, et al. Fructose consumption as a risk factor for non-alcoholic fatty liver disease. *J Hepatol* 2008 Jun;48(6):993–9.

27 Stanhope KL, et al. Consuming fructose-sweetened, not glucose-sweetened, beverages increases visceral adiposity and lipids and decreases insulin sensitivity in overweight/ obese humans. *J Clin Invest* 2009 May; 119(5):1322–34.

28 Taubes, Gary. *Good Calories, Bad Calories.* New York: Anchor Books, 2008: 201.

29 Brown CM, et al. Fructose ingestion acutely elevates blood pressure in healthy young humans. *Am J Physiol Regul Integr Comp Physiol.* 2008 Mar;294(3):R730–7.

30 Stanhope KL, 2009.

31 Choi HK, Willet W, Curhan G. Fructose-rich beverages and risk of gout in women. *JAMA* 2010 Nov 24;304(2):2270–8.

32 Choi HK, Curhan G. Soft drinks, fructose consumption, and the risk of gout in men: prospective cohort study. *BMJ*. 2008 Feb 9;336(7639):309–12.

33 Hennessey, Rachel. Living in color: The potential dangers of artificial dyes. *Forbes* August 27, 2012. www.forbes.com/sites/rachelhennessey/2012/08/27/living-in-color-the-potential-dangers-of-artificial-dyes/

34 Weil, Andrew. Q&A Library: Avoiding hormones in meat and poultry? DrWeil.com. Oct. 31, 2006. www.drweil.com/drw/u/id/QAA400066

35 Tavernise, Sabrina. Farm use of antibiotics defies scrutiny. *The New York Times* Sept. 3 2012. www.nytimes.com/2012/09/04/health/use-of-antibiotics-in-animals-raised-for-food-defies-scrutiny.html?pagewanted=all&_r=0

36 Tavernise, Sabrina, 2012.

37 Environmental Working Group. Pesticides. www.ewg.org/meateatersguide/interactive-graphic/pesticides/

38 U.S. Department of Agriculture Office of Inspector General. FSIS National Residue Program for Cattle. Audit Report 24601–08-KC. March 2010. http://usatoday30.usatoday.com/news/washington/2010–04–12-tainted-meat_N.htm#table

39 U.S. Environmental Protection Agency. What is the TSCA chemical substance inventory? EPA.gov. Updated Sept. 28, 2012. www.epa.gov/oppt/newchems/pubs/invntory.htm

40 U.S. Environmental Protection Agency. TSCA at Twenty. Chemicals in the Environment. Fall 1996. http://nepis.epa.gov/Exe/ZyNET.exe/20001KXT.TXT?ZyActionD=ZyDocument&Client=EPA&Index=1995+Thru+1999&Docs=&Query=&Time=&EndTime=&SearchMethod=1&TocRestrict=n&Toc=&TocEntry=&QField=&QFieldYear=&QFieldMonth=&QFieldDay=&IntQFieldOp=0&ExtQFieldOp=0&XmlQuery=&File=D%3A%5Czyfiles%5CIndex%20Data%5C95thru99%5CTxt%5C00000005%5C20001KXT.txt&User=ANONYMOUS&Password=anonymous&SortMethod=h%7C&MaximumDocuments=1&FuzzyDegree=0&ImageQuality=r75g8/r75g8/x150y150g16/i425&Display=p%7Cf&DefSeekPage=x&SearchBack=ZyActionL&Back=ZyActionS&BackDesc=Results%20page&MaximumPages=1&ZyEntry=1&SeekPage=x&ZyPURL

41 HPV Chemical Hazard Data Availability Study. U.S. Environmental Protection Agency. August 2, 2010. www.epa.gov/hpv/pubs/general/hazchem.htm

42 Duncan, David Ewing. Chemicals within us. *National Geographic* Oct. 2006. http://science.nationalgeographic.com/science/health-and-human-body/human-body/chemicals-within-us/#page=1

43 Good Guide. Pollution Locator: Toxic Chemical Releases. Scorecard: The Pollution Information Site. http://scorecard.goodguide.com/env-releases/us-map.tcl

44 Dichlorodiphenyltrichloroethane (DDT) ubiquity, persistence, and risks. *Environ Health Perspect* 2002 Feb;110(2):125–8.

45 Doheny, Kathleen. Household chemicals linked to heart disease. WebMD.com. Sept. 4, 2012. www.webmd.com/heart-disease/news/20120904/household-chemical-linked-heart-disease

46 Department of Health and Human Services, Centers for Disease Control and Prevention. Fourth National Report on Human Exposure to Environmental Chemicals. Executive Summary. 2009:3. www.cdc.gov/exposurereport/pdf/FourthReport_ExecutiveSummary.pdf

47 Department of Health and Human Services, Centers for Disease Control and Prevention, 2009.

48 Agency for Toxic Substances & Disease Registry. Toxic Substances Portal: Polybrominated biphenyls (PBBs) & Polybrominated Diphenyl Ethers. Sept. 2004. www.atsdr.cdc.gov/toxfaqs/tf.asp?id=900&tid=94#bookmark04

49 Environmental Working Group. Body Burden: The pollution in newborns. Executive Summary. July 14, 2005. www.ewg.org/reports/bodyburden2/execsumm.php

50 New York-Presbyterian Hospital. Cancer surpasses heart disease as number one cause of death in Americans under age 85. *Cancer Prevention Newsletter* Spring 2005, Issue 5. www.nypcancerprevention.com/issue/5/con/features/cancer-surpasses-heart-di.shtml

51 American Cancer Society. Lifetime risk of developing or dying from cancer. Last revised Nov. 29, 2012. www.cancer.org/cancer/cancerbasics/lifetime-probability-of-developing-or-dying-from-cancer

52 American Cancer Society, Last revised Nov. 29, 2012.

53 Davis, Devra. Off target in the war on cancer. *The Washington Post* Nov. 4, 2007:B1–B4. www.washingtonpost.com/wp-dyn/content/article/2007/11/02/AR2007110201648.html

54 Top scientists warn of chemical contamination, rising cancer rates. EurActive.com. May 12, 2004. www.euractiv.com/sustainability/top-scientists-warn-chemical-contamination-rising-cancer-rates/article-117849

55 Weil, Andrew. Weekly Bulletin: Herbal oils thwart germs. DrWeil.com. www.drweil.com/drw/u/WBL02195/Herbal-Oils-Thwart-Germs.html

56 USDA. Pesticide data program. Annual Summary, Calendar Year 2006. Dec. 2007:x. www.ams.usda.gov/AMSv1.0/getfile?dDocName=STELPRDC5064786

57 Environmental Working Group. EWG's 2012 Shopper's Guide to Pesticides in Produce™. EWG.org. June 19, 2012. www.ewg.org/foodnews/summary/

58 Chronic stress and mortality among older adults. *JAMA* 1999 Dec;282(23):2259–2260.

59 Simon, Harvey, reviewer. Stress – Complications. University of Maryland Medical Center. Last reviewed Feb. 13 2009. www.umm.edu/patiented/articles/what_health_consequences_of_stress_000031_3.htm

60 Carnegie Mellon University. Press Release: How stress influences disease: Carnegie Mellon study reveals inflammation as the culprit. Carnegie Mellon University. April 2, 2012. www.cmu.edu/news/stories/archives/2012/april/april2_stressdisease.html

Chapter 3

1 CFR – Code of Federal Regulations Title 21, Volume 2. U.S. Food and Drug Administration. Revised April 1, 2012.www.accessdata.fda.gov/scripts/cdrh/cfdocs/cfCFR/CFRSearch.cfm?CFRPart=111&showFR=1

2 FDA warns consumers against dietary supplement products that may contain digitalis mislabeled as "plantain." International Food Safety Network. June 12, 1997. http://foodsafety.k-state.edu/en/news-details.php?a=4&c=30&sc=218&id=7161

3 U.S. Food and Drug Administration. Guidance for industry: Current Good Manufacturing Practice in manufacturing, packaging, labeling, or holding operations for dietary supplements; small entity compliance guide. Dec. 2010. www.fda.gov/Food/Guidance ComplianceRegulatoryInformation/GuidanceDocuments/SmallBusinessesSmallEntity-ComplianceGuides/ucm238182.htm

4 Tsouderos, Trine. Dietary supplements: Manufacturing troubles widespread, FDA inspections show. *Chicago Tribune.* June 30, 2012. http://articles.chicagotribune.com/2012–06–30/news/ct-met-supplement-inspections-20120630_1_dietary-supplements-inspections-american-herbal-products-association

5 Adams M. Titanium dioxide in vitamins and supplements: Is it safe for human consumption? NaturalNews.com. Sept. 9, 2009. www.naturalnews.com/027000_titanium_dioxide_vitamins.html

Chapter 4

1 Nurmatov U, Devereux G, Sheik A. Nutrients and foods for the primary prevention of asthma and allergy: systematic review and meta-analysis. *J Allergy Clin Immunol* 2011 Mar: 127(3):724–33.

2 Semba RD. The role of vitamin A and related retinoids in immune function. *Nutr Rev* 1998 Jan: 56 (1 Pt 2):S38–48.

3 Huang CR, et al. Serial nerve conduction studies in vitamin B12 deficiency-associated polyneuropathy. *Neurol Sci* 2011 Feb; 32(1):183–6.

4 Bleie Ø, et al. Coronary blood flow in patients with stable coronary artery disease treated long term with folic acid and vitamin B12. *Coron Artery Dis* 2011 Jun; 22(4):270–8.

5 Woolard KJ, et al. Effects of oral vitamin C on monocyte: endothelial cell adhesion in healthy subjects. *Biochem Biophys Res Commun* 2002 Jun 28; 294(5):1161–8.

6 Simon JA, Hudes ES, Perez-Perez GI. Relation of serum ascorbic acid to Helicobacter pylori serology in US adults: the Third National Health and Nutrition Examination Survey. *J Am Coll Nutr.* 2003 Aug;22(4):283–9.

7 Jimenez-Lara AM. Colorectal cancer: potential therapeutic benefits of vitamin D. *Int J Biochem Cell Biol* 2007; 39:672–677.

8 Bischoff-Ferrari HA, et al. Effect of Vitamin D on falls: a meta-analysis. *JAMA* 2004 Apr 28:291(16):1999–2006.

9 Sigounas G, Anagnostou A, Steiner M. dl-alpha-tocopherol induces apoptosis in erythroleukemia, prostate, and breast cancer cells. *Nutr Cancer* 1997; 28(1):30–5.

10 Jiang Q, Wong J, Ames BN. Gamma-tocopherol induces apoptosis in androgen-responsive LNCaP prostate cancer cells via caspase-dependent and independent mechanisms. *Ann NY Acad Sci* 2004 Dec; 1031:399–400.

11 Cockayne S, et al. Vitamin K and the prevention of fracture: systematic review and meta-analysis of randomized controlled trials. *Arch Intern Med* 2006 Jun 26; 166(12):1256–61.

12 Geleijnse JM, et al. Dietary intake of menaquinone is associated with a reduced risk of coronary heart disease: the Rotterdam Study. *J Nutr* 2004 Nov; 134(11): 3100–5.

13 Zemel MB, et al. Regulation of adiposity by dietary calcium. *FASEB J* 2000 Jun; 14(9): 1132–8.

14 Lamson DW, Plaza SM. The safety and efficacy of high-dose chromium. *Altern Med Rev* 2002 Jun; 7(3):218–35.

15 Shay CM, et al. Nutrient and food intakes of middle-aged adults at low risk of cardiovascular disease: the international study of macro-/micronutrients and blood pressure (INTERMAP). *Eur J Nutr* 2012 Dec; 51(8):917–26.

16 Lowe NM, et al. Is there a potential therapeutic value of copper and zinc for osteoporosis? *Proc Nutr Soc* 2002 May; 61(2): 181–5.

17 Joosten MM, Gansevoort RT, Mukamal KJ, van der Harst P, Geleijnse JM, Feskens EJ, Navis G, Bakker SJ; PREVEND Study Group.Urinary and plasma magnesium and risk of ischemic heart disease. *Am J Clin Nutr.* 2013 Jun;97(6):1299–306.

18 Stone C, et al. Role of selenium in HIV infection. *Nutr Rev* 2010 Nov; 68(11):671–81.

19 Chaimowitz NS, et al. A disintegrin and metalloproteinase 10 regulates antibody production and maintenance of lymphoid architecture. *J Immunol* 2011 Nov 15; 187(10): 5114–22.

20 Su KP, et al. Omega-3 fatty acids in major depressive disorder. A preliminary double-blind, placebo- controlled trial. *Eur Neuropsychopharmacol* 2003 Aug;13(4):267–71.

21 Stoll AL, et al. Omega-3 fatty acids and bipolar disorder: a review. *Prostaglandins Leukot Essent Fatty Acids* 1999 May–June; 60(5–6): 329–37.

22 Zanarini MC, Frankenburg FR. Omega-3 fatty acid treatment of women with borderline personality disorder: a double-blind, placebo-controlled pilot study. *Am J Psychiatry* 2003 Jan; 160(1):167–9.

23 Peet M, Stokes C. Omega-3 fatty acids in the treatment of psychiatric disorders. *Drugs.* 2005;65(8):1051–9.

24 Horrobin DF, et al. Eicosapentaenoic acid and arachidonic acid: collaboration and not antagonism is the key to biological understanding. *Prostaglandin Leukot Essent Fatty Acids* 2002 Jan; 66(1):83–90.

25 Richardson AJ, Montgomery P. The Oxford-Durham study: a randomized, controlled trial of dietary supplementation with fatty acids in children with developmental coordination disorder. *Pediatrics* 2005 May; 115(5):1360–6.

26 Van Gelder BM, et al. Fish consumption, n-3 fatty acids, and subsequent 5-y cognitive decline in elderly men: the Zutphen Elderly Study. *Am J Clin Nutr* 2007 Apr; 85(4): 1142–7.

27 Morris MC, Evans DA, Bienias JL, Tangney CC, Bennett DA, Wilson RS, Aggarwal N, Schneider J.

Consumption of fish and n-3 fatty acids and risk of incident Alzheimer disease. *Arch Neurol.* 2003 Jul;60(7):940–6.

28 Durrington PN, et al. An omega-3 polyunsaturated fatty acid concentrate administered for one year decreased triglycerides in simvastatin treated patients with coronary heart disease and persisting hypertriglyceridaemia. *Heart* 2001;85:544–548.

29 Geleijnse JM, et al. Blood pressure response to fish oil supplementation: metaregression analysis of randomized trials. *J Hypertens* 2002;20:1493–1499.

30 Yokoyama M, et al. Effects of eicosapentaenoic acid on major coronary events in hyper-

cholesterolaemic patients (JELIS): a randomised open-label, blinded endpoint analysis. *Lancet* 2007 Mar 31; 369(9567):1090–8.

31 Wilk JB, et al. Plasma and dietary omega-3 fatty acids, fish intake, and heart failure risk in the Physicians' Health Study. *Am J Clin Nutr* 2012 Oct; 96(4):882–8.

32 Marchioli R, et al. Efficacy of n-3 polyunsaturated fatty acids after myocardial infarction: results of GISSI-Prevenzione trial. Gruppo Italiano per lo Studio della Sopravvivenza nell'Infarto Miocardico. *Lipids* 2001; 36Suppl:S119–26.

33 Chrysohoou C, et al. Long-term fish consumption is associated with protection against arrhythmia in healthy persons in a Mediterranean region—the ATTICA study. *Am J Clin Nutr* 2007 May: 85(5):1385–91.

34 Kim YJ, et al. Anti-inflammatory action of dietary fish oil and calorie restriction. *Life Sciences* 2006; 78(21):2523–6.

35 U.S. Department of Health and Human Services, U.S. Department of Agriculture. Dietary Guidelines Advisory Committee Meeting. Meeting Summary. Jan. 28, 2004:34. www.health.gov/dietaryguidelines/dga2005/dgac012004minutes.pdf

36 Kiecolt-Glaser JK. Depressive symptoms, omega-6:omega-3 fatty acids, and inflammation in older adults. *Psychosomatic Medicine* 2007;69:217–224.

37 Kiecolt-Glaser JK, 2007.

38 Hibbeln J, et al. Healthy intakes of n-3 and n-6 fatty acids: estimations considering worldwide diversity. *Amer J Clin Nutr* 2006 Jun;83(6 Suppl):1483S–1493S.

39 Jegtvig, Shereen. How much omega-3 fatty acid is in fish? About.com. Jan 20, 2013. http://nutrition.about.com/od/askyournutritionist/f/calculateomega.htm

40 Fotino AD, Thompson-Paul AM, Bazzano LA. Effect of coenzyme Q10 supplementation on heart failure: a meta-analysis. *Am J Clin Nutr* 2013 Feb; 97(2):268–75.

41 Adarsh K, Kaur H, Mohan V. Coenzyme Q10 (CoQ10) in isolated diastolic heart failure in hypertrophic cardiomyopathy (HCM). *Biofactors* 2008;32(1–4):145–9.

42 Nahas R. Complementary and alternative medicine approaches to blood pressure reduction: An evidence-based review. *Can Fam Physician* 2008 Nov; 54(11): 1529–33.

43 Singh RB, et al. Effect of coenzyme Q10 on risk of atherosclerosis in patients with recent myocardial infarction. *Mol Cell Biochem* 2003 Apr;246(1–2):75–82.

44 Shults CW, et al. Effects of coenzyme q10 in early Parkinson disease: evidence of slowing of the functional decline. *Arch Neurol* 2002;59:1541–1550.

45 Muller T, et al. Coenzyme Q(10) supplementation provides mild symptomatic benefit in patients with Parkinson's disease. *Neurosci Lett* 2003;341:201–204.

46 Hodgson JM, et al. Coenzyme Q(10) improves blood pressure and glycaemic control: a controlled trial in subjects with type 2 diabetes. *Eur J Clin Nutr* 2002;56:1137–1142.

47 Singh RB, et al. Effect of hydrosoluble coenzyme Q 10 on blood pressures and insulin resistance in hypertensive patients with coronary artery disease. *J Human Hypertens* 1999;13:203–208.

48 Porter DA, et al. The effect of oral coenzyme Q10 on the exercise tolerance of middle-aged, untrained men. *Int J Sports Med* 1995 Oct;16(7):421–7.

49 Zheng A, Moritani T. Influence of CoQ10 on autonomic nervous activity and energy

metabolism during exercise in healthy subjects. *J Nutr Sci Vitaminol* (Tokyo). 2008 Aug;54(4):286–90.

50 Kalén A, Appelkvist EL, Dallner G. Age-related changes in the lipid compositions of rat and human tissues. *Lipids* 1989 Jul;24(7):579–84.

51 Ghirlanda G, et al. Evidence of plasma CoQ10-lowering effect by HMG-CoA reductase inhibitors: a double-blind, placebo-controlled study. *J Clin Pharmacol* 1993 Mar;33(3):226–9.

52 Furness JB, Kunze WA, Clerc N. Nutrient tasting and signaling mechanisms in the gut. II. The intestine as a sensory organ: neural, endocrine, and immune responses. *Am J Physiol* 1999 Nov;277(5 Pt 1):G922–8.

53 Rowland I, et al. Current levels of consensus on probiotic science—report of an expert meeting—London, 23 November 2009. *Gut Microbes* 2010 Nov–Dec; 1(6): 436–9.

54 Siitonen S, et al. Effect of *Lactobacillus GG* yoghurt in the prevention of antibiotic associated diarrhoea. *Ann Med* 1990; 22:57–59.

55 De Paula JA, Carmuega E, Weill R. Effect of the ingestion of a symbiotic yogurt on the bowel habits of women with functional constipation. *Acta Gastroenterol Latinoam* 2008;38:16–25.

56 Lesbros-Pantoflickova D, Corthésy-Theulaz I, Blum AL. Heliobacter pylori and probiotics. *J Nutr* 2007 Mar;137(3 Suppl 2):812S–8S.

57 Whelan K, Quigley EM. Probiotics in the management of irritable bowel syndrome and inflammatory bowel disease. *Curr Opin Gastroenterol* 2013 Mar; 29(2):184–9.

58 Whelan K, 2013.

59 American Nutrition Association. The Science of Probiotics. *Nutrition Digest* Spring, 2006. Volume 36, No. 3. http://americannutritionassociation.org/newsletter/science-probiotics

60 Tlaskalová-Hogenová H, et al. Commensal bacteria (normal microflora), mucosal immunity and chronic inflammatory and autoimmune diseases. *Immunol Lett* 2004 May 15;93(2–3):97–108.

61 Brenner DM. Probiotics for the treatment of adult gastrointestinal disorders. American College of Gastroenterology. Patient Education & Resource Center. http://patients.gi.org/topics/probiotics-for-the-treatment-of-adult-gastrointestinal-disorders/

62 Paturi G, et al. Immune enhancing effects of *Lactobacillus acidophilus* LAFTI L10 and *Lactobacillus paracasei* LAFTI L26 in mice. *Int J Food Microbiol.* 2007 Apr 1;115(1):115–8. Epub 2006 Nov 28.

63 Marcos A, et al. The effect of milk fermented by yogurt cultures plus Lactobacillus casei DN-114001 on the immune response of subjects under academic examination stress. *Eur J Nutr.* 2004 Dec;43(6):381–9.

64 Kontiokari T, et al. Dietary factors protecting women from urinary tract infection. *Am J Clin Nutr* 2003 Mar;77(3):600–4.

65 Falagas ME, Betsi GI, Athanasiou S. Probiotics for prevention of recurrent vulvovaginal candidiasis: a review. *J Antimicrob Chemother* 2006 Aug;58(2):266–72.

66 Anukam K, et al. Augmentation of antimicrobial metronidazole therapy of bacterial vaginosis with oral probiotic Lactobacillus rhamnosus GR-1 and Lactobacillus reuteri RC-14: randomized, double-blind, placebo controlled trial. *Microbes Infect* 2006 May;8(6): 1450–4.

67 The restoration of the vaginal microbiota after treatment for bacterial vaginosis with metronidazole or probiotics.Ling Z, Liu X, Chen W, Luo Y, Yuan L, Xia Y, Nelson KE, Huang S, Zhang S, Wang Y, Yuan J, Li L, Xiang C. *Microb Ecol.* 2013 Apr;65(3):773–80.

68 Rossi M, Amaretti A, Raimondi S. Folate production by probiotic bacteria. *Nutrients* 2011 Jan; 3(1):118–34.

69 Rehman A, et al. Effects of probiotics and antibiotics on the intestinal homeostasis in a computer controlled model of the large intestine. *BMC Microbiology* 2012;12:47.

70 Hsieh MH, Versalovic J. The human microbiome and probiotics: Implications for pediatrics. *Curr Probl Pediatr Adolesc Health Care* 2008 Nov–Dec; 38(10): 309–327.

71 Mikelsaar M, et al. Effect of probiotic Heart cheese "Harmony" comprising bacteria L. plantarum TENSIA DSM 21380 on blood pressure and metabolic health indices. [Article in Russian]. *Vopr Pitan* 2012; 81(3):74–81.

72 Chang BJ, et al. Effect of functional yogurt NY-YP901 in improving the trait of metabolic syndrome. *Eur J Clin Nutr* 2011 Nov: 65(11):1250–5.

73 Chen J, et al. Bifidobacterium adolescentis supplementation ameliorates visceral fat accumulation and insulin sensitivity in an experimental model of the metabolic syndrome. *Br J Nutr* 2012 May; 107(10):1429–34.

74 Denipote FG, Trinidade EB, Burini RC. [Probiotics and prebiotics in primary care for colon cancer.] *Arg Gastroenterol* 2010 Jan–Mar;47(1):93–8.

75 El-Nezami HS, et al. Probiotic supplementation reduces a biomarker for increased risk of liver cancer in young men from Southern China. *Am J Clin Nutr* 2006 May; 83(5):1199–203.

76 Naito S, et al. Prevention of recurrence with epirubicin and lactobacillus casei after transurethral resection of bladder cancer. *J Urol* 2008 Feb; 179(2):485–90.

77 Woodmansey EJ. Intestinal bacteria and ageing. *J Appl Microbiol* 2007;102:1178–1186. http://download.bioon.com.cn/upload/month_0911/20091107_53c3e8215cc66e93e53eto-JiihA7HW3O.attach.pdf

78 Tripkovic L, et al. Comparison of vitamin D2 and vitamin D3 supplementation in raising serum 25-hydroxyvitamin D status: a systematic review and meta-analysis. *Am J Clin Nutr* 2012 Jun;95(6):1357–64.

79 Heaney RP, et al. Vitamin D3 is more potent than vitamin D2 in humans. *J Clin Endocrinol Metab* 2011 Mar;96(3):E447–52.

80 Wong RS and Radhakrishan AK. Tocotrienol research: past into present. *Nutr Rev.* 2012 Sep;70(9):483–90.

81 Sakhaee K, et al. Meta-analysis of calcium bioavailability: a comparison of calcium citrate with calcium carbonate. *Am J Ther* 1999 Nov;6(6):313–21.

82 Shults CW, et al. Effects of coenzyme Q10 in early Parkinson disease: evidence of slowing of the functional decline. *Arch Neurol* 2002 Oct;59(10):1541–50.

83 Langsjoen PH, Langsjoen AM. Overview of the use of CoQ10 in cardiovascular disease. *Biofactors* 1999;9(2–4):273–84.

84 Hosoe K, et al. Study on safety and bioavailability of ubiquinol (Kaneka QH(trade mark)) after single and 4-week multiple oral administration to healthy volunteers. *Regul Toxicol Pharmacol* 2006 Aug 17.

Chapter 5

1 Champeau R. Most heart attack patients' cholesterol levels did not indicate cardiac risk. UCLA Newsroom. Jan 11, 2009. http://newsroom.ucla.edu/portal/ucla/majority-of-hospitalized-heart-75668.aspx

2 Homocysteine Studies Collaboration. Homocysteine and risk of ischemic heart disease and stroke: a meta-analysis. *JAMA* 2002 Oct 23–30;288(16):2015–22.

3 Brod SA. Unregulated inflammation shortens human functional longevity. *Inflamm Res* 2000 Nov;49(11):561–70.

4 Morgan D. Low vitamin D raises blood pressure in women: study. Reuters. Sept. 23, 2009. www.reuters.com/article/2009/09/23/us-heart-vitamin-idUSTRE58M6HT20090923

5 Dong Y, et al. A 16-week randomized clinical trial of 2000 international units daily vitamin D3 supplementation in black youth: 25-hydroxyvitamin D, adiposity, and arterial stiffness. *J Clin Endocrinol Metab* 2010 Oct;95(10):4584–91.

6 Wang TJ, et al. Vitamin D deficiency and risk of cardiovascular disease. *Circulation* 2008 Jan 29;117(4):503–11.

7 Attia P. The straight dope on cholesterol – part VII. The Eating Academy. June 13, 2012. http://eatingacademy.com/nutrition/the-straight-dope-on-cholesterol-part-vii

8 Goswami B, et al. Apo-B/apo-AI ratio: a better discriminator of coronary artery disease risk than other conventional lipid ratios in Indian patients with acute myocardial infarction. *Acta Cardiol* 2008 Dec;63(6):749–55

9 Sierra-Johnson J, et al. Concentration of apolipoprotein B is comparable with the apolipoprotein B/apolipoprotein A-I ratio and better than routine clinical lipid measurements in predicting coronary heart disease mortality: findings from a multi-ethnic US population. *Eur Heart J* 2009 Mar;30(6):710–7.

10 de Boer RA, Yu L, Veldhuisen DJ. Galectin-3 in cardiac remodeling and heart failure. *Curr Heart Fail Rep* 2010 March;7(1):1–8. www.ncbi.nlm.nih.gov/pmc/articles/PMC 2831188/

11 Brod SA, 2000.

12 Milne GL, Musiek ES, Morrow JD. F2-isoprostanes as markers of oxidative stress in vivo: an overview. *Biomarkers* 2005 Nov;10 Suppl 1:S10–23.

13 Centers for Disease Control. National diabetes fact sheet: national estimates and general information on diabetes and prediabetes in the United States, 2011. Atlanta, GA: U.S. Department of Health and Human Services, Center for Disease Control and Prevention, 2011. www.cdc.gov/diabetes/pubs/pdf/ndfs_2011.pdf

14 Centers for Disease Control. Diabetes: Successes and opportunities for population-based prevention and control at a glance 2011. Department of Health and Human Services, Center for Disease Control and Prevention, 2011. www.cdc.gov/chronicdisease/resources/publications/AAG/ddt.htm

15 American Heart Association. Cardiovascular disease & diabetes. Jan. 31, 2013. www.heart.org/HEARTORG/Conditions/Diabetes/WhyDiabetesMatters/Cardiovascular-Disease-Diabetes_UCM_313865_Article.jsp

16 Bone fractures can double or triple mortality for up to 10 years. *Garvan Institute* Feb. 4,

2009. www.garvan.org.au/news-events/news/bone-fractures-can-double-or-triple-mortality-for-up-to-10-years.html

17 Rossouw JE. Effect of postmenopausal hormone therapy on cardiovascular risk. *J Hypertens Suppl* 2002 May;20(2):S62–5.

18 Grady D, et al. Effect of postmenopausal hormone therapy on cognitive function: the Heart and Estrogen/progestin Replacement Study. *Am J Med* 2002 Nov;113(7):543–8.

19 Hulley S, et al. Noncardiovascular disease outcomes during 6.8 years of hormone therapy: Heart and Estrogen/progestin Replacement Study follow-up (HERS II). *JAMA* 2002 Jul 3;288(1):58–66.

20 Azoulay C. [Menopause in 2004: "hormone replacement therapy" is not what it used to be anymore]. [Article in French] *Rev Med Interne* 2004 Nov;25(11):806–15.

21 Ragaz J. Adjuvant trials of aromatase inhibitors: determining the future landscape of adjuvant endocrine therapy. *J Steroid Biochem Mol Biol* 2001 Dec;79(1–5):133–41.

22 Rossouw JE, Anderson GL, Prentice RL, LaCroix AZ, Kooperberg C, Stefanick ML, Jackson RD, Beresford SA, Howard BV, Johnson KC, Kotchen JM, Ockene J; Writing Group for the Women's Health Initiative Investigators. Risks and benefits of estrogen plus progestin in healthy postmenopausal women: principal results From the Women's Health Initiative randomized controlled trial. *JAMA.* 2002 Jul 17;288(3):321–33.

23 Antunes CM, Strolley PD, Rosenshein NB, Davies JL, Tonascia JA, Brown C, Burnett L, Rutledge A, Pokempner M, Garcia R. Endometrial cancer and estrogen use. Report of a large case-control study. *N Engl J Med.* 1979 Jan 4;300(1):9–13.

24 Moskowitz D. A comprehensive review of the safety and efficacy of bioidentical hormones for the management of menopause and related health risks. *Altern Med Rev* 2006 Sep;11(3):208–23.

25 Holtorf K. The bioidentical hormone debate: are bioidentical hormones (estradiol, estriol, and progesterone) safer or more efficacious than commonly used synthetic versions in hormone replacement therapy? *Postgrad Med* 2009 Jan;12(1):73–85.

26 Hoffman M. Low testosterone: How to talk to your doctor. *Web MD Men's Health* 2008. http://men.webmd.com/features/low-testosterone-how-to-talk-to-your-doctor

27 Slowik G (ed). Prostate enlargement. ehealthMD.com. Last updated April 23, 2012. http://ehealthmd.com/content/what-causes-prostate-enlarge#axzz2RXmhWZT6

28 Roehrborn CG. Benign prostatic hyperplasia: an overview. *Rev Urol.* 2005;7 Suppl 9:S3-S14.

29 Tammela TL. Endocrine prevention and treatment of prostate cancer.*Mol Cell Endocrinol.* 2012 Sep 5;360(1–2):59–6

30 Setlur SR, Chen CX, Hossain RR, Ha JS, Van Doren VE, Stenzel B, Steiner E, Oldridge D, Kitabayashi N, Banerjee S, Chen JY, Schäfer G, Horninger W, Lee C, Rubin MA, Klocker H, Demichelis F. Genetic variation of genes involved in dihydrotestosterone metabolism and the risk of prostate cancer. *Cancer Epidemiol Biomarkers* Prev. 2010 Jan;19(1):229–39.

31 Abbott RD, et al. Serum estradiol and risk of stroke in elderly men. *Neurology* 2007 Feb 20;68(8):563–8.

32 Phillips GB, Pinkernell BH, Jing TY. The association of hypotestosteronemia with coronary artery disease in men. *Arterioscler Thromb* 1994 May;14(5):701–6.

33 Dunajska K, et al. Evaluation of sex hormone levels and some metabolic factors in men with coronary atherosclerosis. *Aging Male* 2004 Sep;7(3):197–204.

34 Wranicz JK, et al. The relationship between sex hormones and lipid profile in men with coronary artery disease. *Int J Cardiol* 2005 May 11;101(1):105–10.

35 Callou de Sá EQ, Feijó de Sá FC, e Silva Rde S, de Oliveira KC, Guedes AD, Feres F, Verreschi IT. Endogenous oestradiol but not testosterone is related to coronary artery disease in men. *Clin Endocrinol* (Oxf). 2011 Aug;75(2):177–83.

36 Prins GS, Korach KS. The role of estrogens and estrogen receptors in normal prostate growth and disease. *Steroids* 2008 Mar;73(3):233–44.

37 Matsuda T, Abe H, Suda K. Relation between benign prostatic hyperplasia and obesity and estrogen. *Rinsho Byori* 2004 Apr;52(4):291–4.

38 Ho CK, et al. Oestrogen and benign prostatic hyperplasia: effects on stromal cell proliferation and local formation from androgen. *J Endocrinol* 2008 Jun;197(3):483–91.

39 Singh PB, Matanhelia SS, Martin FL. A potential paradox in prostate adenocarcinoma progression: oestrogen as the initiating driver. *Eur J Cancer* 2008 May;44(7):928–36.

40 Giton F, et al. Estrone sulfate (E1S), a prognosis marker for tumor aggressiveness in prostate cancer (PCa). *J Steroid Biochem Mol Biol* 2008 Mar;109(1–2):158–67.

41 Mellström D, et al. Older men with low serum estradiol and high serum SHBG have an increased risk of fractures. *J Bone Miner Res* 2008 Oct;23(10):1552–60.

42 Pernow Y, et al. Bone histomorphometry in male idiopathic osteoporosis. *Calcif Tissue Int* 2009 Jun;84(6):430–8.

43 Barrow K. Is thyroid disease causing your erectile dysfunction? *New York Daily News* Dec. 12, 2010. http://nydailynews.healthology.com/erectile-dysfunction/erectile-dysfunction-information/article3876.htm

44 Seftel A. Testosterone replacement therapy for male hypogonadism: part III. Pharmacologic and clinical profiles, monitoring, safety issues, and potential future agents. *Int J Impot Res* 2007 Jan–Feb;9(1):2–24.

45 Malkin CJ, et al. Low serum testosterone and increased mortality in men with coronary heart disease. *Heart* 2010 Nov;96(22):1821–5.

46 García-Cruz E, Leibar-Tamayo A, Romero J, Piqueras M, Luque P, Cardeñosa O, Alcaraz A. Metabolic Syndrome in Men with Low Testosterone Levels: Relationship with Cardiovascular Risk Factors and Comorbidities and with Erectile Dysfunction. *J Sex Med*. 2013 Jul 30. doi: 10.1111/jsm.12265. [Epub ahead of print]

47 Hyde Z, Norman PE, Flicker L, Hankey GJ, Almeida OP, McCaul KA, Chubb SA, Yeap BB. Low free testosterone predicts mortality from cardiovascular disease but not other causes: the Health in Men Study. *J Clin Endocrinol Metab*. 2012 Jan;97(1):179–89.

48 Wang C, Jackson G, Jones TH, Matsumoto AM, Nehra A, Perelman MA, Swerdloff RS, Traish A, Zitzmann M, Cunningham G. Low testosterone associated with obesity and the metabolic syndrome contributes to sexual dysfunction and cardiovascular disease risk in men with type 2 diabetes. *Diabetes Care*. 2011 Jul;34(7):1669–75.

49 Kapoor D. Testosterone replacement therapy improves insulin resistance, glycaemic control, visceral adiposity and hypercholesterolaemia in hypogonadal men with type 2 diabetes. *Eur J Endocrinol* 2006 Jun;154(6):899–906.

50 Malkin CJ, et al. Testosterone replacement in hypogonadal men with angina improves ischaemic threshold and quality of life. *Heart* 2004 Aug; 90(8):871–6.

51 Heufelder AE. Fifty-two-week treatment with diet and exercise plus transdermal testosterone reverses the metabolic syndrome and improves glycemic control in men with newly diagnosed type 2 diabetes and subnormal plasma testosterone. *J Androl* 2009 Nov–Dec; 30(6):726–33.

52 Malkin CJ, Jones TH, Channer KS. The effect of testosterone on insulin sensitivity in men with heart failure. *Eur J Heart Fail* 2007 Jan;9(1):44–50.

53 Fukui M, et al. Role of endogenous androgen against insulin resistance and athero-sclerosis in men with type 2 diabetes. *Curr Diabetes Rev.* 2007 Feb; 3(1):25–31.

54 LeBrasseur NK, Lajevardi N, Miciek R, Mazer N, Storer TW, Bhasin S. Effects of testosterone therapy on muscle performance and physical function in older men with mobility limitations (The TOM Trial): design and methods. *Contemp Clin Trials.* 2009 Mar; 30(2):133–40.

55 Mitchell JE, et al. Thyroid function in heart failure and impact on mortality. *JCHF* 2013;1(1):48–55. http://heartfailure.onlinejacc.org/article.aspx?articleid=1568322

56 Rhee CM, et al. Hypothyroidism and mortality among dialysis patients. *Clin J Am Soc Nephrol* 2013 Apr;8(4):593–601.

57 Weiss IA, Bloomgarden N, Frishman WH. Subclinical hypothyroidism and cardiovascular risk: recommendations for treatment. *Cardiol Rev.* 2011 Nov-Dec;19(6):291–9.

58 Ghirlanda G, et al. Evidence of plasma CoQ10-lowering effect by HMG-CoA reductase inhibitors: a double-blind, placebo-controlled study. *J Clin Pharmacol* 1993 Mar;33(3):226–9.

59 Rosenfeldt FL, et al. Coenzyme Q10 improves the tolerance of the senescent myocardium to aerobic and ischemic stress: studies in rats and human atrial tissue. *Biofactors* 1999;9(2–4):291–9

60 Hyman M. How hidden food sensitivities make you fat. *Huffington Post.* March 3, 2012. www.huffingtonpost.com/dr-mark-hyman/food-allergy_b_1301271.html

61 Elenkov IJ, Iezzoni DG, Daly A, Harris AG, Chrousos GP. Cytokine dysregulation, inflammation and well-being. *Neuroimmunomodulation* 2005;12(5):255–69

62 Hughes PA, Zola H, Penttila IA, Blackshaw LA, Andrews JM, Krumbiegel D. Immune activation in irritable bowel syndrome: can neuroimmune interactions explain symptoms? *Am J Gastroenterol.* 2013 Jul;108(7):1066–74

63 Di Paola R, Cuzzocrea S. Predictivity and sensitivity of animal models of arthritis. *Autoimmun Rev.* 2008 Oct;8(1):73–5.

64 Wilders-Truschnig M, et al. IgG antibodies against food antigens are correlated with inflammation and intima media thickness in obese juveniles. *Exp Clin Endocrinol Diabetes* 2008 Apr;116(4):241–5.

Chapter 6

1 Hoffman RL. Antioxidants and the Free Radical Theory of Degenerative Disease. In: Wainapel SF, Fast A, editors. *Alternative Medicine and Rehabilitation: A Guide for Practitioners.* New York: Demos Medical Publishing, 2003. www.ncbi.nlm.nih.gov/books/NBK11231/

2 Srikanth V, et al. Advanced glycation endproducts and their receptor RAGE in Alzheimer's disease. *Neurobiol Aging* 2009 May 21.

3 Simm A, et al. Advanced glycation endproducts: a biomarker for age as an outcome predictor after cardiac surgery? *Exp Gerontol* 2007 Jul;42(7):668–75.

4 Zimmerman GA, et al. Neurotoxicity of advanced glycation endproducts during focal stroke and neuroprotective effects of aminoguanidine. *Proc Natl Acad Sci* 1995 Apr 25;92(9):3744–8.

5 Seo AY, et al. New insights into the role of mitochondria in aging: mitochondrial dynamics and more. *J Cell Sci* 2010 Aug 1;123(Pt 15):2533–42.

6 Cui H, Kong Y, Zhang H. Oxidative stress, mitochondrial dysfunction, and aging. *J Signal Transduct* 2012;2012:646354.

7 Dada R, Mahfouz RZ, Kumar R, Venkatesh S, Shamsi MB, Agarwal A, Talwar P, Sharma RK. A comprehensive work up for an asthenozoospermic man with repeated intracytoplasmic sperm injection (ICSI) failure. *Andrologia.* 2011 Oct;43(5):368–72.

8 Menshikova E, et al. Effects of exercise on mitochondrial content and function in aging human skeletal muscle. *J Gerontol A Biol Sci Med Sci* 2006 June;61(6):534–540.

9 Little JP, et al. An acute bout of high-intensity interval training increases the nuclear abundance of PGC-1-alpha and activates mitochondrial biogenesis in human skeletal muscle. *Am J Physiol Regul Integr Comp Physiol* 2011 Jun;300(6):R1303–10.

10 Chowanadisai W, et al. Pyrroloquinoline quinone stimulates mitochondrial biogenesis through cAMP response element–binding protein phosphorylation and increased PGC-1alpha expression. *J Biol Chem* 2010 Jan 1;285(1):142.

11 The University of Utah. Are telomeres the key to aging and cancer? Learn. Genetics. Genetics Science Learning Center. http://learn.genetics.utah.edu/content/begin/traits/telomeres/

12 The University of Utah. Are telomeres the key to aging and cancer? Learn. Genetics. Genetics Science Learning Center. http://learn.genetics.utah.edu/content/begin/traits/telomeres/

13 Hirashima K, Migita T, Sato S, Muramatsu Y, Ishikawa Y, Seimiya H. Telomere length influences cancer cell differentiation in vivo. *Mol Cell Biol.* 2013 Aug;33(15):2988–95.

14 Tiainen AM, et al. Leukocyte telomere length and its relation to food and nutrient intake in an elderly population. *Eur J Clin Nutr* 2012 Dec;66(12):1290–4.

15 Tiainen AM, 2012.

16 Kiecolt-Glaser JK, et al. Omega-3 fatty acids, oxidative stress, and leukocyte telomere length: A randomized controlled trial. *Brain Behav Immun* 2013 Feb;28:16–24.

17 Farzaneh-Far R, Lin J, Epel ES, Harris WS, Blackburn EH, Whooley MA. Association of marine omega-3 fatty acid levels with telomeric aging in patients with coronary heart disease. *JAMA.* 2010 Jan 20;303(3):250–7.

Chapter 7

1 Opportunities and Challenges in Digestive Diseases Research: Recommendations of the National Commission on Digestive Diseases. National Institutes of Health, U.S. Department of Health and Human Services. NIH Publication 08–6514. March, 2009.

www2.niddk.nih.gov/NR/rdonlyres/722FC3D9-B5EC-47AE-8BF5-6DBB8900EAB3/
0/NCDD_04272009_ResearchPlan_CompleteResearchPlan.pdf

2 Inflammatory Bowel Disease. Centers for Disease Control and Prevention. Last reviewed May 1, 2012. www.cdc.gov/ibd/

3 Molodecky NA, et al. Increasing incidence and prevalence of the inflammatory bowel diseases with time, based on systematic review. *Gastroenterol* 2012 Jan;142(1):46–54.

4 Malaty HM, et al. Rising incidence of inflammatory bowel disease among children: A 12-year study. *J Ped Gastroenterol Nutr* 2010 Jan;50(1):27–31.

5 Benjamin J, et al. Glutamine and whey protein improve intestinal permeability and morphology in patients with Crohn's disease: A randomized controlled trial. *Dig Dis Sci* 2012 Apr;57(4):1000–12.

6 Mahmood A, et al. Zinc carnosine, a health food supplement that stabilises small bowel integrity and stimulates gut repair processes. *Gut* 2007 Feb;56(2):168–175.

7 Miyoshi A, et al. Clinical evaluation of Z-103 on gastric ulcer: a multicenter double-blind comparative study with cetrexate hydrochloride. *Jpn Pharmacol Ther* 1992, 20(1):199–223.

8 Gerhardt H, et al. Therapy of active Crohn disease with *Boswellia serrata* extract H 15. *Z Gastroenterol* 2001 Jan;39(1):11–7 [in German].

9 Gupta I, et al. Effects of gum resin of *Boswellia serrata* in patients with chronic colitis. *Planta Med* 2001 Jul;67(5):391–5.

10 Lovell RM, Ford AC. Global prevalence of and risk factors for irritable bowel syndrome: a meta-analysis. *Clin Gastroenterol Hepatol* 2012 Jul;10(7):712–721.e4.

11 Cappello G, et al. Peppermint oil (Mintoil) in the treatment of irritable bowel syndrome: a prospective double blind placebo-controlled randomized trial. *Dig Liver Dis* Jun 2007;39(6):530–536.

12 Merat S, et al. The effect of enteric-coated, delayed-release peppermint oil on irritable bowel syndrome. *Dig Dis Sci* May 2010;55(5):1385–1390.

13 Liu JH, et al. Enteric-coated peppermint-oil capsules in the treatment of irritable bowel syndrome: a prospective, randomized trial. *J Gastroenterol* Dec 1997;32(6):765–768.

14 May B, et al. Efficacy of a fixed peppermint oil/caraway oil combination in non-ulcer dyspepsia. *Arzneimittel-Forschung* Dec 1996;46(12):1149–1153.

15 Walker AF, et al. Artichoke leaf extract reduces symptoms of irritable bowel syndrome in a post-marketing surveillance study. *Phytother Res* Feb 2001;15(1):58–61.

16 Holtmann G, et al. Functional dyspepsia and irritable bowel syndrome - Treatment effects of artichoke-leaf-extract: A placebo-controlled, randomised, multicenter trial. *Gastroenterology* Apr 2003;124(4):A182–A182.

17 Bundy R, et al. Artichoke leaf extract reduces symptoms of irritable bowel syndrome and improves quality of life in otherwise healthy volunteers suffering from concomitant dyspepsia: a subset analysis. *J Altern Complement Med* Aug 2004b;10(4):667–669.

18 Derner DT (reviewer). Understanding the basics of GERD. WebMD.com. Reviewed March 31, 2013. www.webmd.com/heartburn-gerd/understanding-gerd-basics?page=2

19 GERD, Barret's Esophagus and the risk for esophageal cancer. American Society for Gastrointestinal Endoscopy. www.asge.org/index.aspx?id=402&terms=20%20percent

20 Yancy WS Jr, et al. Improvement of gastroesophageal reflux disease after initiation of a low-carbohydrate diet: five brief case reports. *Altern Ther Health Med* 2001 Nov–Dec; 7(6):120, 116–9.

21 Austin GL, et al. A very low-carbohydrate diet improves gastroesophageal reflux and its symptoms. *Dig Dis Sci* 2006 Aug;51(8):1307–12.

22 Larkworthy W, Holgate PF. Deglycyrrhizinized liquorice in the treatment of chronic duodenal ulcer. A retrospective endoscopic survey of 32 patients. *Practitioner* 1975 Dec;215(1290):787–92.

23 Morgan AG, et al. Cimetidine: an advance in gastric ulcer treatment? *Br Med J* 1978 Nov 11;2(6148):1323–6.

24 Morgan AG, et al. Comparison between cimetidine and Caved-S in the treatment of gastric ulceration, and subsequent maintenance therapy. *Gut* 1982 Jun;23(6):545–51.

25 Morgan AG, Pacsoo C, McAdam WA. Maintenance therapy: a two year comparison between Caved-S and cimetidine treatment in the prevention of symptomatic gastric ulcer recurrence. *Gut* 1985 Jun;26(6):599–602.

26 Gaddipati JP, et al. Picroliv modulates the expression of insulin-like growth factor (IGF)-I, IGF-II and IGF-I receptor during hypoxia in rats. *Cell Mol Life Sci* 1999 Oct 15;56(3–4):348–55.

27 Li P, Matsunaga K, Ohizumi Y. Nerve growth factor-potentiating compounds from Picrorhizae Rhizoma. *Biol Pharm Bull* 2000 Jul;23(7):890–2.

28 Singh AK, et al. Picroliv accelerates epithelialization and angiogenesis in rat wounds. *Planta Med* 2007 Mar;73(3):251–6.

29 Salthouse TA. When does age-related cognitive decline begin? *Neurobiol Aging* 2009 April; 30(4):507–514.

30 Whalley LJ. Brain ageing and dementia: what makes the difference? *Brit J Psych* 2002;181:369–371.

31 Cognitive impairment: A call for action, now! Centers for Disease Control and Prevention. Feb. 2011. www.cdc.gov/aging/pdf/cognitive_impairment/cogimp_policy_final.pdf

32 Mecocci P, et al. Oxidative damage to mitochondrial DNA shows marked age-dependent increases in human brain. *Ann. Neurol* 1993 Oct; 34(4):609–16.

33 Peng H, et al. HIV-1-infected and/or immune-activated macrophage-secreted TNF-alpha affects human fetal cortical neural progenitor cell proliferation and differentiation. *Glia* 2008 Jun;56(8):903–16.

34 Monje ML, Toda H, Palmer TD. Inflammatory blockade restores adult hippocampal neurogenesis. *Science* 2003 Dec; 302(5651):1760–5.

35 Cognition & Memory: How Hormones Influence Our Minds. Connections: An Educational Resource of Women's International Pharmacy. Jan. 2013. www.womensinternational.com/pdf/cognition.pdf

36 Drake EB, et al. Associations between circulating sex steroid hormones and cognition in normal elderly women. *Neurology* 2000 Feb 8;54(3):599–603.

37 Pederen BK, et al. Role of exercise-induced brain-derived neurotrophic factor production in the regulation of energy homeostasis in mammals. *Exp. Physiol* 2009 Dec; 94(12):1153–60.

38 McIntyre RS, et al. Brain volume abnormalities and neurocognitive deficits in diabetes mellitus: points of pathophysiological commonality with mood disorders? *Adv Ther* 2010 Feb; 27(2):63–80.

39 Biessels GJ, et al. Risk of dementia in diabetes mellitus: a systematic review. *Lancet Neurol* 2006 Jan;5(1):64–74.

40 Abbatecola AM, et al. Adiposity predicts cognitive decline in older persons with diabetes: a 2-year follow-up. *PLoS One* 2010 Apr 23;5(4):e10333.

41 Walther K, et al. Structural brain differences and cognitive functioning related to body mass index in older females. *Hum Brain Mapp* 2010 Jul; 31(7):1052–64.

42 Kerwin DR, et al. Interaction between body mass index and central adiposity and risk of incident cognitive impairment and dementia: results from the Women's Health Initiative Memory Study. *J Am Geriatr Soc* 2011 Jan;59(1):107–12.

43 Krikorian R, et al. Blueberry supplementation improves memory in older adults. *J Agric Food Chem* 2010 Apr 14;58(7):3996–4000.

44 Joseph JA, et al. Reversals of age–related declines in neuronal signal transduction, cognitive, and motor behavioral deficits with blueberry, spinach, or strawberry dietary supplementation. *J Neurosci* 1999 Sep 15;19(18):8114–21.

45 Malin DH, et al. Short-term blueberry-enriched diet prevents and reverses object recognition memory loss in aging rats. *Nutrition* 2011 Mar;27(3):338–42.

46 Papandreou MA, et al. Effect of a polyphenol-rich wild blueberry extract on cognitive performance of mice, brain antioxidant markers and acetylcholinesterase activity. *Behav Brain Res* 2009 Mar 17;198(2):352–8.

47 Papandreou MA, 2009.

48 Casadesus G, et al. Modulation of hippocampal plasticity and cognitive behavior by short-term blueberry supplementation in aged rats. *Nutr Neurosci* 2004 Oct–Dec; 7(5–6):309–16.

49 Stull AJ, et al. Bioactives in blueberries improve insulin sensitivity in obese, insulin-resistant men and women. *J Nutr* 2010 Oct;140(10):1764–8.

50 Kidd PM. Alzheimer's disease, amnestic mild cognitive impairment, and age-associated memory impairment: current understanding and progress toward integrative prevention. *Altern Med Rev* 2008 Jun;13(2):85–115.

51 Kato-Kataoka A, et al. Soybean-derived phosphatidylserine improves memory function of the elderly Japanese subjects with memory complaints. *J Clin Biochem Nutr* 2010 Nov; 47(3):246–55.

52 Vakhapova V, et al. Phosphatidylserine containing omega-3 fatty acids may improve memory abilities in non-demented elderly with memory complaints: a double-blind placebo-controlled trial. *Dement Geriatr Cogn Disord* 2010; 29(5):467–74.

53 Richter Y, et al. The effect of phosphatidylserine-containing omega-3 fatty acids on memory abilities in subjects with subjective memory complaints: a pilot study. *Clin Interv Aging* 2010 Nov 2;5:313–6.

54 Amenta F, et al. Association with the cholinergic precursor choline alphoscerate and the cholinesterase inhibitor rivastigmine: An approach for enhancing cholinergic neurotransmission. *Mech Ageing Dev* 2006 Feb; 127(2):173–9.

55 Parnetti L, Amenta F, Gallai V. Choline alphoscerate in cognitive decline and in acute cerebrovascular disease: an analysis of published clinical data. Mech Ageing Dev. 2001 Nov;122(16):2041–55.

56 Ng T, et al. Curry consumption and cognitive function in the elderly. Am J Epidemiol. 2006 Nov 1;164(9):898–906.

57 Frautschy SA, et al. Phenolic anti-inflammatory antioxidant reversal of Abeta-induced cognitive deficits and neuropathology. Neurobiol Aging. 2001 Nov; 22(6):993–1005.

58 Lim GP, et al. The curry spice curcumin reduces oxidative damage and amyloid pathology in an Alzheimer transgenic mouse. J Neurosci. 2001 Nov 1; 21(21):8370–7.

59 2011 Alzheimer's Disease Facts and Figures. Alzheimer's & Dementia. Volume 7, Issue 2. www.alz.org/downloads/facts_figures_2011.pdf

60 2011 Alzheimer's Disease Facts and Figures. Alzheimer's & Dementia. Volume 7, Issue 2. www.alz.org/downloads/facts_figures_2011.pdf

61 Miklossy J. Emerging roles of pathogens in Alzheimer disease. Expert Rev Mol Med. 2011 Sep 20;13:e30. doi: 10.1017/S1462399411002006.

62 Vest RS, Pike CJ. Gender, sex steroid hormones, and Alzheimer's disease. Horm Behav. 2013 Feb;63(2):301–7. doi: 10.1016/j.yhbeh.2012.04.006.

63 Mayo W, et al. Individual differences in cognitive aging: Implication of pregnenolone sulfate. Prog Neurobiol. 2003 Sep;71(1):43–8.

64 Nanfaro F, et al. Pregnenolone sulfate infused in lateral septum of male rats impairs novel object recognition memory. Pharmacol Rep. 2010 Mar-Apr;62(2):265–72.

65 Mayo W, et al. Pregnenolone sulfate enhances neurogenesis and PSA-NCAM in young and aged hippocampus. Neurobiol Aging. 2005 Jan;26(1):103–14.

66 Lim GP, 2001.

67 DiSilvestro RA, et al. Diverse effects of a low dose supplement of lipidated curcumin in healthy middle aged people. Nutr J. 2012 Sep 26;11:79.

68 Wang XD, et al. Modulation of NMDA receptor by huperzine A in rat cerebral cortex. Zhongguo Yao Li Xue Bao. 1999 Jan;20(1):31–5.

69 Wang BS, et al. Efficacy and safety of natural acetylcholinesterase inhibitor huperzine A in the treatment of Alzheimer's disease: An updated meta-analysis. J Neural Transm. 116.4 (2009): 457–65.

70 Amaducci L. Phosphatidylserine in the treatment of Alzheimer's disease: Results of a multicenter study. Psychopharmacol Bull. 1988;24:130–134.

71 Crook T, et al. Effects of phosphatidylserine in Alzheimer's disease. Psychopharmacol Bull. 1992;28:61–66.

72 Engel RR, et al. Double-blind cross-over study of phosphatidylserine vs. placebo in patients with early dementia of the Alzheimer type. Eur Neuropsychopharmacol. 1992; 2:149–155.

73 Nagy Z, et al. Meta-analysis of Cavinton. Praxis. 1988 Sep 15; 7(9):63–8.

74 Szatmari SZ, Whitehouse PJ. Vinpocetine for cognitive impairment and dementia. Cochrane Database Syst Rev. 2003; (1):CD003119.

75 Pereira C, Agostinho P, Oliveira CR. Vinpocetine attenuates the metabolic dysfunction induced by amyloid beta-peptides in PC12 cells. Free Radic Res. 2000 Nov; 33(5):497–506.

76 Kiss B, Cai NS, Erdo SL. Vinpocetine preferentially antagonizes quisqualate/AMPA receptor responses: evidence from release and ligand binding studies. Eur J Pharmacol. 1991 Dec 10; 209(1–2):109–12.

77 Osawa M, Maruyama S. Effects of TCV-3B (vinpocetine) on blood viscosity in ischemic cerebrovascular diseases. Ther Hung. 1985; 33:7–12.

78 Kuzuya F. Effects of vinpocetine on platelet aggregability and erythrocyte deformability. Ther Hung. 1985; 33:22–34.

79 Feher G, et al. Effect of parenteral or oral vinpocetine on the hemorheological parameters of patients with chronic cerebrovascular diseases. Phytomedicine. 2009 Mar; 16(2–3):111–7.

80 Dopamine and Parkinson's. News-Medical.Net. Aug. 10, 2008. www.news-medical .net/news/2008/08/10/40602.aspx

81 Shen W, et al. Dichotomous dopaminergic control of striatal synaptic plasticity. Science. 2008 Aug 8;321(5890):848–51.

82 Statistics on Parkinson's. Parkinson's Disease Foundation. www.pdf.org/en/parkinson _statistics

83 Góngora–Alfaro JL. Caffeine as a preventive drug for Parkinson's disease: epidemiologic evidence and experimental support. [Article in Spanish] Rev Neurol. 2010 Feb 16–28;59(4):221–9.

84 Parkinsons. Foundation for Mitochondrial Medicine. http://mitochondrialdiseases .org/parkinsons/

85 Zhang H, et al. Combined R-alpha-lipoic acid and acetyl-L-carnitine exerts efficient preventative effects in a cellular model of Parkinson's disease. J Cell Mol Med. 2010 Jan;14(1–2):215–25.

86 Chowanadisai W, et al. Pyrroloquinoline quinone stimulates mitochondrial biogenesis through cAMP response element-binding protein phosphorylation and increased PGC-1a expression. J Biol Chem. 2010 Jan 1;285(1):142–52.

87 Koikeda T, Neremo M, Masuda K. Pyrroloquinoline quinone disodium salt improves higher brain function. Medical Consultation and New Remedies. 2011. 48(5): 1.

88 Jin F, et al. Neuroprotective effect of resveratrol on 6-OHDA-induced Parkinson's disease in rats. Eur J Pharmacol. Dec 14 2008;600(1–3):78–82.

89 Levites Y, et al. Green tea polyphenol (–)-epigallocatechin-3-gallate prevents N-methyl-4-phenyl-1,2,3,6-tetrahydropyridine-induced dopaminergic neurodegeneration. J Neurochem. Sep 2001;78(5):1073–1082.

90 Levites Y, et al. Involvement of protein kinase C activation and cell survival/ cell cycle genes in green tea polyphenol (-)-epigallocatechin 3-gallate neuroprotective action. J Biol Chem. Aug 23 2002;277(34):30574–30580.

91 Choi JY, et al. Prevention of nitric oxide-mediated 1-methyl-4-phenyl-1,2,3,6-tetrahydropyridine-induced Parkinson's disease in mice by tea phenolic epigallocatechin 3-gallate. Neurotoxicology. Sep 2002;23(3):367–374.

92 Takada Y, et al. Acetyl-11-keto-beta-boswellic acid potentiates apoptosis, inhibits inva-

sion, and abolishes osteoclastogenesis by suppressing NF-kappa B and NF-kappa B-regulated gene expression. J Immunol. 2006 Mar 1;176(5):3127–40.

93 Shakibaei M, et al. Suppression of NF-kappaB activation by curcumin leads to inhibition of expression of cyclo-oxygenase-2 and matrix metalloproteinase-9 in human articular chondrocytes: Implications for the treatment of osteoarthritis. Biochem Pharmacol. 2007 May 1;73(9):1434–45.

94 Pan J, et al. Curcumin inhibition of JNKs prevents dopaminergic neuronal loss in a mouse model of Parkinson's disease through suppressing mitochondria dysfunction. Transl Neurodegener. 2012 Aug 20;1(1):16.

95 Kazmi S, et al. The effects of Boswellia resin extract on dopaminergic cell line, SK-N-SH, against MPP+-induced neurotoxicity. Basic and Clinical Neuroscience. 2011;3(1):16–21. http://bcn.tums.ac.ir/browse.php?a_id=192&slc_lang=en&sid=1&ftxt=1

96 Ojha RP, et al. Neuroprotective effect of curcuminoids against inflammation-mediated dopaminergic neurodegeneration in the MPTP model of Parkinson's disease. J Neuroimmune Pharmacol. 2012 Sep;7(3):609–18.

97 HP-200 in Parkinson's Disease Study Group. An alternative medicine treatment for Parkinson's disease: results of a multicenter clinical trial. J Altern Complement Med. 1995;1:249–55.

98 Vayda AB, et al. Treatment of Parkinsons disease with the cowhage plant - Mucuna pruriens (Bak). Neurol India. 1978;36:171–6.

99 Nagashayana N, et al. Association of L-dopa with recovery following ayurveda medication in Parkinson's disease. J Neurol Sci. 2000;176:124–7.

100 Katzenschlager R, et al. Mucuna pruriens in Parkinson's disease: a double blind clinical and pharmacological study. J Neurol Neurosurg Psychiatry. 2004 Dec;75(12):1672–7.

101 Top scientists warn of chemical contamination, rising cancer rates. EurActiv.com. May 13 2004. www.euractiv.com/sustainability/top-scientists-warn-chemical-contamination-rising-cancer-rates/article-117849

102 Brody JE. How cancer rose to the top of the charts. The New York Times. Feb. 1, 2005. www.nytimes.com/2005/02/01/health/01brod.html?pagewanted=all

103 Lifetime risk of developing or dying from cancer. American Cancer Society. Reviewed Nov. 29, 2012. www.cancer.org/cancer/cancerbasics/lifetime-probability-of-developing-or-dying-from-cancer

104 Lifetime risk of developing or dying from cancer. American Cancer Society. Reviewed Nov. 29, 2012. www.cancer.org/cancer/cancerbasics/lifetime-probability-of-developing-or-dying-from-cancer

105 Keck A-S, Finley JW, Cruciferous vegetables: cancer protective mechanisms of glucosinolate hydrolysis products and selenium. Integr Cancer Ther. 2004 Mar;3(1):5–12.

106 Akiyama T, et al. Genistein, a specific inhibitor of tyrosine-specific protein kinases. J Biol Chem. 1987;262(12):5592–5595.

107 Dashwood RH, Breinholt V, Bailey GS. Chemopreventive properties of chlorophyllin: inhibition of aflatoxins B1 (AFB1)-DNA binding in vivo and anti-mutagenic activity against AFB1 and two heterocyclic amines in the salmonella mutagenicity assay. Carcinogenesis. 1991;12(5):939–942.

108 Egner PA, et al. Chlorophyllin intervention reduces aflatoxin-DNA adducts in individuals at high risk for liver cancer. Proc Natl Acad Sci U S A. 2001;98(25):14601–14606.

109 Mandal, Ananya. Metastasis: What is metastasis? NewsMedical.net. www.news-medical.net/health/Metastasis-What-is-Metastasis.aspx

110 Platt D, Raz A. Modulation of the lung colonization of B16-F1 melanoma cells by citrus pectin. J Natl Cancer Inst. 1992 Mar 18;84(6):438–42.

111 What are the key statistics about breast cancer? American Cancer Society. Reviewed Aug. 23, 2012. www.cancer.org/cancer/breastcancer/detailedguide/breast-cancer-key-statistics

112 What are the key statistics about prostate cancer? American Cancer Society. Reviewed Feb. 27, 2012. www.cancer.org/cancer/prostatecancer/detailedguide/prostate-cancer-key-statistics

113 What are the key statistics about lung cancer? American Cancer Society. Reviewed Feb. 17, 2012. www.cancer.org/cancer/lungcancer-non-smallcell/detailedguide/non-small-cell-lung-cancer-key-statistics

114 Jatoi A, et al. Is voluntary vitamin and mineral supplementation associated with better outcome in non-small cell lung cancer patients? Results from the Mayo Clinic lung cancer cohort. Lung Cancer. 2005 Jul;49(1):77–84.

115 Liver cancer survival rates. American Cancer Society. Reviewed July 19, 2012. www.cancer.org/cancer/livercancer/overviewguide/liver-cancer-overview-survival-rates

116 Breast cancer survival statistics. Cancer Research UK. Reviewed Oct. 5, 2012. www.cancerresearchuk.org/cancer-info/cancerstats/types/breast/survival/breast-cancer-survival-statistics

117 Survival rates for prostate cancer. American Cancer Society. Reviewed Feb. 27, 2012. www.cancer.org/cancer/prostatecancer/detailedguide/prostate-cancer-survival-rates

118 What are the key statistics about liver cancer? American Cancer Society. Reviewed June 21, 2012. www.cancer.org/cancer/livercancer/detailedguide/liver-cancer-what-is-key-statistics

119 What are the key statistics about brain cancer? American Cancer Society. Reviewed Oct. 9, 2012. www.cancer.org/cancer/braincnstumorsinadults/detailedguide/brain-and-spinal-cord-tumors-in-adults-key-statistics

120 Survival rates for selected adult brain and spinal cord tumors. American Cancer Society. Reviewed Oct. 9, 2012. www.cancer.org/cancer/braincnstumorsinadults/detailedguide/brain-and-spinal-cord-tumors-in-adults-survival-rates

121 What are the key statistics about colorectal cancer? American Cancer Society. Reviewed May 24, 2012. www.cancer.org/cancer/colonandrectumcancer/detailedguide/colorectal-cancer-key-statistics

122 Chronic fatigue syndrome: Diagnosis. Centers for Disease Control and Prevention. Last reviewed May 14, 2012. www.cdc.gov/cfs/diagnosis/index.html

123 Chronic fatigue syndrome: Diagnosis. Centers for Disease Control and Prevention. Last reviewed May 14, 2012. www.cdc.gov/cfs/diagnosis/index.html

124 MedlinePlus. Chronic fatigue syndrome. Reviewed Jan. 11, 2013. www.nlm.nih.gov/medlineplus/chronicfatiguesyndrome.html

125 Walsh CM, et al. A family history study of chronic fatigue syndrome. *Psychiatr Genet.* 2001 Sep;11(3):123–8.

126 Buchwald D, et al. A twin study of chronic fatigue. *Psychosom Med.* 2001 Nov-Dec;63(6):936–43.

127 Bansal AS, et ak. Chronic fatigue syndrome, the immune system and viral infection. *Brain Behav Immun.* 2012 Jan;26(1):24–31.

128 Stejskal VD, et al. Metal-specific lymphocytes: biomarkers of sensitivity in man. *Neuro Endocrinol Lett.* 1999;20(5):289–298.

129 Himmel PB, Seligman TM. A pilot study employing Dehydroepiandrosterone (DHEA) in the treatment of chronic fatigue syndrome. J Clin Rheumatol. 1999 Apr;5(2):56–9.

130 Forsyth LM, et al. Therapeutic effects of oral NADH on the symptoms of patients with chronic fatigue syndrome. Ann Allergy Asthma Immunol. 1999 Feb;82(2):185–91.

131 Plioplys AV, Plioplys S. Amantadine and L-carnitine treatment of chronic fatigue syndrome. Neuropsychobiology. 1997;35(1):16–23.

132 Bounous G, Molson J. Competition for glutathione precursors between the immune system and the skeletal muscle: pathogenesis of chronic fatigue syndrome. Med Hypotheses. 1999 Oct;53(4):347–9.

133 Wang PY, Zhu XL, Lin ZB. Antitumor and immunomodulatory effects of polysaccharides from broken-spore of *Ganoderma lucidum*. Front Pharmacol. 2012;3:135.

134 Jeurink PV, et al. Immunomodulatory capacity of fungal proteins on the cytokine production of human peripheral blood mononuclear cells. Int Immunopharmacol. 2008 Aug;8(8):1124–33.

135 Kingsbury KJ, et al. Contrasting plasma free amino acid patterns in elite athletes: association with fatigue and infection. Br J Sports Med. 1998b Mar;32(1):25–32.

136 Maes M, Leunis J-C. Normalization of leaky gut in chronic fatigue syndrome (CFS) is accompanied by a clinical improvement: effects of age, duration of illness and the translocation of LPS from gram-negative bacteria. Neuro Endocrinol Lett. 2008;29(6):902–10.

137 Miyoshi A, et al. Clinical evaluation of Z-103 on gastric ulcer: a multicenter double-blind comparative study with cetrexate hydrochloride. Jpn Pharmacol Ther. 1992, 20(1):199–223.

138 National Resource Council. *Relieving Pain in America, A Blueprint for Transforming Prevention, Care, Education and Research.* Washington, DC: The National Academies Press, 2011. http://books.nap.edu/openbook.php?record_id=13172&page=1.

139 Connolly DA, et al. Efficacy of a tart cherry juice blend in preventing symptoms of muscle damage. Br J Sports Med. 2006 Aug;40(8):679–83.

140 Kim KM, Kim MJ, Kang JS. Absorption, distribution, metabolism, and excretion of decursin and decursinol angelate from Angelica gigas Nakai. J Microbiol Biotechnol. 2009;19(12):1569–1572.

141 Kim JH, et al. Decursin inhibits induction of inflammatory mediators by blocking nuclear factor-kappaB activation in macrophages. Mol Pharmacol. 2006 Jun;69(6):1783–90.

142 Seo YJ, et al. The analgesic effect of decursinol. Arch Pharm Res. 2009;32(6):937–943.

143 Choi SS, et al. Antinociceptive mechanisms of orally administered decursinol in the mouse. Life Sci. 2003 Jun 13;73(4):471–85.

144 Seo YJ, et al. The analgesic effect of decursinol. Arch Pharm Res. 2009 Jun;32(6):937–43.

145 Chrubasik S, Weiser T, Beime B. Effectiveness and safety of topical capsaicin cream in the treatment of chronic soft tissue pain. Phytother Res. 2010;24(12):1877–1885.

146 McCleane G. Topical application of doxepin hydrochloride, capsaicin and a combination of both produces analgesia in chronic human neuropathic pain: a randomized, double-blind, placebo-controlled study. Br J Clin Pharmacol. 2000;49:574–579.

147 England J, et al. The capsaicin 8% patch for peripheral neuropathic pain. Br J Nurs. 2011;20(15):926–931.

148 Deal CL, et al. Treatment of arthritis with topical capsaicin: A double blind trial. Clin Ther. 1991;13:383–395.

149 McCarty DJ, et al. Treatment of pain due to fibromyalgia with topical capsaicin: A pilot study. Semin Arthritis Rheum. 1994;23(suppl 3):41–47.

150 Yeon KY, et al. Curcumin produces an antihyperalgesic effect via antagonism of TRPV1. J Dent Res. 2010;89(2):170–174.

151 Agarwal KA, et al. Efficacy of turmeric (curcumin) in pain and postoperative fatigue after laparoscopic cholecystectomy: a double-blind, randomized placebo-controlled study. Surg Endosc. 2011;25(12):3805–3810.

152 Deodhar SD, Sethi R, Srimal RC. Preliminary study on antirheumatic activity of curcumin (diferuloyl methane). Indian J Med Res. 1980 Apr; 71:632–4.

153 Chandran B, Goel A. A randomized, pilot study to assess the efficacy and safety of curcumin in patients with active rheumatoid arthritis. Phytother Res. 2012 Nov;26(11):1719–25.

154 Daneman D. Type 1 diabetes. *Lancet*. 2006 Mar 11;367(9513):847–58.

155 National Diabetes Fact Sheet, 2011. Centers for Disease Control and Prevention. Jan. 26, 2011. www.cdc.gov/diabetes/pubs/pdf/ndfs_2011.pdf

156 National Diabetes Fact Sheet, 2011. Centers for Disease Control and Prevention. Jan. 26, 2011. www.cdc.gov/diabetes/pubs/pdf/ndfs_2011.pdf

157 National Diabetes Fact Sheet, 2011. Centers for Disease Control and Prevention. Jan. 26, 2011. www.cdc.gov/diabetes/pubs/pdf/ndfs_2011.pdf

158 Stratton IM, et al. Association of glycaemia with macrovascular and microvascular complications of type 2 diabetes (UKPDS 35): Prospective observational study. BMJ. 2000 Aug 12;321(7258):405–12.

159 Stoecker BJ, et al. Cinnamon extract lowers blood glucose in hyperglycemic subjects. FASEB J. 2010 Apr; 24 (Meeting Abstract Supplement) 722.1.

160 Lu T, et al. Cinnamon extract improves fasting blood glucose and glycosylated hemoglobin level in Chinese patients with type 2 diabetes. Nutr Res. 2012 Jun;32(6):408–12.

161 Mang B, et al. Effects of a cinnamon extract on plasma glucose, HbA, and serum lipids in diabetes mellitus type 2. Eur J Clin Invest. 2006 May; 36(5):340–4.

162 Ghosh D, et al. Role of chromium supplementation in Indians with type 2 diabetes mellitus. J Nutr Biochem. 2002 Nov; 13(11):690–697.

163 Mertz W. Chromium in human nutrition: a review. J Nutr. 1993 Apr; 123(4):626–33.

164 Bagchi M, et al. Efficacy and toxicological assessment of a novel, niacin-bound chromium in ameliorating metabolic disorders. July 2004. Presented at the 10th International Congress of Toxicology-Finland.

165 Anderson RA, et al. Elevated intakes of supplemental chromium improve glucose and insulin variables in individuals with type 2 diabetes. Diabetes. 1997 Nov; 46(11):1786–91.

166 Kamenova P. Improvement of insulin sensitivity in patients with type 2 diabetes mellitus after oral administration of alpha-lipoic acid. Hormones (Athens). 2006 Oct–Dec;5(4):251–8.

167 Jacob S, et al. Enhancement of glucose disposal in patients with type 2 diabetes by alpha-lipoic acid. Arzneimittelforschung. 1995 Aug;45(8):872–4.

168 Fukino Y, et al. Randomized controlled trial for an effect of green tea-extract powder supplementation on glucose abnormalities. Eur J Clin Nutr. 2008 Aug; 62(8):953–60.

169 Park JH, et al. Green tea extract with polyethylene glycol-3350 reduces body weight and improves glucose tolerance in db/db and high-fat diet mice. Naunyn schmiedebergs Arch Pharmacol. 2013 Apr 27. [Epub ahead of print]

170 Bogdanski P, et al. Green tea extract reduces blood pressure, inflammatory biomarkers, and oxidative stress and improves parameters associated with insulin resistance in obese, hypertensive patients. Nutr Res. 2012 Jun; 32(6):421–7.

171 Yan H, Harding JJ. Carnosine protects against the inactivation of esterase induced by glycation and a steroid. Biochim Biophys Acta. 2005 Jun 30; 1741(1–2):120–6.

172 McFarland GA, Holliday R. Retardation of the senescence of cultured human diploid fibroblasts by carnosine. Exp. Cell Res. 1994 Jun;212(2):167–75.

173 Gualano B, et al. Reduced muscle carnosine content in type 2, but not in type 1 diabetic patients. *Amino Acids*. 2012 Jul;43(1):21–4.

174 Lee YT, et al. Histidine and carnosine delay diabetic deterioration in mice and protect human low density lipoprotein against oxidation and glycation. Eur J Pharmacol. 2005 Apr 18; 513(1–2):145–50.

175 Yan H, et al. Effect of carnosine, aminoguanidine, and aspirin drops on the prevention of cataracts in diabetic rats. Mol Vis. 2008; 14:2282–91.

176 Pfister F, et al. Oral carnosine supplementation prevents vascular damage in experimental diabetic retinopathy. Cell Physiol Biochem. 2011; 28(1):125–36.

177 Kamei J, et al. Preventive effect of L-carnosine on changes in the thermal nociceptive threshold in streptozotocin-induced diabetic mice. Eur J Pharmacol. 2008 Dec 14; 600(1–3):83–6.

178 Barski OA, et al, Bhatnagar A, Srivastava S. Dietary carnosine prevents early atherosclerotic lesion formation in apolipoprotein e-null mice. Arterioscler Thromb Vasc Biol. 2013 Jun;33(6):1162–70.

179 Bitsch R, et al. Bioavailability assessment of the lipophilic benfotiamine as compared to a water-soluble thiamin derivative. Ann Nutr Metab. 1991;35(5):292–6.

180 Greb A, Bitsch R. Comparative bioavailability of various thiamine derivatives after oral administration. Int J Clin Pharmacol Ther. 1998 Apr; 36(4):216–21.

181 Stracke H, Lindemann A, Federlin K. A benfotiamine-vitamin B combination in treatment of diabetic polyneuropathy. Exp Clin Endocrinol Diabetes. 1996; 104(4):311–6.

182 Haupt E, Ledermann H, Kopcke W. Benfotiamine in the treatment of diabetic polyneuropathy—a three-week randomized, controlled pilot study (BEDIP study). Int J Clin Pharmacol Ther. 2005 Feb; 43(2):71–7.

183 Stirban A, et al. Benfotiamine prevents macro- and microvascular endothelial dysfunction and oxidative stress following a meal rich in advanced glycation end products in individuals with type 2 diabetes. Diabetes Care. 2006 Sep; 29(9):2064–71.

184 Ganea E, Rixon KC, Harding JJ. Binding of glucose, galactose and pyridoxal phosphate to lens crystallins. Biochim Biophys Acta. 1994 Jul 18; 1226(3):286–90.

185 Okada AM, Ayabe Y. Effects of aminoguanidine and pyridoxal phosphate on glycation reaction of aspartate aminotransferase and serum albumin. J Nutr Sci Vitaminol. 1995 Feb; 41(1):43–50.

186 Higuchi O, et al. Aminophospholipid glycation and its inhibitor screening system: a new role of pyridoxal 5′-phosphate as the inhibitor. J Lipid Res. 2006 May; 47(5):964–74.

187 Rosenblat M, Hayek T, Aviram M. Anti-oxidative effects of pomegranate juice (PJ) consumption by diabetic patients on serum and on macrophages. Atherosclerosis. 2006 Aug; 187(2):363–71.

188 Li Y, et al. Punica granatum flower extract, a potent alpha-glucosidase inhibitor, improves postprandial hyperglycemia in Zucker diabetic fatty rats. J Ethnopharmacol. 2005 Jun 3; 99(2):239–44.

189 Esmaillzadeh A, et al. Concentrated pomegranate juice improves lipid profiles in diabetic patients with hyperlipidemia. J Med Food. 2004;7(3):305–8.

190 Mesias M, et al. Antiglycative effect of fruit and vegetable seed extracts: inhibition of AGE formation and carbonyl-trapping abilities. J Sci Food Agric. 2013 Jun; 93(8):2037–44.

191 Mahesh T, Menon VP. Quercetin allievates oxidative stress in streptozotocin-induced diabetic rats. Phytother Res. 2004 Feb;18(2):123–7. 2008; 14:2282–91

192 Narita Y, Inouye KJ. Kinetic analysis and mechanism on the inhibition of chlorogenic acid and its components against porcine pancreas alpha-amylase isozymes I and II. J Agric Food Chem. 2009;57:9218–25.

193 Henry-Vitrac C, et al. Contribution of chlorogenic acids to the inhibition of human hepatic glucose-6-phosphatase activity in vitro by Svetol, a standardized decaffeinated green coffee extract. J Agric Food Chem. 2010 Apr 14;58(7):4141–4144.

194 Nagendran MV. Effect of green coffee bean extract (GCE), high in chlorogenic acids, on glucose metabolism. Poster presentation number: 45-LB-P. Obesity 2011, the 29th Annual Scientific Meeting of the Obesity Society. Orlando, Florida. October 1–5, 2011.

195 Obiro WC, Zhang T, Jiang B. The nutraceutical role of the Phaseolus vulgaris alpha-amylase inhibitor. Br J Nutr. 2008 Jul; 100(1):1–12.

196 Tormo MA, et al. White bean amylase inhibitor administered orally reduces glycaemia in type 2 diabetic rats. Br J Nutr. 2006 Sep; 96(3):539–44.

197 Udani JK, et al. Lowering the glycemic index of white bread using a white bean extract. Nutr J. 2009 Oct 28;8:52.

198 Vinson J, Hassan A, Shuta D. Investigation of an amylase inhibitor on human glucose absorption after starch consumption. Open Nutraceuticals J. 2009;2:88–91.

199 Dilwari JB, et al. Reduction of postprandial plasma glucose by Bengal gram dal (Cicer arietinum) and rajmah (Phaseolus vulgaris). Am J Clin Nutr. 1981 Nov; 34(11):2450–3.

200 What is COPD? National Heart, Lung, and Blood Institute. U.S. Department of Health & Human Services. www.nhlbi.nih.gov/health/health-topics/topics/copd/

201 What is COPD? National Heart, Lung, and Blood Institute. U.S. Department of Health & Human Services. www.nhlbi.nih.gov/health/health-topics/topics/copd/

202 Smokers, take note: An apple a day may reduce risk of common lung ailment. U.S. Apple Association. http://applepolyphenols.com/news/usapple_may082001.htm

203 Bao MJ, et al. Apple polyphenol protects against cigarette smoke-induced acute lung injury. Nutrition. 2013 Jan;29(1):235–43.

204 Abdel-Tawab M, Werz O, Schubert-Zsilavecz M. Boswellia serrata: an overall assessment of in vitro, preclinical, pharmacokinetic and clinical data. Clin Pharmacokinet. 2011;50(6):349–69.

205 Siddiqui MZ. Boswellia serrata, a potential antiinflammatory agent: an overview. Indian J Pharm Sci. 2011 May;73(3):255–61.

206 Gupta I, et al. Effects of Boswellia serrata gum resin in patients with bronchial asthma: results of a double-blind, placebo-controlled, 6-week clinical study. Eur J Med Res. 1998;3(11):511–4.

207 Maryanoff BE, et al. Dual inhibition of cathepsin G and chymase is effective in animal models of pulmonary inflammation. Am J Respir Crit Care Med. 2010;181(3):247–53.

208 De Benedetto F, et al. Long-term oral n-acetylcysteine reduces exhaled hydrogen peroxide in stable COPD. Pulm Pharmacol Ther 2005;18:41–47.

209 Sadowska AM. N-Acetylcysteine mucolysis in the management of chronic obstructive pulmonary disease. Ther Adv Respir Dis. 2012 Jun;6(3):127–35.

210 Dekhuijzen PN, van Beurden WJ. The role for N-acetylcysteine in the management of COPD. Int J Chron Obstruct Pulmon Dis. 2006;1(2):99–106.

211 Stav D, Raz M. Effect of N-acetylcysteine on air trapping in COPD: a randomized placebo-controlled study. Chest. 2009 Aug;136(2):381–6.

212 Foschino Barbaro MP, et al. Oxygen therapy at low flow causes oxidative stress in chronic obstructive pulmonary disease: Prevention by N-acetyl cysteine. Free Radic Res. 2005;39(10):1111–8.

213 Heart disease facts. Centers for Disease Control and Prevention. www.cdc.gov/heartdisease/facts.htm

214 Attia P. The straight dope on cholesterol – part VII. The Eating Academy. June 13, 2012. http://eatingacademy.com/nutrition/the-straight-dope-on-cholesterol-part-vii

215 Kontush A, Chantepie S, Chapman MJ. Small, dense HDL particles exert potent protection of atherogenic LDL against oxidative stress. *Arterioscler Thromb Vasc Biol.* 2003 Oct 1;23(10):1881–8.

216 Liu J, et al. Chinese red yeast rice(Monascus purpureus) for primary hyperlipidemia: a meta-analysis of randomized controlled trials. Chin Med. 2006;1(1):4.

217 Ulbricht C, et al. Guggul for hyperlipidemia: a review by the Natural Standard Research Collaboration. Complement Ther Med. 2005 Dec;13(4):279–290.

218 Roza JM, Xian-Liu Z, Guthrie N. Effect of citrus flavonoids and tocotrienols on serum cholesterol levels in hypercholesterolemic subjects. Altern Ther. 2007 Nov/Dec;13(6):44–48.

219 Morgan JM, et al. Effects of extended-release niacin on lipoprotein subclass distribution. Am J Cardiol. 2003 Jun.;91(12):1432–1436.

220 Zema MJ. Gemfibrozil, nicotinic acid and combination therapy in patients with isolated hypoalphalipoproteinemia: a randomized, open-label, crossover study. J Am Coll Cardiol. 2000 Mar.;35(3):640–646.

221 Duggal JK, et al. Effect of niacin therapy on cardiovascular outcomes in patients with coronary artery disease. J Cardiovasc Pharmacol Ther. 2010 Jun;15(2):158–166.

222 Kim HJ, et al. Influence of amla (Emblica officinalis Gaertn.) on hypercholesterolemia and lipid peroxidation in cholesterol-fed rats. J Nutr Sci Vitaminol (Tokyo). 2005 Dec;51(6):413–8.

223 Yokozawa T, et al. Amla (Emblica officinalis Gaertn.) prevents dyslipidaemia and oxidative stress in the ageing process. Br J Nutr. 2007 Jun;97(6):1187–95.

224 Akhtar MS, et al. Effect of Amla fruit (Emblica officinalis Gaertn.) on blood glucose and lipid profile of normal subjects and type 2 diabetic patients. Int J Food Sci Nutr. 2011 Sep;62(6):609–16.

225 Ramprasath VR, Jones PJ. Anti-atherogenic effects of resveratrol. Eur J Clin Nutr. 2010 Jul;64(7):660–8.

226 Rocha KK, et al. Weekend ethanol consumption and high-sucrose diet: resveratrol effects on energy expenditure, substrate oxidation, lipid profile, oxidative stress and hepatic energy metabolism. Alcohol Alcohol. 2011 Jan–Feb;46(1):10–6.

227 Ganji V, Kafai MR. Population reference values for plasma total homocysteine concentrations in US adults after the fortification of cereals with folic acid. Am J Clin Nutr. 2006;84:989–994.

228 Saposnik G, et al. Homocysteine-lowering therapy and stroke risk, severity, and disability: additional findings from the HOPE 2 trial. Stroke. 2009;40:1365–1372.

229 Bønaa KH. NORVIT: Randomized trial of homocysteine-lowering with B-vitamins for secondary prevention of cardiovascular disease after acute myocardial infarction. Program and Abstracts from the European Society of Cardiology Congress 2005; September 3–7, 2005; Stockholm, Sweden. Hot Line II.

230 Ebbing M, et al. Mortality and cardiovascular events in patients treated with homocysteine-lowering B vitamins after coronary angiography: a randomized controlled trial. JAMA. 2008;300:795–804.

231 Homocysteine Studies Collaboration. Homocysteine and risk of ischemic heart disease and stroke: a meta-analysis. JAMA. 2002;288:2015–2022.

232 Broxmeyer L. Heart disease: the greatest 'risk' factor of them all. Med Hypotheses. 2004;62:773–779.

233 Schwab U, et al. Betaine supplementation decreases plasma homocysteine concentrations but does not affect body weight, body composition, or resting energy expenditure in human subjects. Am J Clin Nutr. 2002;76:961–967.

234 Pearson TA, et al. Markers of inflammation and cardiovascular disease: application to clinical and public health practice: A statement for healthcare professionals from the Centers for Disease Control and Prevention and the American Heart Association. Circulation. 2003 Jan 28;107(3):499–511.

235 Toss H, et al. Prognostic influence of increased fibrinogen and C-reactive protein levels in unstable coronary artery disease. FRISC Study Group. Fragmin during Instability in Coronary Artery Disease. Circulation. 1997 Dec 16;96(12):4204–10.

236 Fibrinogen assays. Practical-Heamostasis.com. www.practical-haemostasis. com/Screening%20Tests/fibrinogen.html

237 Hsia CH, et al. Nattokinase decreases plasma levels of fibrinogen, factor VII, and factor VIII in human subjects. Nutrition Research. 2009;29:190–96.

238 Pais E, et al. Effects of nattokinase, a pro-fibrinolytic enzyme, on red blood cell aggregation and whole blood viscosity. Clin Hemorheol Microcir. 2006;35(1–2):139–42.

239 Kim JY, et al. Effects of nattokinase on blood pressure: a randomized, controlled trial. Hypertens Res. 2008 Aug;31(8):1583–88.

240 Chesney CM, et al. Effect of niacin, warfarin, and antioxidant therapy on coagulation parameters in patients with peripheral arterial disease in the Arterial Disease Multiple Intervention Trial (ADMIT). Am Heart J. 2000 Oct;140(4):631–6.

241 Philipp CS, et al. Effect of niacin supplementation on fibrinogen levels in patients with peripheral vascular disease. Am J Cardiol. 1998 Sep 1;82(5):697–9, A9.

242 Johansson JO, et al. Nicotinic acid treatment shifts the fibrinolytic balance favourably and decreases plasma fibrinogen in hypertriglyceridaemic men. J Cardiovasc Risk. 1997 Jun;4(3):165–71.

243 Bordia AK. The effect of vitamin C on blood lipids, fibrinolytic activity and platelet adhesiveness in patients with coronary artery disease. Atherosclerosis. 1980 Feb;35(2): 181–7.

244 Taubes G. Good Calories, Bad Calories. Anchor Books: New York, 2008:158.

245 Sarwar N, et al. Triglyceride-mediated pathways and coronary disease: collaborative analysis of 101 studies. Lancet. 2010 May 8;375(9726):1634–9.

246 Taubes G, 2008.

247 Eslick GD, et al. Benefits of fish oil supplementation in hyperlipidemia: a systematic review and meta-analysis. Int J Cardiol. 2009 Jul 24;136(1):4–16.

248 Colquhoun D, et al. Review of evidence: Fish, fish oils, n-3 polyunsaturated fatty acids and cardiovascular health. Heart Foundation. 2008 Aug. www.heartfoundation.org.au/ SiteCollectionDocuments/Fish-FishOils-revie-of-evidence.pdf

249 Solà R, et al. Soluble fibre (Plantago ovata husk) reduces plasma low-density lipoprotein (LDL) cholesterol, triglycerides, insulin, oxidised LDL and systolic blood pressure in hypercholesterolaemic patients: A randomised trial. Atherosclerosis. 2010 Aug;211 (2):630–7.

250 Narita Y, Inouye KJ. Kinetic analysis and mechanism on the inhibition of chlorogenic

acid and its components against porcine pancreas alpha-amylase isozymes I and II. J Agric Food Chem. 2009;57:9218–25.

251 Henry-Vitrac C, et al. Contribution of chlorogenic acids to the inhibition of human hepatic glucose-6-phosphatase activity in vitro by Svetol, a standardized decaffeinated green coffee extract. J Agric Food Chem. 2010 Apr 14;58(7):4141–4144.

252 Shimoda H, Seki E, Aitani M. Inhibitory effect of green coffee bean extract on fat accumulation and body weight gain in mice. BMC Complement Alt Med. 2006;6:9–18.

253 Kones R. Rosuvastatin, inflammation, C-reactive protein, JUPITER, and primary prevention of cardiovascular disease—a perspective. Drug Des Devel Ther 2010;4:383–413.

254 Schnohr P. Coronary heart disease risk factors ranked by importance for the individual and community. A 21 year follow-up of 12000 men and women from The Copenhagen City Heart Study. Eur Heart J. 2002 Apr;23(8):620–626.

255 Kshirsagar AV, et al. Blood pressure usually considered normal is associated with an elevated risk of cardiovascular disease. Am J Med. 2006 Feb;119(2):133–41.

256 Lewington S, et al. Age-specific relevance of usual blood pressure to vascular mortality: a meta-analysis of individual data for one million adults in 61 prospective studies. Lancet. 2002 Dec 14; 360(9349):1903–1913.

257 Sivaprakasapillai B, et al. Effect of grape seed extract on blood pressure in subjects with the metabolic syndrome. Metabolism. 2009 Dec;58(12):1743–6.

258 Aviram M, Dornfeld L. Pomegranate juice consumption inhibits serum angiotensin converting enzyme activity and reduces systolic blood pressure. Atherosclerosis. 2001 Sep;158(1):195–198.

259 Aviram M, et al. Pomegranate juice consumption for 3 years by patients with carotid artery stenosis reduces common carotid intima-media thickness, blood pressure and LDL oxidation. Clin Nutr. 2004 Jun;23(3):423–433.

260 Jauhiainen T, Korpela R. Milk peptides and blood pressure. J Nutr. 2007;137(3):825S–829S.

261 Vermeirssen V, et al. Angiotensin-I converting enzyme (ACE) inhibitory peptides derived from pea and whey protein. Meded Rijksuniv Gent Fak Landbouwkd Toegep Biol Wet. 2002;67(4):27–30.

262 Vermeirssen V, et al. Release of angiotensin I converting enzyme (ACE) inhibitory activity during in vitro gastrointestinal digestion: from batch experiment to semicontinuous model. J Agric Food Chem. 2003 Sep 10;51(19):5680–7.

263 Manso MA, Lopez-Fandino R. Angiotensin I converting enzyme-inhibitory activity of bovine, ovine, and caprine kappa-casein macropeptides and their tryptic hydrolysates. J Food Prot. 2003 Sep;66(9):1686–92

264 About lower extremity arterial disease. New York-Presbyterian. http://nyp.org/services/lower-extremity-arterial-disease.html

265 Strong JP, et al. Prevalence and extent of atherosclerosis in adolescents and young adults. JAMA. 1999 Feb 24;281(8):727–35.

266 Aviram M, et al. Pomegranate juice consumption for 3 years by patients with carotid artery stenosis reduces common carotid intima-media thickness, blood pressure and LDL oxidation. Clin Nutr. 2004 Jun;23(3):423–33.

267 Aviram M, et al. Pomegranate juice consumption reduces oxidative stress, atherogenic modifications to LDL, and platelet aggregation: studies in humans and in atherosclerotic apolipoprotein E-deficient mice. Am J Clin Nutr. 2000 May;71(5):1062–76.

268 Mertens-Talcott SU, et al. Absorption, metabolism, and antioxidant effects of pomegranate (Punica granatum l.) polyphenols after ingestion of a standardized extract in healthy human volunteers. J Agric Food Chem. 2006 Nov 15; 54(23):8956–61.

269 Fuhrman B, Volkova N, Aviram M. Pomegranate juice inhibits oxidized LDL uptake and cholesterol biosynthesis in macrophages. J Nutr Biochem. 2005 Sep; 16(9):570–6.

270 Wei EP, et al. Superoxide generation and reversal of acetylcholine-induced cerebral arteriolar dilation after acute hypertension. Circ Res. 1985; 57:781–7.

271 Rubanyi GM, Vanhoutte PM. Superoxide anions and hyperoxia inactivate endothelium-derived relaxing factor. Am J Physiol Heart Circ Physiol. 1986; 250: H822–7.

272 Landmesser U, et al. Vascular oxidant stress and endothelial dysfunction in patients with chronic heart failure: role of xanthine-oxidase and extracellular superoxide dismutase. Circulation. 2002; 106:3073–8.

273 Cloarec M, et al. GliSODin, a vegetal sod with gliadin, as preventative agent vs. atherosclerosis, as confirmed with carotid ultrasound-B imaging. Allerg Immunol. (Paris). 2007 Feb; 39(2):45–50.

274 Durak A, et al. Effects of garlic extract supplementation on blood lipid and antioxidant parameters and atherosclerotic plaque formation process in cholesterol-fed rabbits. J Herb Pharmcother. 2002; 2(2):19–32.

275 Budoff MJ, et al. Inhibiting progression of coronary calcification using aged garlic extract in patients receiving statin therapy: a preliminary study. Prev Med. 2004 Nov; 39(5):985–91.

276 Budoff, M. Aged garlic extract retards progression of coronary artery calcification. J Nutr. 2006 Mar;136(3 Suppl):741S–4S.

277 Koscielny J, et al. The antiatherosclerotic effect of Allium sativum. Atherosclerosis. 1999 May;144(1):237–49.

278 Schurgers LJ, et al. Post-translational modifications regulate matrix Gla protein function: importance for inhibition of vascular smooth muscle cell calcification. J Thromb Haemost. 2007 Dec; 5(12):2503–11.

279 Tsukamoto Y, et al. Intake of fermented soybean (natto) increases circulating vitamin K2 (menaquinone-7) and gamma-carboxylated osteocalcin concentration in normal individuals. J Bone Miner Metab. 2000; 18(4):216–22.

280 Kawashima H, et al. Effects of vitamin K2 (menatetrenone) on atherosclerosis and blood coagulation in hypercholesterolemic rabbits. Jpn J Pharmacol. 1997 Oct; 75(2):135–43.

281 Spronk HM, et al. Tissue-specific utilization of menaquinone-4 results in the prevention of arterial calcification in warfarin-treated rats. J Vasc Res. 2003 Nov–Dec; 40(6):531–7.

282 Buelens JWJ, et al. High dietary menaquinone intake is associated with reduced coronary calcification. Atherosclerosis. 2009 Apr; 203(2):489–93.

283 Geleijnse JM, et al. Dietary intake of menaquinone is associated with a reduced risk of coronary heart disease: the Rotterdam Study. J Nutr. 2004 Nov;134(11):3100–5.

284 Heart failure facts. Centers for Disease Control and Prevention. Last reviewed Oct. 17, 2012. www.cdc.gov/dhdsp/data_statistics/fact_sheets/fs_heart_failure.htm

285 Heart failure facts. Centers for Disease Control and Prevention. Last reviewed Oct. 17, 2012. www.cdc.gov/dhdsp/data_statistics/fact_sheets/fs_heart_failure.htm

286 McCullough PA, et al. Confirmation of a heart failure epidemic: findings from the Resource Utilization Among Congestive Heart Failure (REACH) study . J Am Coll Cardiol. 2002;39:60–69.

287 Werbach MR. Nutritional Influences on Illness. [book on CD-ROM] Tarzana, CA: Third Line Press; 1998.

288 Morisco C, Trimarco B, Condorelli M. Effect of coenzyme Q 10 therapy in patients with congestive heart failure: a long-term multicenter randomized study. Clin Investig. 1993;71(suppl 8):S134–S136.

289 Schwinger RH, et al. Crataegus special extract WS 1442 increases force of contraction in human myocardium cAMP-independently. J Cardiovasc Pharmacol. 2000 May; 35(5):700–7.

290 Pittler MH, Guo R, Ernst E. Hawthorn extract for treating chronic heart failure. Cochrane Database Syst Rev. 2008; (1):CD005312.

291 Tauchert M. Efficacy and safety of crataegus extract WS 1442 in comparison with placebo in patients with chronic stable New York Heart Association class-III heart failure. Am Heart J. 2002 May; 143(5):910–5.

292 Holubarsch CJ, et al. The efficacy and safety of Crataegus extract WS 1442 in patients with heart failure: the SPICE trial. Eur J Heart Fail. 2008 Dec; 10(12):1255–63.

293 Bharani A, Ganguly A, Bhargava KD. Salutary effect of Terminalia Arjuna in patients with severe refractory heart failure. Int J Cardiol. 1995 May; 49(3):191–9.

294 Dwivedi S, Jauhari R. Beneficial effects of Terminalia arjuna in coronary artery disease. Indian Heart J. 1997 Sep–Oct; 49(5):507–10.

295 Chowanadisal W, et al. Pyrroloquinoline quinone stimulates mitochondrial biogenesis through cAMP response element-binding protein phosphorylation and increased PGC-1alpha expression. J Biol Chem. 2010 Jan 1; 285(1):142–52.

296 Karamandilis G, et al. Defective DNA replication impairs mitochondrial biogenesis in human failing hearts. Circ Res. 2010 May 14; 106(9): 1541–8.

297 Insufficient sleep is a public health epidemic. Centers for Disease Control and Prevention. Reviewed March 14, 2013. www.cdc.gov/features/dssleep/

298 Gangwisch JE, et al. Inadequate sleep as a risk factor for obesity: Analyses of the NHANES I. Sleep. 2005;28:1289–96.

299 Tasali E, et al. Slow–wave sleep and the risk of type 2 diabetes in humans. Proc Natl Acad Sci USA. 2008 Jan 22;105(3):1044–9.

300 Huget J. Defense against colds: plenty of sleep. *The Washington Post*. Jan. 9, 2009.

301 Cohen S, et ak. Sleep habits and susceptibility to the common cold. *Arch Intern Med*. 2009 Jan 12;169(1):62–7

302 Office of Medical Center Communications. Skipping sleep may signal problems for

coronary arteries. The University of Chicago Medical Center. Dec. 24, 2008. www.uchospitals.edu/news/2008/20081224-sleep.html

303 King CR, et al. Short sleep duration and incident coronary artery calcification. *JAMA*. 2008 Dec 24;300(24):2859–66.

304 Kakizaki M, et al. Sleep duration and the risk of breast cancer: the Ohsaki Cohort Study. *Br J Cancer*. 2008 Nov 4;99(9):1502–5.

305 Humphreys K. The more you sleep, the longer you live. SFGate.com. Sept. 2, 2007. www.sfgate.com/cgi-bin/article.cgi?f=/c/a/2007/09/02/CMR2RF6AK.DTL

306 Humphreys K, 2007.

307 Paul MA, et al. Sleep-inducing pharmaceuticals: a comparison of melatonin, zaleplon, zopiclone, and temazepam. Aviat Space Environ Med. 2004;75:512–519.

308 Rogers NL, Kennaway DJ, Dawson D. Neurobehavioural performance effects of daytime melatonin and temazepam administration. J Sleep Res. 2003;12:207–212.

309 van Geijlswijk IM, et al. Dose finding of melatonin for chronic idiopathic childhood onset insomnia: a RCT. Psychopharmacology (Berl). 2010 Oct;212(3): 379–91.

310 Garfinkel D, et al. Efficacy and safety of prolonged-release melatonin in insomnia patients with diabetes: A randomized, double-blind, crossover study. Diabetes, Metab Syndr Obes. 2011;4:307–13.

311 Kim JH, et al. Efficacy of as1-casein hydrolysate on stress-related symptoms in women. Eur J Clin Nutr. 2007;61: 536–541.

312 Saint-Hilaire Z, et al. Effects of a bovine alpha S1-casein tryptic hydrosylate (CTH) on sleep disorder in Japanese general population. Open Sleep J. 2009;2:26–32.

313 Durlach J, et al. Biorhythms and possible central regulation of magnesium status, phototherapy, darkness therapy and chronopathological forms of magnesium depletion. Magnes Res. 2002 Mar;15(1–2):49–66.

314 Omiya K, et al. Heart-rate response to sympathetic nervous stimulation, exercise, and magnesium concentration in various sleep conditions. Int J Sport Nutr Exerc Metab. 2009 Apr;19(2):127–35.

315 Rondanelli M, et al. The effect of melatonin, magnesium and zinc on primary insomnia in long-term care facility residents in Italy: A double-blind, placebo-controlled clinical trial. J Amer Geriatr Soc. 2011 Jan;59(1): 82–90.

316 Hornyak M, et al. Magnesium therapy for periodic leg movements-related insomnia and restless legs syndrome: an open pilot study. Sleep. 1998 Aug 1;21(5):501–5.

317 Abdou A, et al. Relaxation and immunity enhancement effects of Gamma-Aminobutyric acid (GABA) administration in humans. BioFactors. 2006:26:201–8.

318 An estimated 1 in 10 U.S. adults report depression. Centers for Disease Control and Prevention. Last reviewed April 20, 2012. www.cdc.gov/features/dsdepression/

319 An estimated 1 in 10 U.S. adults report depression. Centers for Disease Control. Last reviewed April 20, 2012. www.cdc.gov/features/dsdepression/

320 Andrews G, Pouton R, Skoog I. Lifetime risk of depression: restricted to a minority or waiting for most? BJ Pysch. 2005; 187:495–6.

321 Nauert R. Brain imaging shows brain changes in depression. PsychCentral. com.

Reviewed Sept. 2, 2010. http://psychcentral.com/news/2010/09/02/brain-imaging-shows-brain-changes-in-depression/17541.html

322 Bremner JD. Structural changes in the brain in depression and relationship to symptom recurrence. CNS Spect. 2002 Feb;7(2):129–30, 135–9.

323 What causes depression? Harvard Health Publications, Harvard Medical School. www.health.harvard.edu/newsweek/what-causes-depression.htm

324 What causes depression? Harvard Health Publications, Harvard Medical School. www.health.harvard.edu/newsweek/what-causes-depression.htm

325 Ganji V, et al. Serum vitamin D concentrations are related to depression in young adult US population: the Third National Health and Nutrition Examination Survey. Int Arch Med. 2010 Nov 11;3:29.

326 Hoogendijk WJ, et al. Depression is associated with decreased 25-hydroxyvitamin D and increased parathyroid hormone levels in older adults. Arch Gen Psychiatry. 2008 May;65(5):508–12.

327 Ganji V, 2010.

328 Kaye WH, et al. Effects of acute tryptophan depletion on mood in bulimia nervosa. Biol Psychiatry. 2000 Jan 15;47(2):151–7.

329 Neumeister A, et al. Effects of tryptophan depletion vs. catecholamine depletion in patients with seasonal affective disorder in remission with light therapy. Arch Gen Psychiatry. 1998;55:524–30.

330 Byerley WF, et al. 5-hydroxytryptophan: a review of its antidepressant efficacy and adverse effects. J Clin Psychopharmacol. 1987;7:127–137.

331 Poldinger W, Calanchini B, Schwarz W. A functional-dimensional approach to depression: Serotonin deficiency as a target syndrome in a comparison of 5-hydroxytryptophan and fluvoxamine. Psychopathology. 1991;24:53–81.

332 Bell KM, et al. S-adenosylmethionine blood levels in major depression: changes with drug treatment. Acta Neurol Scand Suppl. 1994;154:15–18.

333 Papakostas GI, et al. S-adenosyl methionine (SAMe) augmentation of serotonin reuptake inhibitors for antidepressant nonresponders with major depressive disorder: a double-blind randomized clinical trial. Am J Psychiatry. 2010; 167:942–8.

334 Delle Chiaie R, Pancheri P, Scapicchio P. MC3: multicentre, controlled efficacy and safety trial of oral S-adenosyl-methionine (SAMe) vs. oral imipramine in the treatment of depression [abstract]. Int J Neuropsychopharmcol. 2000;3(suppl 1):S230.

335 De Vanna M, Rigamonti R. Oral S-adenosyl-L-methionine in depression. Curr Ther Res. 1992;52:478–485.

336 Bressa GM. S-adenosyl-l-methionine (SAMe) as antidepressant: meta-analysis of clinical studies. Acta Neurol Scand Suppl. 1994;154:7–14.

337 Facts & Statistics. Anxiety and Depression Association of America. www.adaa.org/about-adaa/press-room/facts-statistics

338 Facts & Statistics. Anxiety and Depression Association of America. www.adaa.org/about-adaa/press-room/facts-statistics

339 Armstrong DJ, et al. Vitamin D deficiency is associated with anxiety and depression in fibromyalgia. Clin Rhematol. 2007 Apr;26(4):551–4.

340 Robinson OJ, et al. Acute tryptophan depletion increases translational indices of anxiety but not fear: serotonergic modulation of the bed nucleus of the stria terminalis? *Neuropsychopharmacology.* 2012 Jul;37(8):1963–71.

341 van Veen JF, et al. Tryptophan depletion affects the autonomic stress response in generalized social anxiety disorder. *Psychoneuroendocrinology.* 2009 Nov;34(10):1590–4.

342 Kahn RS, et al. Effect of a serotonin precursor and uptake inhibitor in anxiety disorders; a double-blind comparison of 5-hydroxytryptophan, clomipramine and placebo. *Int Clin Psychopharmacol.* 1987 Jan;2(1):33–45.

343 Kobayashi K, et al. Effects of L-theanine on the release of alpha-brain waves in human volunteers. Nippon Nögei Kagakukaighi. 1998:72(2):153–7.

344 Higashiyama A, et al. Effects of L-theanine on attention and reaction time response. Journal of Functional Foods. 2011:3(3):171–8.

345 Kimura K, Ozeki M, Juneja LR, Ohira H. L-Theanine reduces psychological and physiological stress responses. Biol Psychol. 2007 Jan;74(1):39–45.

346 Awad R, et al: Effects of traditionally used anxiolytic botanicals on enzymes of the gamma-aminobutyric acid (GABA) system. Can J Physiol Pharmacol. 2007;85(9):933–42

347 Kennedy D, Little W, Scholey A. Attenuation of laboratory-induced stress in humans after acute administration of Melissa officinalis (lemon balm). Psychosom Med. 2004 Jul–Aug;66:607–613.

348 Sartori SB, et al. Magnesium deficiency induces anxiety and HPA axis dysregulation: modulation by therapeutic drug treatment. *Neuropharmacology.* 2012 Jan;62(1):304–12.

349 Hayes, Carolyn. Magnesium Miracle. New York: Ballantine Books, 2007:47.

350 Hanus M, Lafon J, Mathieu M. Double-blind, randomised, placebo-controlled study to evaluate the efficacy and safety of a fixed combination containing two plant extracts (Crataegus oxyacantha and Eschscholtzia californica) and magnesium in mild-to-moderate anxiety disorders. Curr Med Res Opin. 2004 Jan;20(1):63–71.

351 Carroll D, et al. The effects of an oral multivitamin combination with calcium, magnesium, and zinc on psychological well-being in healthy young male volunteers: a double-blind placebo-controlled trial. Psychopharmacology (Berl). 2000 Jun;150(2):220–5.

352 De Souza MC, et al. A synergistic effect of a daily supplement for 1 month of 200 mg magnesium plus 50 mg vitamin B6 for the relief of anxiety-related premenstrual symptoms: a randomized, double-blind, crossover study. J Womens Health Gend Based Med. 2000 Mar;9(2):131–9.

353 The heavy burden of arthritis in the U.S. Arthritis Foundation. Updated March 20, 2012. www.arthritis.org/files/images/AF_Connect/Departments/Public_Relations/Arthritis-Prevalence-Fact-Sheet—3-7-12.pdf

354 The heavy burden of arthritis in the U.S. Arthritis Foundation. Updated March 20, 2012. www.arthritis.org/files/images/AF_Connect/Departments/Public_Relations/Arthritis-Prevalence-Fact-Sheet—3-7-12.pdf

355 Fouladbakhsh J. Complementary and alternative modalities to relieve osteoarthritis symptoms: A review of the evidence on several therapies often used for osteoarthritis management. Orthop Nurs. 2012;31(2):115–121.

356 Poolsup N, et al. Glucosamine long–term treatment and the progression of knee

osteoarthritis: systematic review of randomized controlled trials. Ann Pharmacother. 2005 Jun;39(6):1080–7.

357 Palmieri B, Lodi D, Cappone S. Osteoarthritis and degenerative joint disease: local treatment options update. Acta Biomed. 2010 Sep; 81(2):94–100.

358 Huang SL, Ling PX, Zhang TM. Oral absorption of hyaluronic acid and phospholipids complexes in rats. World Gastroenterol. 2007 Feb 14; 13(6):945–9.

359 Kalman DS, et al. Effect of a natural extract of chicken combs with a high content of hyaluronic acid (Hyal-Joint) on pain relief and quality of life in subjects with knee osteoarthritis: a pilot randomized double-blind placebo-controlled trial. Nutr J. 2008 Jan 21; 7:3

360 Bergin BJ, et al. Oral hyaluronan gel reduces post operative tarsocrural effusion in the yearling thoroughbred. Equine Vet J. 2006 Jul;38(4):375–8.

361 Debbi EM, et al. Efficacy of methylsulfonylmethane supplementation on osteoarthritis of the knee: a randomized controlled study. BMC Complement Altern Med. 2011 Jun 27;11:50.

362 Usha PR, Naidu MU. Randomised, Double-Blind, Parallel, Placebo-Controlled Study of Oral Glucosamine, Methylsulfonylmethane and their Combination in Osteoarthritis. Clin Drug Investig. 2004;24(6):353–63.

363 Hill P, Brantley H, Van Dyke M. Some properties of keratin biomaterials: kerateines. Biomaterials. 2010 Feb;31(4):585–93.

364 Fakfakh N, et al. Wool-waste valorization: production of protein hydrolysate with high antioxidative potential by fermentation with a new keratinolytic bacterium, Bacillus pumilus A1. J Appl Microbiol. 2013 May 11; doi: 10.1111/jam.12246. [Epub ahead of print]

365 Aitken R. Technical Summary of Cynatine FLX Clinical Trial. 2010.

366 New findings suggest keratin ingredient Cynatine FLX activates joint defense enzymes. Nov. 10, 2005. Keratec press release. www.marketwire.com/press-release/new-findings-suggest-keratin-ingredient-cynatine-flx-activates-joint-defense-enzymes-665164.htm

367 Kahan A, et al. Long-term effects of chondroitins 4 and 6 sulfate on knee osteoarthritis: the study on osteoarthritis progression prevention, a two-year, randomized, double-blind, placebo-controlled trial. Arthritis Rheum. 2009 Feb;60(2):524–33.

368 Wildi LM , et al. Chondroitin sulphate reduces both cartilage volume loss and bone marrow lesions in knee osteoarthritis patients starting as early as 6 months after initiation of therapy: a randomised, double-blind, placebo-controlled pilot study using MRI. Ann Rheum Dis 2011;70:982–989.

369 Gabay C, et al. Symptomatic effects of chondroitin 4 and chondroitin 6 sulfate on hand osteoarthritis: A randomized, double-blind, placebo-controlled clinical trial at a single center. Arthritis Rheum. 2011 Nov;63(11):3383–91.

370 Hardy ML, et al. S-adenosyl-L-methionine for treatment of depression, osteoarthritis, and liver disease. Evid Rep Technol Asses (Summ). 2003 Aug;(64):1–3.

371 Kim J, et al. Comparative clinical trial of S-adenosylmethionine versus nabumetone for the treatment of knee osteoarthritis: an 8-week, multicenter, randomized, double-blind, double-dummy, Phase IV study in Korean patients. Clin Ther. 2009 Dec;31(12):2860–72.

372 De Silva V, et al. Evidence for the efficacy of complementary and alternative medicine in the management of osteoporosis: a systematic review. Rheumatology (Oxford). 2011 May;50(5):911–20.

373 Soeken KL, et al. Safety and efficacy of S-adenosylmethionine (SAMe) for osteoarthritis. J Fam Pract. 2002 May;51(5):425–30.

374 Hosea Blewett HJ. Exploring the mechanisms behind S-adenosylmethionine (SAMe) in the treatment of osteoarthritis. Crit Rev Food Sci Nutr. 2008 May;48(5):458–63.

375 Belcaro G, et al. Efficacy and safety of Meriva(R), a curcumin-phosphatidylcholine complex, during extended administration in osteoarthritis patients. Altern Med Rev. 2010;15(4):337–344.

376 Belcaro G, et al. Product-evaluation registry of Meriva(R), a curcumin-phosphatidylcholine complex, for the complementary management of osteoarthritis. Panminerva Med. 2010;52(2 Suppl 1):55–62.

377 Shakibaei M, et al. Suppression of NF-kappaB activation by curcumin leads to inhibition of expression of cyclo-oxygenase-2 and matrix metalloproteinase-9 in human articular chondrocytes: Implications for the treatment of osteoarthritis. Biochem Pharmacol. 2007 May 1;73(9):1434–45.

378 Takada Y, et al. Acetyl-11-keto-beta-boswellic acid potentiates apoptosis, inhibits invasion, and abolishes osteoclastogenesis by suppressing NF-kappa B and NF-kappa B-regulated gene expression. J Immunol. 2006 Mar 1;176(5):3127–40.

379 Siddiqui MZ. Boswellia serrata, a potential antiinflammatory agent: an overview. Indian J Pharm Sci. 2011 May;73(3):255–61.

380 Kimmatkar N, et al. Efficacy and tolerability of Boswellia serrata extract in treatment of osteoarthritis of knee—a randomized double blind placebo controlled trial. Phytomedicine. 2003;10(1):3–7.

381 Sengupta K, et al. A double blind, randomized, placebo controlled study of the efficacy and safety of 5-Loxin for treatment of osteoarthritis of the knee. Arthritis Res Ther. 2008;10(4):30.

382 Sengupta K, et al. Comparative efficacy and tolerability of 5-Loxin and Aflapin against osteoarthritis of the knee: a double blind, randomized, placebo controlled clinical study. Int J Med Sci. 2010;7(6):366–77.

383 Kim KM, Kim MJ, Kang JS. Absorption, distribution, metabolism, and excretion of decursin and decursinol angelate from Angelica gigas Nakai. J Microbiol Biotechnol. 2009 Dec;19(12):1569–72.

384 Song JS, et al. Pharmacokinetic characterization of decursinol derived from Angelica gigas Nakai in rats. Xenobiotica. 2011 Oct;41(10):895–902.

385 Choi SS, et al. Antinociceptive profiles of crude extract from roots of Angelica gigas NAKAI in various pain models. Biol Pharm Bull. 2003 Sep;26(9):1283–8.

386 Kim JH, et al. Decursin inhibits induction of inflammatory mediators by blocking nuclear factor-kappaB activation in macrophages. Mol Pharmacol. 2006 Jun;69(6):1783–90.

387 Seo YJ, et al. The analgesic effect of decursinol. Arch Pharm Res. 2009 Jun;32(6):937–43.

388 Shin S, et al. Ethanol extract of *Angelica gigas* inhibits croton oil-induced inflammation by suppressing the cyclooxygenase-prostaglandin pathway. J Vet Sci. 2010 Mar;11(1):43–50.

389 Guise TA. Bone loss and fracture risk associated with cancer therapy. Oncologist. 2006 Nov–Dec;11(10):1121–31.

390 Center JR, et al. Mortality after all major types of osteoporotic fracture in men and women: an observational study. Lancet. 1999 Mar 12;353(9156):878–82.

391 Cummings SR, Black DM, Rubin SM. Lifetime risks of hip, Colles', or vertebral fracture and coronary heart disease among white postmenopausal women. Arch Intern Med. 1989 Nov;149(11):2445–8.

392 Cawthorn PM. Gender differences in osteoporosis and fractures. Clin Orthop Relat Res. 2011 Jul;469(7):1900–5.

393 Facts and statistics. International Osteoporosis Foundation. www.iofbonehealth.org/facts-statistics#category-14

394 Facts and statistics. International Osteoporosis Foundation. www.iofbonehealth.org/facts-statistics#category-14

395 Seeman E. The dilemma of osteoporosis in men. Am J Med. 1995 Feb 27;98(2A):76S–88S.

396 Osteoporosis: risk factors. Mayo Clinic. Dec. 13, 2011. www.mayoclinic.com/health/osteoporosis/DS00128/DSECTION=risk-factors

397 Cherniack EP, Levis S, Troen BR. Hypovitaminosis D: a widespread epidemic. Geriatrics. 2008 Apr;63(4): 24–30.

398 Lips P, et al. Reducing fracture risk with calcium and vitamin D. Clin Endocrinol (Oxf). 2010 Sep;73(3):277–85.

399 Hernandez JL, et al. Metabolic syndrome and bone metabolism: the Camargo Cohort study. Menopause. 2010 Sep–Oct;17(5):955–61.

400 McClung M. Is altered bone health part of the metabolic syndrome? Menopause. 2010 Sep–Oct;17(5):900–1.

401 Hein G, et al. Advanced glycation end product modification of bone proteins and bone remodelling: hypothesis and preliminary immunohistochemical findings. Ann Rheum Dis. 2006 Jan;65(1):101–4.

402 Valcourt U, et al. Non-enzymatic glycation of bone collagen modifies osteoclastic activity and differentiation. J Biol Chem. 2007 Feb 23;282(8):5691–703.

403 Graham LS, et al. Oxidized lipids enhance RANKL production by T lymphocytes: implications for lipid-induced bone loss. Clin Immunol. 2009 Nov;133(2):265–75.

404 Maziere C, et al. Oxidized low density lipoprotein inhibits phosphate signaling and phosphate-induced mineralization in osteoblasts. Involvement of oxidative stress. Biochim Biophys Acta. 2010 Nov;1802(11):1013–9.

405 Chang J, et al. Inhibition of osteoblastic bone formation by nuclear factor-kappaB. Nat Med. 2009 Jun;15(6):682–9.

406 Lee WT, et al. A randomized double-blind controlled calcium supplementation trial, and bone and height acquisition in children. Br J Nutr. 1995 Jul; 74(1):125–39.

407 Courtiex D, et al. Cumulative effect of calcium supplementation and physical activity on bone accretion in premenarchal children: a double-blind randomised placebo-controlled trial. Int J Sports Med. 2005 Jun; 26(5):332–8.

408 Winters-Stone KM, Snow CM. One year of oral calcium supplementation maintains cortical bone density in young adult female runners. Int J Sport Nutr Exerc Metab. 2004 Feb; 14(1):7–17.

409 Going S, et al. Effects of exercise on bone mineral density in calcium-replete post-menopausal women with and without hormone replacement therapy. Osteoporos Int. 2003 Aug; 14(8):637–43.

410 Ortolani S, Scotti A, Cherubini R. Rapid suppression of bone resorption and parathyroid hormone secretion by acute oral administration of calcium in healthy adult men. J Endocrinol Invest. 2003 Apr; 26(4):353–8.

411 Wagner G, et al. Effects of various forms of calcium on body weight and bone turnover markers in women participating in a weight loss program. J Am Coll Nutr. 2007 Oct; 26(5):456–61.

412 Lau EM, et al. Milk supplementation of the diet of postmenopausal Chinese women on a low calcium intake retards bone loss. J Bone Miner Res. 2001 Sep; 16(9):1704–9.

413 Holick MF. Optimal vitamin D status for the prevention and treatment of osteoporosis. Drugs Aging. 2007;24(12):1017–29.

414 Dawson-Hughes B, et al. Effect of calcium and vitamin D supplementation on bone density in men and women 65 years of age or older. N Engl J Med. 1997;337:670–676.

415 Dawson-Hughes B, et al. Effect of vitamin D supplementation on wintertime and overall bone loss in healthy postmenopausal women. Ann Intern Med. 1991;115:505–512.

416 Ginde AA, Liu MC, Camargo CA Jr. Demographic differences and trends of vitamin D insufficiency in the US population, 1988–2004. Arch Intern Med. 2009 Mar 23;169 (6): 626–32.

417 Hegsted MD. Fractures, calcium, and the modern diet. Am J Clin Nutr. 2001 Nov;74(5):571–573.

418 Aydin H, et al. Short-term oral magnesium supplementation suppresses bone turnover in postmenopausal osteoporotic women. Biol Trace Elem Res. 2010 Feb;133(2):136–43.

419 Sojka JE, Weaver CM. Magnesium supplementation and osteoporosis. Nutr Rev. 1995 Mar;53(3):71–4.

420 Schurgers LJ, et al. Role of vitamin K and vitamin K-dependent proteins in vascular calcification. Z Kardiol. 2001;90 Suppl 3:57–63.

421 Okura T, et al. Undercarboxylated osteocalcin is a biomarker of carotid calcification in patients with essential hypertension. Kidney Blood Press Res. 2010;33(1):66–71.

422 Sogabe N, et al. Effects of long-term vitamin K(1) (phylloquinone) or vitamin K(2) (menaquinone-4) supplementation on body composition and serum parameters in rats. Bone. 2011 May 1;48(5):1036–42.

423 Schurgers LJ, et al. Vitamin-K containing dietary supplements: comparison of synthetic vitamin K1 and natto-derived menaquinone-7. Blood. 2007 Apr;109(8):3279–83.

424 Takino Y, et al. Zinc l-pyrrolidone carboxylate inhibits the UVA-induced production of matrix metalloproteinase-1 by in vitro cultured skin fibroblasts, whereas it enhances their collagen synthesis. Int J of Cosmet Sci. 2012 Feb;34(1):23–8.

425 Reffitt DM, et al. Orthosilicic acid stimulates collagen type 1 synthesis and osteoblastic differentiation in human osteoblast-like cells in vitro. Bone. 2003 Feb;32(2):127–35.

426 Jugdaohsingh R, et al. Dietary silicon intake is positively associated with bone mineral density in men and premenopausal women of the Framingham Offspring cohort. J Bone Miner Res. 2004 Feb;19(2):297–307.

427 Calomme M, et al. Partial prevention of long-term femoral bone loss in aged ovariectomized rats supplemented with choline-stabilized orthosilicic acid. Calcif Tissue Int. 2006 Apr;78(4):227–32.

428 Rivas A, et al. Association between dietary antioxidant quality score (DAQs) and bone mineral density in Spanish women. Nutr Hosp. 2012 Dec;27)6):1886–93.

429 Elmstahl S, et al. Increased incidence of fractures in middle-aged and elderly men with low intakes of phosphorus and zinc. Osteoporos Int. 1998;8(4):333–40.

430 Nielsen FH, et al. Effect of dietary boron on mineral, estrogen, and testosterone metabolism in postmenopausal women. FASEB J. 1987 Nov;1(5):394–7.

431 Hegsted M, et al. Effect of boron on vitamin D deficient rats. Biol Trace Elem Res. 1991 Mar;28(3):243–55.

432 Unpublished study

433 Bu SY, et al. Dried plum polyphenols inhibit osteoclastogenesis by downregulating NFATc1 and inflammatory mediators. Calcif Tissue Int. 2008 Jun;82(6):475–88.

434 Franklin M, et al. Dried plum prevents bone loss in a male osteoporosis model via IGF-I and the RANK pathway. Bone. 2006 Dec;39(6):1331–42.

435 Bu SY, Hunt TS, Smith BJ. Dried plum polyphenols attenuate the detrimental effects of TNF-alpha on osteoblast function coincident with up-regulation of Runx2, Osterix and IGF-I. J Nutr Biochem. 2009 Jan;20(1):35–44.

436 Arjmandi BH, et al. Dried plums improve indices of bone formation in postmenopausal women. J Womens Health Gend Based Med. 2002 Jan;11(1):61–8.

437 Bu SY, et al. Comparison of dried plum supplementation and intermittent PTH in restoring bone in osteopenic orchidectomized rats. Osteoporos Int. 2007 Jul;18(7):931–42.

438 Deyhim F, et al. Dried plum reverses bone loss in an osteopenic rat model of osteoporosis. Menopause. 2005 Nov;12(6):755–62.

439 Kondo K. Beer and health: preventive effects of beer components on lifestyle-related diseases. Biofactors. 2004;22(1–4):303–10.

440 Effenberger KE, et al. Regulation of osteoblastic phenotype and gene expression by hop-derived phytoestrogens. J Steroid Biochem Mol Biol. 2005 Sep;96(5):387–99.

441 Stevens JF, Page JE. Xanthohumol and related prenylflavonoids from hops and beer: to your good health! Phytochemistry. 2004 May;65(10):1317–30.

442 Overweight and obesity statistics. Weight-control Information Network, National Institute of Diabetes and Digestive and Kidney Diseases (NIDDK). Last modified March 12, 2013. http://win.niddk.nih.gov/statistics/

443 Stevens GA, et al. National, regional, and global trends in adult overweight and obesity prevalences. Popul Health Metr. 2012 Nov;20:10(1):22.

444 Obesity. Medline Plus, U.S. National Library of Medicine, National Institutes of Health. Last reviewed Jan. 22, 2013. www.nlm.nih.gov/medlineplus/obesity.html

445 Overweight and obesity: Health consequences. SurgeonGeneral.gov, U.S. Department of

Health & Human Services. www.surgeongeneral.gov/library/calls/obesity/fact_consequences.html

446 Lee CD, et al. Cardiorespiratory fitness, body composition, and all-cause and cardiovascular disease mortality in men. Amer J Clin Nutr. 1999 March;69(3):373–380.

447 Insulin resistance and prediabetes. National Diabetes Information Clearinghouse (NDIC), National Institute of Diabetes and Digestive and Kidney Diseases (NIDDK), National Institutes of Health (NIH). Last updated Jan. 22, 2013. http://diabetes.niddk.nih.gov/dm/pubs/insulinresistance/#causes

448 Keene M. Serotonin and the biology of bingeing. Eating Disorders: A Reference Sourcebook. Ed. Lemberg R. Cohn L., Oryx Press; 1998:51.

449 Vinson JA, Burnham BR, Nagendran MV. Randomized, double-blind, placebo-controlled, linear dose, crossover study to evaluate the efficacy and safety of a green coffee bean extract in overweight subjects. Diabetes, Metab Syndr Obes. 2012;5:21–7.

450 Kamenova P. Improvement of insulin sensitivity in patients with type 2 diabetes mellitus after oral administration of alpha-lipoic acid. Hormones (Athens). Oct–Dec 2006;5(4):251–8.

451 Jacob S, et al. Enhancement of glucose disposal in patients with type 2 diabetes by alpha-lipoic acid. Arzneimittelforschung. 1995 Aug;45(8):872–4.

452 Maeda H, et al. Fucoxanthin from edible seaweed, Undaria pinnatifida, shows antiobesity effect through UCP1 expression in white adipose tissues. Biochem Biophys Res Commun. 2005;332(2):6–6.

453 Abidov M, et al. The effects of Xanthigen in the weight management of obese premenopausal women with non-alcoholic fatty liver disease and normal liver fat. Diabetes Obes Metab. 2010;12(1):72–81.

454 Oben JE, Ngondi JL, Blum K. Inhibition of Irvingia gabonensis seed extract (OB131) on adipogenesis as mediated via down regulation of the PPARgamma and Leptin genes and up-regulation of the adiponectin gene. Lipids Health Dis. 2008;7:44.

455 Ngondi JL, Oben JE, Minka SR. The effect of Irvingia gabonensis seeds on body weight and blood lipids of obese subjects in Cameroon. Lipids Health Dis. 2005 May 25;4:12

456 Ngondi JL, et al. IGOB131, a novel seed extract of the West African plant Irvingia gabonensis, significantly reduces body weight and improves metabolic parameters in overweight humans in a randomized double-blind placebo controlled investigation. Lipids Health Dis. 2009 Mar 2;8:7.

457 Oben JE, et al. The use of a Cissus quadrangularis/Irvingia gabonensis combination in the management of weight loss: a double-blind placebo-controlled study. Lipids Health Dis. 2008 Mar 31;7:12.

458 Ngondi JL, 2009.

459 Wolfe BE, Metzger ED, Stollar, C. The effects of dieting on plasma tryptophan concentration and food intake in healthy women. Physiol Behav. 1997;61(4):537–41.

460 Hrboticky N, Leiter LA, Anderson GH. Effects of L-tryptophan on short term food intake in lean men. Nutr Res. 1985;5(6):595–607.

461 Cavaliere H, Medeiros-Neto G. The anorectic effect of increasing doses of L-tryptophan in obese patients. Eat Weight Disord. 1997 Dec;2(4):211–5.

Index

ACE, 194
Acesulfame, 9
Acetyl-L-carnitine, 156, 161
Acid reflux, 151
Active hexose correlated
    compound (AHCC), 168
Additives, artificial, 42
Adenosine triphosphate (ATP), 61,
    144, 209
Adipocytes, 215, 217
Adipogenesis, 217
Adiponectin, 215, 217
Adrenal glands, 124
Adrenaline, 25, 206
Advanced glycation end products
    (AGEs), 143, 177, 179, 180
Age-related cognitive decline
    (ARCD), 153–156
Aging, 63, 115, 116, 118, 125, 129,
    139–146, 153–156, 214–215, 237
Agriculture, 14–15
Air fresheners, 21, 98
Air quality, 98
AKBA, 183, 209
ALA. See Alpha-linolenic acid
    (ALA).
Alcohol, 63, 102
Allergens, 48, 131
Allergies, food, 131

Alpha-linolenic acid (ALA), 66, 68,
    72, 130
Alpha tocopherol. See Vitamin E.
Alzheimer's disease, 87, 156–159
American Cancer Society, 83
American Heart Association, 59,
    192
Amino acids, 116
    branched chain, 168
Amylase, 181, 192
Anaphylaxis, 131
Aneurysms, 90
Antibiotics, 14–15, 16, 26, 63
Antioxidants, 20, 116, 129, 141–142,
    160, 179, 180, 183, 186
Anxiety, 76, 203–206
Anxiety and Depression
    Association of America, 204
APO A-1, 112
APO-B, 112
APO-B100, 111
Apolipoproteins, 111–112
Appetite, 215, 217
Apple polyphenols, 153, 183
ARCD. See Age-related cognitive
    decline (ARCD).
Arjuna, 198
Arteries, 109, 110, 184, 194–195,
    212

Ashwagandha, 206
Aspartame, 8–9, 10
Astaxanthin, 76
Asthma, 99
Astragalus, 167
Atherosclerosis, 193, 194–197
ATP. *See* Adenosine triphosphate (ATP).

Bacopa, 156
Bacteria, 62–63
Bait and switch, 45–46
Baldness, 124
BDE-47, 19
Benfotiamine. *See* Vitamin B$_1$.
Berberine, 169
Beta-amyloid protein, 157, 158
Beta-carotene, 64–65, 116
Beverages, carbonated, 102
BHA. *See* Butylated hydroxyanisole (BHA).
BHRT. *See* Bioidentical hormone replacement therapy (BHRT).
Bioidentical hormone replacement therapy (BHRT), 140–141
Blood-brain barrier (BBB), 154
Blood clotting, 109, 123, 189, 195
Blood pressure, 11, 25, 75, 85, 89–90, 109, 172, 190
  high, 192–194
Blood sugar, 10, 24, 25, 61, 85, 117–118, 154, 176, 177, 179, 181, 192, 214
Blood vessels, 75, 89–90, 192–193, 194
Blueberries, 86, 155, 181
BNP. *See* B-type natriuretic peptide (BNP).
Body Mass Index (BMI), 89, 99
Bone formula, 75
Bones, 75, 96–97, 118–120, 206, 210–213

Boron, 166, 212
Boswellia, 149, 161, 166, 169, 170, 183, 209
Bowel movements, 150
BPA, 19, 22
Brain, 75, 86–87, 153–161
  proteins, 157
  waves, 201, 205
Bromelain, 143
Bronchitis, chronic, 182
B-type natriuretic peptide (BNP), 112–113
Butter, 146
Butylated hydroxyanisole (BHA), 7

Caffeine, 102, 160
Calcium, 47, 55, 71, 97, 211
Calcium collagen chelate, 212
Calcium phosphate, 119
Calories, 214
Cancer, 7, 8–9, 14, 18, 20–21, 63, 75, 82–83, 123, 161–170
  brain, 169
  breast, 165
  colon, 170
  liver, 168
  lung, 167
  prostate, 125, 166
Cans, 33
Capsaicin, 176, 190
Carbohydrates, 102, 117, 152, 191, 214, 215, 216
Carcinogens, 11, 12–13, 162
Cardiovascular disease. *See* Heart disease.
Carlson Laboratories, 241
Carnosine, 135, 144, 179–180
Cartilage, 206, 208–209
Cataracts, 100
Cathespin, 183
Cattle, 14–15, 17

Cells
   damage to, 20, 141, 144
   fat. *See* Adipocytes.
   foam, 195
   health of, 120
   natural killer, 161
Certificates of analysis (C of As),
   41, 42–44
CFS. *See* Chronic fatigue syndrome
   (CFS).
Chemicals, 19, 20, 162
   HPV (high-produce volume),
   17–18
   VOC (volatile organic
   compounds), 21, 98
Chia seeds, 66, 68
Chlorogenic acid (CGA), 181
Chlorophyllin, 164
Cholesterol, 7, 81, 85, 109, 110,
   184–187
   high-density lipoprotein (HDL),
   109, 110, 111, 112, 184, 186–187
   low-density lipoprotein (LDL),
   109, 110, 111, 112, 184–186, 195,
   196
   very low-density lipoprotein
   (VLDL), 111
Chondroitin sulfate, 208–209
Chromium, 55, 75, 179
Chrondrocytes, 208
Chronic fatigue syndrome (CFS),
   105, 171–174
Chronic obstructive pulmonary
   disease (COPD), 181–183
Circulatory system, 80–81
Coal tar, 11
Coenzyme Q10 (CoQ10), 29, 38,
   60–61, 144, 185, 198, 237
   absorption of, 68–69
   dosage, 72, 129
   forms, 68
Coenzymes, 60

Colitis, ulcerative, 148, 149
Collagen, 119, 143, 212, 213
Colonoscopies, 170
Colony-forming units (CFUs), 47,
   72
Colors, artificial, 11–13
Congestive heart failure, 197–199
Constipation, 150
ConsumerLab.com, 38, 41
COPD. *See* Chronic obstructive
   pulmonary disease (COPD).
Copper, 5, 55
CoQ10. *See* Coenzyme Q10
   (CoQ10).
Coriolus, 164
Cortisol, 24, 25, 215
Cosmetics, 22
Country Life, 240
Creatine, 161
C-reactive protein (CRP), 81, 109,
   132
Crohn's disease, 147–149
C-telopeptides, 119
Curcumin, 75, 135, 156, 158, 161,
   164, 176, 209
Curry, 156
Cyclooxygenase, 209
Cysteine, 116, 187

Dairy products, 14–17
Davis, Donald R., 3, 5
DDT, 18
Decursinol, 175, 209
Dehydroepiandrosterone sulfate
   (DHEA-S), 124
Dementia, 153–156
Dental amalgam toxicity, 172
Deoxypyridinoline (DPD), 120
Depression, 76, 201–203
DHA. *See* Docosahexaenoic acid
   (DHA).
DHEA, 91, 93, 173, 217

DHEA-S. *See* Dehydroepiandrosterone sulfate (DHEA-S).
DHT. *See* Dihydrotestosterone
   (DHT).
Diabetes, 75, 84–85, 117–118,
   154–155, 168, 176–181, 214
   type 1, 176
   type 2, 176–177
Diarrhea, 149, 151
Diet, 81, 83, 85, 86, 88, 95, 98, 102,
   103, 145–146, 191–192
   anti-inflammatory, 101, 103
   low-carbohydrate, 152
   low-glycemic, 100
   standard American, 58, 63
   vegetarian, 66, 68
Dietary Supplement Health and
   Education Act (DSHEA), 36
Digestion, 62–63
Digestive tract. *See* Gastrointestinal
   tract (GI).
Dihydrotestosterone (DHT), 91,
   124
Diosmin, 76
Diseases
   age-related/chronic, 20–21, 25,
      58, 109, 115, 142, 143
   bowel and gut, 147–153
   brain, 153–161
   infectious, 172
   mood disorder, 201–206
   nutrition deficient, 52, 53
   prevention of, 29
   See also Alzheimer's disease;
      Cancer; Chronic fatigue
      syndrome; Chronic obstructive
      pulmonary disease (COPD);
      Diabetes; Heart disease;
      Insomnia; Osteoarthritis; Pain,
      chronic; Parkinson's disease.
DL-phenylalanine, 176
D-mannose, 76

DNA, 144, 145, 161–162, 164
Docosahexaenoic acid (DHA), 66,
   68
Dopamine, 159
D-ribose, 76, 199
DSHEA. *See* Dietary Supplement
   Health and Education Act
   (DSHEA).
DuPont, 23
Dyes, food. *See* Colors, artificial.

Ears, 76
Eden Organic, 22
EGCG, 161, 179
Eicosapentaenoic acid (EPA), 66, 68
Electrons, 20, 141
Emphysema, 181–182
Endothelium, 110, 184, 195
Endrocine system, 172
Energy, 76, 173
   cellular, 60–61, 144–145
Enterocytes, 148, 174
Environmental Working Group, 22
EPA. *See* Eicosapentaenoic acid
   (EPA).
Esophagus, 151
Estradiol, 122, 124–125, 154
Estrogen, 91, 93, 97, 122, 163, 210,
   213
European Medicines Agency, 11
European Union, 12, 21
Excipients, 48
Excitotoxins and excitotoxicity, 9,
   158
Exercise, 61, 81, 83, 85, 95, 103, 105,
   106, 145, 207
   aerobic, 89
   low-impact, 101
   weight-bearing, 97
Extracts
   acai, 142
   aged garlic, 75, 196

artichoke leaf (ALE), 76, 151, 186
aronia, 142
astragalus, 146
black tea theaflavin, 142, 143, 186
blueberry, 75, 142, 155
Boswellia, 76, 143
cinnamon, 75, 179
cranberry, 75, 76
cruciferous vegetable, 75, 163
curcumin, 75, 143
dark chocolate, 142, 187
dried plum, 212
elderberry, 142
ginger, 176, 190
grape seed, 75, 194
green coffee bean (CGA), 75, 181, 192, 216
green tea, 142, 160, 167, 179, 187, 217
hibiscus, 76
honeysuckle, 142
Irvingia, 76
mangosteen, 217
olive leaf, 75, 194
pomegranate juice, 75, 142, 180, 194, 196
Picrorhiza, 76
Reishi mushroom, 75, 146, 164, 173
saffron, 76, 176, 203, 206, 217
tart cherry, 76, 142, 175
thymus, 75
turmeric, 135
white kidney bean, 181
Eyes, 76

Fat, 214
belly, 11, 155
Fatigue, 76, 127
Fats, 151
saturated, 17, 192
trans, 6–7
Fertilizers, synthetic, 3
Fiber, 81, 85, 102, 103, 181, 192
Fibrinogen, 81, 109, 189–191
Fibromyalgia, 107
Fish, 66
5-HTP, 76, 203, 205
5-Hydroxytryptophan. *See* 5-HTP.
5-lipoxygenase (5-LOX), 183, 209
Flax, 66, 68, 72
Flooring, 22
Folate, 2, 187
Food chain, 6–23
Foods, 6
canned, 22
heating of, 22
nutrient intake from, 2, 4, 5–6, 26
packaging, 23
processed, 6–13
storage, 22
sensitivities to, 130–135
washing, 23
Fractures, bone, 210
Framingham Offspring Study, 188
Free radicals, 19–20, 115, 131, 141–142, 154, 160, 178
Fructose, 10–11
Fruits, 1–2, 3, 5–6, 22–23, 26, 83, 86, 88, 89, 98, 116, 146, 183
Fucoxanthin, 76, 217

GABA, 76, 201, 205, 206
Gaia Herbs, 241
Galectin-3, 113
Gamma E tocopherol. *See* Vitamin E.
Gamma linolenic acid (GLA), 174, 176
Gamma-aminobutryric acid (GABA). *See* GABA.
Garden of Life, 241

Gastroesophageal reflux disease (GERD), 151–153
Gastrointestinal tract (GI), 62–63, 76, 131–132, 147–153, 174
Generalized anxiety disorder (GAD). *See* Anxiety.
GERD. *See* Gastroesophageal reflux disease (GERD).
Ginkgo biloba, 159, 197
Glaucoma, 100
Glucosamine sulfate, 75, 208
Glucose. *See* Blood sugar.
Glucose-6-phosphate, 181, 192
Glutamine, 148–149
Glutathione, 76, 116, 142, 168, 173, 208
Glycation, 118, 143–144, 177, 179–180
Glycerol-3-phosphate dehydrogenase, 215
Glyceryl phosphoryl choline (GPC), 156
Glycogen, 176
Glycosaminoglycans, 208
Glycyrrhizin, 153
Good Manufacturing Practices (GMPs), 37, 39–40
Gout, 11
Grains, 14, 15, 17
Guggulipids, 185

Hawthorn, 198
HBA1c. *See* Hemoglobin, glycated (HbA1c).
Heart, 61, 75, 80–81, 108–109, 197
Heart attacks, 189–190, 195
Heart disease, 59, 108–110, 112–113, 123, 183–199
Heartburn, 151
Hemoglobin, glycated (HbA1c), 177
Hepatitis, 103

HFCS. *See* High-fructose corn syrup (HFCS).
High-fructose corn syrup (HFCS), 9–10
Hippocampus, 25
Histamines, 131
HIV/AIDS, 103
Holy basil, 151
Homocysteine, 81, 109, 187–189
Hops, 213
Hormone replacement therapy (HRT), 123
    See also Bioidentical hormone replacement therapy (BHRT).
Hormones, 14, 26, 90–93, 140–141, 154
    bioidentical, 140
    female, 122–124
    male, 124–126
    steroidal, 140, 154
    synthetic, 140
Horsetail, 75
Huperzine A, 156, 158
Hyaluronic acid (HA), 208
Hydrogenation, 7
Hyperinsulinemia, 214
Hypertension. *See* Blood pressure, high.

IBD. *See* Inflammatory bowel disease (IBD).
IBS. *See* Irritable bowel syndrome (IBS).
Ideal daily intake (IDI), 52, 53–56, 71
IgG. *See* Immunoglobulin G (IgG).
Immune system, 25, 62, 63, 75, 132, 172, 173
Immunoglobulin E (IgE), 131, 133
Immunoglobulin G (IgG), 131, 132, 133, 135
Indian gooseberry, 186–187

Infections, 103
    bladder, 76
Inflammation, 25, 58, 76, 94–95,
    109, 114–115, 132, 142–143, 145,
    148–149, 154, 160, 161, 183, 207,
    209
Inflammatory bowel disease (IBD),
    148–149
Inositol, 203
Insomnia, 199–201
Insulin, 117, 176, 214
Insulin resistance, 11, 63, 118, 154,
    176, 179, 214, 216
International Fish Oil Standards,
    67
International Osteoporosis
    Foundation, 210
International units (IU), 47
Intra-abdominal pressure, 151–152
Iodine, 76
Irritable bowel syndrome (IBS),
    149–151
Irvingia gabonensis, 217
Isoleucine-prolyl-proline (IPP), 194
Isoprostanes, 115, 116
Isothiocynates, 163

Jarrow Formulas, 242
Jensen, Bernard, 5
Joints, 75, 101, 206, 207

Keratin, 208
Kidneys, 75
Knees, 208
Korean angelica, 175, 209

Labels, 46–49, 56
Lactate dehydrogenase (LD), 120
L-arginine, 194, 197
L-carnitine, 145, 173, 181, 197
L-dopa, 161
Leaky gut syndrome, 131, 149, 174

Lemon balm, 76, 201, 205
Leptin, 215
Licorice, 135, 153
Life Extension, 43, 79, 137, 140,
    242–243
Lignans, 165
Lipoic acid, 160, 179
    See also R-lipoic acid.
Lipoproteins, 112
Lovastatin, 184
LP(a), 111
L-theanine, 205
L-tyrosine, 76
Lungs, 75
Lutein, 76
Lycopene, 166

Macular degeneration, 100
Magnesium, 2, 55, 206, 212
Magnesium ascorbate, 150
Magnesium citrate, 76, 201
Magnesium-L-threonate, 75
Meat, 14–17, 98, 109
Medical inventories, 30–31, 237
    family, 73–74, 136
    personal, 74–77, 79, 136
Meditation, 105
Melatonin, 149, 151, 153, 161, 169,
    200
Memory, 7, 25, 87–88
Memory games, 88
Menopause, 123
Meriva, 209
Metabolic disorders, 75, 84–85
Metabolic syndrome. See Insulin
    resistance.
Metabolism, 124, 126, 141
Metastasis, 164
Methionine, 116, 187, 209
Methyl-folate, 170, 188
Methylsulfonylmethane (MSM),
    75, 208

Milk. *See* Dairy products.
Milk peptides, 194, 200–201
Milk thistle. *See* Silymarin.
Minerals, 4–5, 53–54, 66, 71
Mitochondria, 61, 144–145, 160, 199
Mitoschronial DNA (mtDNA), 144
Modified citrus pectin (MCP), 164
Monacolins, 184–185
Monascus purpureus, 184
Morris, Glenn, 15
MSM. *See* Methylsulfonylmethane
    (MSM).
Mucuna pruriens, 161
Muscles, 76

N-acetyl-cysteine (NAC), 75, 117,
    142, 161, 172, 174, 181, 183,
    189
NADH, 173
National Cancer Institute (NCI), 8
National Organic Program, 16
Natto, 190
Nattokinase, 190
Neotame, 10
Nerves, 75, 86–87
Netels, 165
Neurodegeneration, 9
Neurotransmittors, 158, 159, 202,
    205
New Chapter, 243–244
NF-kappaB, 161, 209
Niacin, 186, 190
Nonsteroidal anti-inflammatory
    drugs (NSAIDs), 158
Nose, 76
NOW Foods, 240
NPA Natural Seal, 22

Obesity, 76, 83, 85, 89, 132, 155, 168,
    206, 213–217
Oils
    borage, 68
    fish, 59, 67, 71, 81, 130, 135, 146,
        192
    flaxseed, 72, 130
    peppermint, 151
    pomegranate seed, 217
    thyme, 21
Omega-3 fatty acids, 17, 29, 57–59,
    86, 88, 95, 130, 135, 143, 192,
    237
    dosage, 71
    forms, 66–68
    ratio to Omega-6 fatty acids, 59
Omega-6 fatty acids, 58–59
Osteoarthritis, 206–209
Osteoporosis, 97, 101, 118–120,
    210–213
Oxidants. *See* Free radicals.
Oxidative stress, 19–21, 115–117,
    141–142, 145, 153, 160, 172, 173,
    177, 178, 180
Oxygen, 154

Pain, chronic, 76, 101, 106–107,
    174–176, 208
Panax ginseng, 75, 159, 183
Pans, 23
Parkinson's disease, 61, 87, 159–161
Passionflower, 201
Pesticides, 5, 15, 20, 22, 26
PFOA, 18–19, 23
Phosphatidylserine (PS), 156, 158
Phospholipase A-2 (Lp-PLA2),
    113–114
Phospholipids, 154, 208, 209
Phthalates, 22
Phytoestrogens, 163
Phytosterols, 45, 185
Picrorhiza kurroa, 135, 153
Plants, 98
Plaques
    arterial, 113–114, 189, 194, 195
    brain, 157

Plastics, 22
Policosinol, 186
Pollution, 20
Polycystic ovarian syndrome, 123
Polyenylphosphatidylcholine
    (PPC), 168
Polyphenols, 153, 183, 212
PON-1, 196
Popcorn, 23
Poultry, 14–17
PQQ. *See* Pyrroloquinoline quinine
    (PQQ).
Prebiotics, 69
Pregnenolone, 91, 93, 123, 124, 158
Preservatives, artificial, 7
Probiotics, 29, 47, 62–64, 237
    benefits, 70
    dosage, 72
    preservation of potency, 70–71
Produce, 1–2
    organic, 4–5, 22–23
Progesterone, 93, 122
Propionyl-L-carnitine, 76
Propyl gallate, 7
Prostate, 124
Prostate-specific antigen (PSA), 125
Proteins, 5, 81, 85, 106
PSA. *See* Prostate-specific antigen
    (PSA).
Puberty, 14
Pygeum, 44–45, 166
Pyridoxal-5-phosphate. *See*
    Vitamin B$_6$.
Pyrroloquinoline quinine (PQQ),
    145, 160, 198–199

Quercetin, 167, 180
Quizzes, medical, 31, 77–107, 136,
    237
    blood pressure and blood
        vessels, 89–90
    bones, 96–97
    brain and nerves, 86–87
    cancer, 82–83
    chronic fatigue, 104–105
    chronic infections, 103
    diabetes and metabolic
        disorders, 84–85
    eyes, 99–100
    fibromyalgia and pain
        syndromes, 106–107
    heart and circulation, 80–81
    hormone imbalances (men),
        90–91
    hormone imbalances (women),
        92–93
    inflammatory conditions, 94–95
    joints, 101
    kidneys and urinary tract, 102
    memory, 87–88
    respiratory, 98–99
Raft forming alginate, 153
Rainbow Light Nutritional
    Systems, 240
Recommended daily intake (RDI),
    53–54, 57, 59
Recommended dietary allowance
    (RDA), 52–54, 56
Red yeast rice (RYR), 184–185
Remethylation, 187
Respiratory system, 98, 181
Resting metabolic rate (RMR),
    214–215, 217
Resveratrol, 146, 156, 160, 169, 183,
    187, 197
Rhodiola, 76, 174
R-lipoic acid, 75, 142, 174, 179, 216
RMR. *See* Resting metabolic rate
    (RMR).
Robillard, Norm, 152
Rutgers University, 4

Saccharin, 8
Saccharomyces boulardii, 149, 151

SAMe, 76, 81, 189, 203, 206, 209
Satiety, 215
Saw palmetto, 166
Scents, 22
Selective estrogen modulators, 213
Selenium, 56, 75, 116
Sensitivities, food, 130–135
Serotonin, 203, 205, 215, 217
7-Keto-DHEA. *See* DHEA.
Sex hormone binding globulin
    (SHBG), 91, 123, 125
SHBG. *See* Sex hormone binding
    globulin (SHBG).
Shilajit, 60
Shower curtains, 22
Silica, 212
Silymarin, 168
Skin, 76
Sleep, 105, 199–201
Smoking, 20, 63, 98, 99, 167, 182
Social life, 88
SOD. *See* Superoxide dismutase
    (SOD).
Sodium nitrate, 7
Soil, 2–4, 5, 26
Source Naturals, 239
Soy, 3, 163–164
Sphaeranthus indicus, 217
St. John's wort, 203
Statins, 61, 129, 185
Stomach, 151–152
Stress, 202, 205, 206, 215
    chronic, 23–25, 26, 63
Stress response, 23–24, 215
Strokes, 189–190, 195
Substance P, 176
Sucralose, 10
Sugar, 10
Sulforaphane, 169, 183
Sulfur, 208
Sunglasses, 100
Superbugs, 15

Superoxide dismutase (SOD), 142,
    196, 208
Supplement pyramid, 27–33,
    74–76, 78, 235–236
    case studies, 219–234
    disease, 147–217
    foundation level, 28–29, 51–72,
    237
    optimization level, 28, 32–33,
    139–146
    personalization level, 28, 29–32,
    73–137, 219–234, 235–236
Supplements, nutritional (dietary),
    36, 75–76, 245–270
    additives, 42
    adulteration, 38, 45
    anxiety, 76
    blood pressure and blood
        vessels, 75, 90
    body systems listing, 75–76
    bones and joints, 75, 97, 101
    brain and nerves, 75, 87
    cancer, 75, 83
    choosing, 35–50
    chronic infections, 103
    chronic fatigue, 105
    companies, 239–244
    composition, 40
    cost, 36, 47, 56
    daily values, 48
    depression, 76
    descriptions, 245–270
    diabetes and metabolic
        disorders, 75, 85
    elements, 37–39
    energy, low/fatigue, 76, 105
    eyes, ears, nose and throat, 76,
    100
    fibromyalgia and pain
        syndromes, 107
    gastrointestinal system, 75
    heart, 75, 81

hormone imbalances (men), 91
hormone imbalances (women), 93
identity, 37
immune problems, 75
inactive ingredients, 48, 64–66
inflammatory and pain syndromes, 76, 95
kidneys and urinary tract, 75, 102
labeling, 46–49
lungs, 75
memory, 88
men, 91
muscles and skin, 76
organic, 37
overweight and obesity, 76
potencies, 38, 47
purity, 37–38, 65
quality, 35–50
raw materials, 40, 45–46
reasons to take, 1–26
respiration, 90
scams, 44–46
serving size, 47
standardization, 47–48
storage, 49
testing of, 40–41, 45
thyroid, low, 76
urinary and bladder infections, 76
vetting, 39–42
women, 93
See also Supplement pyramid.
Sweeteners, artificial, 8–11
Sytrinol, 185

Tangles, 157
Taurine, 116, 199
Teflon, 18, 23
Telomeres, 145–146
Testosterone, 91, 93, 97, 123, 124

Tests, laboratory, 31–32, 107–135, 137
alkaline phosphatase, 119
apolipoprotein, 111–112
basal temperature, 127
bone, 118–120
B-type natriuretic peptide (BNP), 112–113
cardiac, 108–114
cellular, 120
comprehensive metabolic panel (chemistry/CBC), 108, 137
CoQ10, 68, 129
C–telopeptide, 119
deoxypyridinoline (DPD) cross-link urine, 120
food safe allergy, 130–136
galectin-3, 112–113
glucose tolerance, 117–118
hemoglobin A1C, 118
hormone (female), 93, 121–124, 137
hormone (male), 91, 124–126, 137
inflammation panel, 114–115
isoprostane, 115–117, 137
lactate dehydrogenase (LD) isoenzyme, 120
nutrient, 128–135, 137
Omega Score, 130
phospholipase A-2 (Lp-PLA2), 113–114
thyroid, 91, 93, 126–128, 137
VAP, 110–111
Vitamin D, 103, 106
Thermogenesis, 217
3-Oacetyl-11-keto-ß-boswellic acid (AKBA). *See* AKBA.
Throat, 76
Thyroid, 76, 91, 93, 124, 126
Thyroid stimulating hormone (TSH), 124, 126, 127

Thyroxine (T4), 127–128
Toxic Substances Control Act, 18
Toxins, environmental, 17–23, 26, 162
Transsulfuration, 187
Triglycerides, 10, 59, 81, 109, 191–192, 215
Triiodothyronine (T3), 127
Trimethylglycine (TMG), 188–189
Tryptophan, 76, 116, 201, 203, 217
TSH. *See* Thyroid stimulating hormone (TSH).
Turmeric, 156
Twinlab, 244
Tyrosine, 116

U.S. Department of Agriculture (USDA), 1, 2, 15
U.S. Environmental Protection Agency (EPA), 15
U.S. Food and Drug Administration (FDA), 8, 37, 39–40
U.S. National Academy of Science (NAS), 52
Ubiquinol, 68
Ubiquinone, 68
UCPI, 217
Ulcers, 149, 152–153
Underdosing, 44–45
Uric acid, 11
Urinary tract, 75, 76

Valerian, 76, 206
Valyl-propyl-proline (VPP), 194

Vegetables, 1–2, 4, 5–6, 22–23, 26, 81, 83, 85, 86, 88, 89, 98, 106, 117, 146, 183
cruciferous, 163
Veins, varicose/spider, 90
Vinpocetine, 159
Vitamin A, 2, 55, 65, 165
Vitamin B-complex, 65, 81
Vitamin B_1, 75, 143, 180
Vitamin B_2, 5
Vitamin B_6, 3, 144, 180, 187, 188
Vitamin B_{12}, 55, 75, 187, 188
Vitamin C, 2, 5, 55, 56, 65, 116, 150, 186, 190
Vitamin D, 38, 55, 65, 75, 95, 97, 103, 110, 202–203, 205, 211
Vitamin E, 2, 55, 65, 66, 75, 76, 116, 159, 168, 169
Vitamin K_2, 55, 196, 211, 212
Vitamins
dosages, 52–54, 55–56, 71, 190
ingredients, 64–66
multi/mineral, 29, 51–56, 237
natural vs. synthetic, 64–65
Watercress, 164
Weight, 76, 83, 85, 89, 101, 132, 155, 213–217
Women's Health Initiative (WHI), 123
Wormwood, 149

Zeaxanthin, 76
Zinc, 2, 56, 116, 212
Zinc-carnosine, 76, 149, 152–153, 174

About the Authors

Michael A. Smith, M.D., is the senior health scientist and online personality for Life Extension, the world's leading organization dedicated to extending the healthy human life span. He is an author and blogger, creates and conducts webinars, and appears in informational health and wellness videos.

He was a recurring guest on *The Suzanne Show* with Suzanne Somers on the Lifetime Network, appeared on *Gem of the Caribbean*, a television show dedicated to disease prevention, and is seen in several regional infomercials as an expert guest. He is also heard on numerous syndicated national health radio shows. He hosts *Healthy Talk* radio on www.RadioMD.com.

A graduate of the University of Texas, Southwestern Medical Center in Dallas, Texas, Dr. Smith completed an internship in internal medicine at the University of Utah and three years of a residency in radiology at UT Southwestern Medical Center.

Sara Lovelady has been a professional health writer specializing in nutritional supplements for nearly twenty years. She has written numerous health-related articles for both print and websites including *Delicious Living*, *Aisle 7* (previously *HealthNotes*), *Healthy Living*, *Holistic Primary Care*, *WholeFoods*, *Nutrition Business Journal* and *Natural Foods Merchandiser*.